T0348623

Innovations in the Management of Neuroendocrine Tumors

Editor

ASHLEY GROSSMAN

ENDOCRINOLOGY AND METABOLISM CLINICS OF NORTH AMERICA

www.endo.theclinics.com

Consulting Editor
ADRIANA G. IOACHIMESCU

September 2018 • Volume 47 • Number 3

ELSEVIER

1600 John F. Kennedy Boulevard • Suite 1800 • Philadelphia, Pennsylvania, 19103-2899

http://www.theclinics.com

ENDOCRINOLOGY AND METABOLISM CLINICS OF NORTH AMERICA Volume 47, Number 3
September 2018 ISSN 0889-8529, ISBN 13: 978-0-323-64105-0

Editor: Stacy Eastman
Developmental Editor: Meredith Madeira

Endocrinology and Metabolism Clinics of North America (ISSN 0889-8529) is published quarterly by Elsevier Inc., 360 Park Avenue South, New York, NY 10010-1710. Months of issue are March, June, September, and December. Periodicals postage paid at New York, NY and additional mailing offices. Subscription prices are USD 357.00 per year for US individuals, USD 721.00 per year for US institutions, USD 100.00 per year for US students and residents, USD 447.00 per year for Canadian individuals, USD 893.00 per year for Canadian institutions, USD 490.00 per year for international individuals, USD 893.00 per year for international institutions, and USD 245.00 per year for international and Canadian and foreign students/residents. To receive student/resident rate, orders must be accompanied by name of affiliated institution, date of term, and the signature of program/residency coordinator on institution letterhead. Orders will be billed at individual rate until proof of status is received. Foreign air speed delivery is included in all *Clinics* subscription prices. All prices are subject to change without notice. **POSTMASTER:** Send address changes to *Endocrinology and Metabolism Clinics of North America*, Elsevier Health Sciences Division, Subscription Customer Service, 3251 Riverport Lane, Maryland Heights, MO 63043. **Customer Service: Telephone: 1-800-654-2452** (U.S. and Canada); **1-314-447-8871** (outside U.S. and Canada). **Fax: 1-314-447-8029. E-mail: journalscustomerservice-usa@elsevier.com (for print support); journalsonlinesupport-usa@elsevier.com (for online support).**

Reprints. For copies of 100 or more, of articles in this publication, please contact the Commercial Rights Department, Elsevier Inc., 360 Park Avenue South, New York, NY 10010-1710; phone: +1-212-633-3874; fax: +1-212-633-3820; E-mail: reprints@elsevier.com.

Endocrinology and Metabolism Clinics of North America is covered in *MEDLINE/PubMed (Index Medicus), EMBASE/Excerpta Medica, Current Contents/Clinical Medicine, Current Contents/Life Sciences, Science Citation Index, ISI/BIOMED, BIOSIS,* and *Chemical Abstracts.*

Contributors

CONSULTING EDITOR

ADRIANA G. IOACHIMESCU, MD, PhD, FACE
Professor of Medicine (Endocrinology) and Neurosurgery, Emory University School of Medicine, Atlanta, Georgia, USA

EDITOR

ASHLEY GROSSMAN, BA, BSC, MD, FRCP, FMEDSCI
Consultant Endocrinologist, Neuroendocrine Tumour Unit, Royal Free Hospital, Professor of Neuroendocrinology, Barts and the London School of Medicine, London, United Kingdom; Professor of Endocrinology, Green Templeton College, University of Oxford, Oxford, United Kingdom

AUTHORS

KRYSTALLENIA I. ALEXANDRAKI, MD
1st Department of Propaedeutic Internal Medicine, National and Kapodistrian University of Athens, Athens, Greece

TAYMEYAH AL-TOUBAH, MPH
Department of GI Oncology, H. Lee Moffitt Cancer Center and Research Institute, Tampa, Florida, USA

ANNA ANGELOUSI, MD
1st Department of Propaedeutic Internal Medicine, National and Kapodistrian University of Athens, Athens, Greece

ERIC BAUDIN, MD
Endocrine Oncology, Gustave Roussy, Villejuif, France

LISA BODEI, MD, PhD
Memorial Sloan Kettering Cancer Center, New York, New York, USA

MARTYN E. CAPLIN, BSc (Hons), DM, FRCP
Neuroendocrine Tumour Unit, Royal Free Hospital, London, United Kingdom

DAVID L. CHAN, MBBS, FRACP
Department of Medical Oncology, Sunnybrook Health Sciences Centre, Toronto, Ontario, Canada; Department of Medical Oncology, Royal North Shore Hospital, St Leonards, New South Wales, Australia

ELEFTHERIOS CHATZELLIS, MD
1st Department of Propaedeutic Internal Medicine, National and Kapodistrian University of Athens, Athens, Greece

KYUNG-MIN CHUNG, PhD
Wren Laboratories, Branford, Connecticut, USA

ASHLEY KIERAN CLIFT, BA, MBBS
Academic Clinical Fellow and Honorary Research Associate, Department of Surgery and Cancer, Imperial College London, Hammersmith Hospital Campus, London, United Kingdom

JOSEPH DAVAR, MRCP, MD, PhD
Carcinoid Heart Disease Clinic, Department of Cardiology, Royal Free Hospital, London, United Kingdom

WOUTER W. DE HERDER, MD, PhD
Professor of Endocrine Oncology, Department of Internal Medicine, Sector of Endocrinology, ENETS Center of Excellence for Neuroendocrine Tumors, Erasmus MC, Rotterdam, The Netherlands

IGNAT DROZDOV, MD, PhD
Wren Laboratories, Branford, Connecticut, USA

PATRICK M. FORDE, MB BCh
Upper Aerodigestive Cancer Program, Assistant Professor, Department of Oncology, Sidney Kimmel Comprehensive Cancer Center, Johns Hopkins School of Medicine, Baltimore, Maryland, USA

DESHKA S. FOSTER, MD
Department of Surgery, Stanford University School of Medicine, Stanford, California, USA

ANDREA FRILLING, MD, PhD
Chair in Endocrine Surgery and Consultant Surgeon, Department of Surgery and Cancer, Imperial College London, Hammersmith Hospital Campus, London, United Kingdom

MICHAIL GALANOPOULOS, MD
Gastroenterology Registrar, Department of Gastroenterology, Evangelismos Hospital, Athens, Greece

SIMONA GROZINSKY-GLASBERG, MD
Neuroendocrine Tumor Unit, Department of Endocrinology, Hadassah-Hebrew University Medical Center, Jerusalem, Israel

CHRISTINE L. HANN, MD, PhD
Upper Aerodigestive Cancer Program, Assistant Professor, Department of Oncology, Sidney Kimmel Comprehensive Cancer Center, Johns Hopkins School of Medicine, Baltimore, Maryland, USA

AIMEE R. HAYES, BSc (Med), MBBS (Hons), MMed (Clin Epi), FRACP
Neuroendocrine Tumour Unit, Royal Free Hospital, London, United Kingdom

ANTHONY P. HEANEY, MD, PhD
Departments of Medicine and Neurosurgery, David Geffen School of Medicine, University of California, Los Angeles, Los Angeles, California, USA

FREDIANO INZANI, MD, PhD
Pathology Consultant, Department of Anatomic Pathology, Roma ENETS Center of Excellence, Gynecological and Breast Pathology Unit, IRCCS Fondazione Policlinico Universitario A. Gemelli, Roma, Italy

TETSUHIDE ITO, MD, PhD
Professor of Medicine, Neuroendocrine Tumor Center, Fukuoka Sanno Hospital,
International University of Health and Welfare, Fukuoka, Japan

ROBERT T. JENSEN, MD
Digestive Diseases Branch, NIDDK, National Institutes of Health, Bethesda, Maryland,
USA

GREGORY KALTSAS, MD, FRCP
1st Department of Propaedeutic Internal Medicine, National and Kapodistrian University
of Athens, Athens, Greece

MARK KIDD, PhD
Wren Laboratories, Branford, Connecticut, USA

KATE E. LINES, BSc, PhD
Radcliffe Department of Medicine, Oxford Centre for Diabetes, Endocrinology and
Metabolism (OCDEM), University of Oxford, Churchill Hospital, Oxford, United Kingdom

PAUL BENJAMIN LOUGHREY, MD
Departments of Ophthalmology, and Endocrinology and Diabetes, Royal Victoria
Hospital, Belfast, United Kingdom

ANNA MALCZEWSKA, MD
Department of Endocrinology and Neuroendocrine Tumors, Medical University of Silesia,
Katowice, Poland

SOMER MATAR, BS
Wren Laboratories, Branford, Connecticut, USA

TIM MEYER, MD, PhD
Department of Oncology, UCL Cancer Institute, University College London, London,
United Kingdom

**IRVIN M. MODLIN, MB ChB, MD (Hon causa), PhD, DSc, MA (Hon Causa), FRCS (Ed),
FRCS (Eng), FCS (RSA)**
Emeritus Professor, Gastroenterological and Endoscopic Surgery, Yale School
of Medicine, New Haven, Connecticut, USA; FRCS Edinburgh, Edinburgh,
United Kingdom

JEFFREY A. NORTON, MD
Department of Surgery, Stanford University School of Medicine, Stanford, California, USA

KJELL ÖBERG, MD, PhD
Professor, Department of Endocrine Oncology, Uppsala University Hospital, Uppsala,
Sweden

AUREL PERREN, MD
Department of Pathology, University of Bern, Bern, Switzerland

GIANLUIGI PETRONE, MD, PhD
Pathology Consultant, Department of Anatomic Pathology, Roma ENETS Center of
Excellence, Anatomic Pathology Unit, IRCCS Fondazione Policlinico Universitario A.
Gemelli, Roma, Italy

GUIDO RINDI, MD, PhD
Department of Anatomic Pathology, Roma ENETS Center of Excellence, Anatomic Pathology Unit, IRCCS Fondazione Policlinico Universitario A. Gemelli, Institute of Pathology, Università Cattolica-IRCCS Fondazione Policlinico Universitario A. Gemelli, Roma, Italy

FRANCESCA MARIA RIZZO, MD
Department of Oncology, UCL Cancer Institute, University College London, London, United Kingdom

SIMRON SINGH, MD, MPH, FRCPC
Department of Medical Oncology, Sunnybrook Health Sciences Centre, Department of Medicine, University of Toronto, Odette Cancer Centre, Toronto, Ontario, Canada

HALFDAN SORBYE, MD
Departments of Oncology and Clinical Science, Haukeland University Hospital, Bergen, Norway

STAVROS SOUGIOULTZIS, MD
Department of Pathophysiology, National and Kapodistrian University of Athens, Athens, Greece

MARK STEVENSON, BSc, PhD
Radcliffe Department of Medicine, Oxford Centre for Diabetes, Endocrinology and Metabolism (OCDEM), University of Oxford, Churchill Hospital, Oxford, United Kingdom

JONATHAN STROSBERG, MD
Department of GI Oncology, H. Lee Moffitt Cancer Center and Research Institute, Tampa, Florida, USA

ANDERS SUNDIN, MD, PhD
Professor, Department of Radiology, Molecular Imaging, Institution of Surgical Sciences, Uppsala University, Uppsala University Hospital, Uppsala, Sweden

RAJESH V. THAKKER, MD, ScD, FRCP, FMedSci, FRS
May Professor of Medicine, Radcliffe Department of Medicine, Oxford Centre for Diabetes, Endocrinology and Metabolism (OCDEM), University of Oxford, Churchill Hospital, Oxford, United Kingdom

CHRISTOS TOUMPANAKIS, MD, PhD, FRCP, FEBGH
Consultant in Gastroenterology and Neuroendocrine Tumours, Neuroendocrine Tumour Unit, ENETS Centre of Excellence, Royal Free Hospital, London, United Kingdom

DONGYUN ZHANG, PhD
Department of Medicine, David Geffen School of Medicine, University of California, Los Angeles, Los Angeles, California, USA

Contents

individual tumor in real time. The assay meets the 3 critical requirements of an optimal biomarker: diagnostic accuracy, prognostic value, and predictive therapeutic assessment. NETest performance metrics are sensitivity and specificity and in head-to-head comparison are 4-fold to 10-fold more accurate than chromogranin A. NETest accurately identifies completeness of surgery and response to somatostatin analogs. Clinical registry data demonstrate significant clinical utility in watch/wait programs.

Somatostatin receptor imaging constitutes an integral part in neuroendocrine tumor visualization and should, because of its vastly superior performance, use ^{68}Ga-DOTA-somatostatin analogue-PET/computed tomography rather than scintigraphy; it is particularly valuable for detecting metastases to lymph nodes, bone, peritoneum, and liver, which may be missed by morphologic imaging. ^{18}FDG-PET/computed tomography is better suited for G3 and high-G2 neuroendocrine tumors. ^{18}FDG-PET/computed tomography provides prognostic information. Alternative available PET tracers are ^{18}F-DOPA and ^{11}C-5-hydroxytryptophan. To take full advantage of the technique, PET/computed tomography should include diagnostic intravenous contrast-enhanced computed tomography. PET/MRI is currently mainly investigational.

Pancreatic neuroendocrine tumors (PNETs) arise sporadically or as part of familial syndromes. Genetic studies of hereditary syndromes and whole exome sequencing analysis of sporadic NETs have revealed the roles of some genes involved in PNET tumorigenesis. The multiple endocrine neoplasia type 1 (MEN1) gene is most commonly mutated. Its encoded protein, menin, has roles in transcriptional regulation, genome stability, DNA repair, protein degradation, cell motility and adhesion, microRNA biogenesis, cell division, cell cycle control, and epigenetic regulation. Therapies targeting epigenetic regulation and MEN1 gene replacement have been reported to be effective in preclinical models.

Long-acting depot formulations of the currently available somatostatin analogues are considered the first-line treatment for control of hormonal excess by hormone-producing neuroendocrine tumors of the gastrointestinal tract and pancreas. These drugs are currently also considered the first-line treatment for tumor control of both hormone-producing and non–hormone-producing neuroendocrine tumors of the gastrointestinal tract and pancreas. These drugs need coupling and interaction with specific somatostatin receptor subtypes, which are expressed on the cells of neuroendocrine tumors of the gastrointestinal tract and pancreas.

Paul Benjamin Loughrey, Dongyun Zhang, and Anthony P. Heaney

Neuroendocrine tumors, including carcinoids, are rare and insidiously growing tumors. Related to their site of origin, tumors can be functional, causing various forms of the carcinoid syndrome, owing to the overproduction of serotonin, histamine, or other bioactive substances. They often invade adjacent structures or metastasize to the liver and elsewhere. Treatment includes multimodal approaches, including cytoreductive surgery, locoregional embolization, cytotoxic therapy, peptide receptor radionuclide therapy, and various targeted therapies with goals of symptom relief and control of tumor growth. This article summarizes current and emerging approaches to management and reviews several promising future therapies.

Jeffrey A. Norton, Deshka S. Foster, Tetsuhide Ito, and Robert T. Jensen

This article reviews the role of surgical and medical management in patients with Zollinger-Ellison syndrome (ZES) due to a gastrin-secreting neuroendocrine tumor (gastrinoma). It concentrates on the status at present and also briefly reviews the changes over time in treatment approaches. Generally, surgical and medical therapy are complementary today; however, in some cases, such as patients with ZES and multiple endocrine neoplasia type 1, the treatment approach remains controversial.

David L. Chan and Simron Singh

The role of chemotherapy in neuroendocrine tumors (NETs) has evolved with the development of other effective systemic therapies. At the same time, the evolving classification of NETs by grade has allowed for prognostic stratification. Chemotherapy is not routinely used for grade 1 to 2 NETs, but capecitabine (CAPTEM) or streptozotocin-based regimens may be used, particularly for pancreatic NETs. In contrast, poorly differentiated grade 3 NETs are usually treated with platinum doublet chemotherapy. There is no consensus for the treatment of well-differentiated G3 NETs, but platinum doublets or CAPTEM are reasonable options.

Taymeyah Al-Toubah and Jonathan Strosberg

Peptide receptor radionuclide therapy is a form of systemic radiotherapy shown to be effective in treating neuroendocrine tumors expressing somatostatin receptors. The NETTER-1 trial was the first randomized phase 3 clinical trial evaluating a radiolabeled somatostatin analog and demonstrated significant improvement in progression-free survival among patients with midgut neuroendocrine tumors treated with ^{177}Lu-DOTATATE versus high-dose octreotide. This article discusses the evolution of peptide receptor radionuclide therapy, side effects, and potential future treatment approaches.

as early symptoms and signs have low sensitivity for the disease. Cardiac surgery, in appropriate cases, is the only definitive therapy for advanced carcinoid heart disease, and it improves patient symptoms and survival. Management of carcinoid heart disease is complex, and multidisciplinary assessment of cardiac status, hormonal syndrome, and tumor burden is critical in guiding optimal timing of surgery.

High grade gastroenteropancreatic neuroendocrine neoplasms are well-differentiated neuroendocrine tumors or poorly differentiated small/large cell neuroendocrine carcinoma. Distinguishing these entities relies on different genetic backgrounds and resulting different biology. The new classification creates several problems. Almost all clinical treatment data on neuroendocrine neoplasms do not stratify between well and poorly differentiated, providing insufficient help in treatment selection. Treatment of gastroenteropancreatic neuroendocrine neoplasms should differentiate between well-differentiated neuroendocrine tumors and neuroendocrine carcinoma and depends on primary tumor site, stage, proliferation rate, and clinical course. This article addresses how to diagnose and treat gastroenteropancreatic neuroendocrine neoplasms, focusing on well-differentiated neuroendocrine tumors versus neuroendocrine carcinomas.

Carcinoids of the lung and thymus are rare thoracic cancers. In general, lung carcinoid tumors have a favorable prognosis, particularly when diagnosed at an early stage and treated with surgical resection. Thymic neuroendocrine tumors may be associated with multiple endocrine neoplasia-1 syndrome, tend to have a more aggressive natural history, and relatively frequently secrete ectopic adrenocorticotropic hormone.

The concept of neuroendocrine tumors (NETs) began in the 1900s with Oberndorfer's description of carcinoid tumors, followed by specific cytotoxic agents and the identification of somatostatin. NETs diagnosis was confirmed by World Health Organization classification. Histopathology included immunohistochemistry with specific antibodies. Imaging was refined with molecular imaging. Somatostatin is the leading agent for controlling clinical symptoms related to hormone production. Increasing interest in these tumors, previously thought rare, led to increased incidence and prevalence. Between 1960 and 1970, the true NET concept was established with the development of radioimmunoassays for peptides and hormones and imaging with computerized tomography.

ENDOCRINOLOGY AND METABOLISM CLINICS OF NORTH AMERICA

Foreword

Management of Neuroendocrine Tumors in the Twenty-First Century

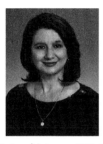

Adriana G. Ioachimescu, MD, PhD, FACE
Consulting Editor

The "Innovation in the Management of Neuroendocrine Tumors" issue of the *Endocrinology and Metabolism Clinics of North America* is well timed to reflect the significant progress in this field. The guest editor is Dr Ashley Grossman, Professor of Endocrinology at University of Oxford, Barts and the London School of Medicine. Dr Grossman is a distinguished international expert in neuroendocrinology and author of the recent European Neuroendocrine Tumors Society consensus guidelines released in 2017.

Neuroendocrine tumors (NETs) represent a heterogeneous group of neoplasms with variable prognosis and behavior that have been increasingly detected in recent years. The diagnosis and management entail collaboration between specialists in endocrinology, surgery, radiology, nuclear medicine, medical oncology, and radiation oncology. Care for the NET patients requires a thorough understanding of pathophysiology, accurate risk stratification, and involvement of a multidisciplinary team.

One of the challenges regarding effective management of NETs consists of a paucity of biomarkers to monitor outcomes and response to treatment. The multianalyte liquid biopsy (NETest) is a promising step forward. NETest has higher diagnostic, prognostic, and predictive therapeutic accuracy than chromogranin A. Molecular genetic studies are important for pancreatic and thymic NETs that may occur in the context of hereditary syndrome mutations of menin (MEN1) or sporadic MEN1 mutations. New therapeutic approaches are under development, including Men1 gene replacement therapy, epigenetic modulators, and antagonists of Wnt signaling.

Somatostatin receptor imaging is an essential part of the NET diagnostic process. The technique has undergone significant improvement since addition of the ^{68}Galium-DOTA-somatostatin analogue-PET/CT. In addition, the somatostatin receptor status predicts the tumor response to peptide receptor radiotherapy (PRRT). The

Endocrinol Metab Clin N Am 47 (2018) xiii–xiv
https://doi.org/10.1016/j.ecl.2018.05.005
0889-8529/18/© 2018 Published by Elsevier Inc.
endo.theclinics.com

NETTER-1 phase 3 clinical trial showed efficacy of PRRT in midgut NETs. Somatostatin receptor ligands, first developed in 1980, remain the mainstay treatment for control of the hormonal excess associated with NET and for tumor control in gastrointestinal and pancreatic NET.

The 2017 World Health Organization (WHO) classification of NET introduced some changes. New categories include the high-grade (G3) well-differentiated NETs and the mixed NET non-NET neoplasms. The high-grade (WHO 3) gastroenteropancreatic neoplasms represent a challenge due to difficulties to distinguish well-differentiated from poorly differentiated tumors based solely on morphologic criteria.

The articles were carefully chosen to reflect specific advances in management of different types of NET. Gastrinomas are important to recognize early as the majority of these neoplasms are malignant; patients may also have other tumors as part of MEN1 syndrome. Carcinoid tumors associate a variety of biochemical syndromes and often invade adjacent structures and metastasize to the liver. Carcinoid heart disease is a major comorbidity; treatment is comprehensive, targeting the hormonal syndrome, tumor burden, and cardiac status. Lung carcinoid tumors have a good outcome after surgery when localized. Thymic carcinoid tumors tend to be more aggressive and often associate ectopic ACTH secretion. Appendiceal carcinoids are heterogenous and rare. Surgery is an adequate treatment; however, the risk of metastasis is difficult to predict. Liver metastases of NET are common and impact survival; liver surgery with curative or cytoreductive intent in properly selected patients has been shown to improve outcomes. The role of chemotherapy in NET has evolved along with the introduction of other systemic therapies.

I hope you will find this issue of the *Endocrinology and Metabolism Clinics of North America* informative and helpful in your practice. I thank Dr Grossman for guest editing this very exciting issue and the authors for their excellent contributions. I also would like to acknowledge the Elsevier editorial staff for their support.

Adriana G. Ioachimescu, MD, PhD, FACE
Emory University School of Medicine
1365 B Clifton Road, Northeast, B6209
Atlanta, GA 30322, USA

E-mail address:
aioachi@emory.edu

Preface

NET-Working for the Future

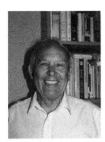

Ashley Grossman, BA, BSC, MD, FRCP, FMEDSCI
Editor

Neuroendocrine tumors (NETs) have increased dramatically in incidence in recent years, a change in part due to better recognition and more accurate pathologic and diagnostic techniques. This extraordinary change has only partially been matched by the increasing awareness of these tumors by clinicians. In previous years, such tumors were seen in isolation by a variety of different medical specialties, including surgeons, gastroenterologists, oncologists, endocrinologists, and many others. Furthermore, they were often inadequately treated due to a lack of both local expertise and awareness of their optimal management, and indeed, because of a lack of effective therapies. There is now a much better understanding of their natural history, a dramatic improvement in imaging and other diagnostic techniques, a realization of the importance of joint management by a multidisciplinary team, and a surge in large-scale clinical trials. Finally, a more detailed analysis of their molecular biology has led to new targeted therapies. This is therefore, in my opinion, an ideal time to summarize where we are in terms of clinical practice. I am delighted that a highly distinguished international group of scientists and clinicians have helped to provide a totally contemporary guide for clinician with this issue. The articles range from diagnostic techniques, especially histopathologic and liquid biopsies, to radiologic surveillance and surgical developments, plus the latest ideas on chemotherapy and radiolabeled treatment. We have also included the vexing problems of appendiceal and gastric carcinoids, and the importance of carcinoid heart disease. In addition, there is discussion of bronchopulmonary and thymic NETs, which are increasingly being seen at NET centers. Finally, it is always useful to see the history of our field: if we do not know how we have got here, we will not have the best idea of how to move forward.

Many of the articles overlap to some extent, and some of the recommendations given by different authors may not always be congruent. I have deliberately allowed for these overlaps and disagreements, which are inevitable in an evolving field. Only time will tell which therapeutic paradigms are robust and consensual. I am truly grateful

Endocrinol Metab Clin N Am 47 (2018) xv–xvi
https://doi.org/10.1016/j.ecl.2018.05.004
0889-8529/18/© 2018 Published by Elsevier Inc.

to all the authors for the time and trouble they have taken in contributing to this issue of *Endocrinology and Metabolism Clinics of North America.*

This issue should be of value to all clinicians, in any specialty, who may come in to regular, or even occasional, contact with patients with NETs, and who may be involved in the treatment of these fascinating disorders. I particularly hope it will enthuse younger clinicians to take up the challenge of improving the care of our patients.

Ashley Grossman, BA, BSC, MD, FRCP, FMEDSCI
Neuroendocrine Tumour
Royal Free Hospital
Pond Street
London NW3 2QG, UK

E-mail address:
Ashley.Grossman@ocdem.ox.ac.uk

The New World Health Organization Classification for Pancreatic Neuroendocrine Neoplasia

Frediano Inzani, MD, PhD[a,b,c], Gianluigi Petrone, MD, PhD[a,b,d], Guido Rindi, MD, PhD[a,b,d,e],*

KEYWORDS

- Neuroendocrine neoplasm • Neuroendocrine tumor • Neuroendocrine carcinoma
- Ki67 • World Health Organization • American Joint Cancer Committee

KEY POINTS

- The World Health Organization (WHO) in 2017 classification emphasizes the concept of separate neuroendocrine tumor (NET) and neuroendocrine carcinoma (NEC) families for pancreatic neuroendocrine neoplasms (panNENs).
- NENs comprise both NET and NEC.
- NETs are G1-G3 with increasingly aggressive behavior.
- NEC are by default G3 with highly aggressive behavior.
- The American Joint Cancer Committee in 2017 applied this classification to NENs of the entire gastro-enteric tract and pancreas.

INTRODUCTION

Neuroendocrine neoplasms (NENs) are found throughout the body in all organs, although they are more common in the lung, the digestive tract, and the pancreas.[1,2] By definition the neuroendocrine neoplasm is made by cancer cells expressing

Disclosure Statement: G. Rindi declares that he has received speaker's fee by Novartis Pharma and Ipsen Pharma. The other authors have nothing to disclose. In part supported by internal university grants (Università Cattolica line D.1/2014-R412500215 and D.1 2015-R412500333) and by the Associazione Italiana Ricerca sul Cancro - AIRC IG 2013 14696 to G. Rindi.

[a] Department of Anatomic Pathology, IRCCS Fondazione Policlinico Universitario A. Gemelli, Largo A. Gemelli, 8, Roma I-00168, Italy; [b] Roma ENETS Center of Excellence, IRCCS Fondazione Policlinico Universitario A. Gemelli, Largo A. Gemelli, 8, Roma I-00168, Italy; [c] Gynecological and Breast Pathology Unit, IRCCS Fondazione Policlinico Universitario A. Gemelli, Largo A. Gemelli, 8, Roma I-00168, Italy; [d] Anatomic Pathology Unit, IRCCS Fondazione Policlinico Universitario A. Gemelli, Largo A. Gemelli, 8, Roma I-00168, Italy; [e] Institute of Pathology, Università Cattolica-IRCCS Fondazione Policlinico Universitario A. Gemelli, Largo A. Gemelli, 8, Roma I-00168, Italy
* Corresponding author. Institute of Anatomic Pathology, Università Cattolica-IRCCS Fondazione Policlinico Universitario A. Gemelli, Largo A. Gemelli, 8, Roma I-00168, Italy.
E-mail address: guido.rindi@unicatt.it

Endocrinol Metab Clin N Am 47 (2018) 463–470
https://doi.org/10.1016/j.ecl.2018.04.008
0889-8529/18/© 2018 Elsevier Inc. All rights reserved.

endo.theclinics.com

markers of neuroendocrine differentiation including chromogranin A and synaptophysin (also called general markers of neuroendocrine differentiation), as well as hormones (also called [organ] specific markers of neuroendocrine differentiation), and transcription factors, which are tissue-specific and assimilate the cancer cell to its normal neuroendocrine cell counterpart.[3]

THE PATIENT OUTCOME

Predicting outcome for patients with NENs is usually difficult, with the notable exception of the high-grade carcinomas comprising the small cell carcinoma of the lung (SCLC) and the poorly differentiated neuroendocrine carcinoma (NEC) of the digestive tract and pancreas.[4–6] These aggressive cancers are usually diagnosed when at a high stage and drive patients to death at a rapid pace not comparable to any other epithelial cancer of both the respiratory and the digestive systems. On the contrary, the behavior of well-differentiated neuroendocrine neoplasms has always been considered as poorly predictable. This fact is embedded in the iconic definition of carcinoid, coined in 1907 by Siegfried Oberndorfer for the well-differentiated neuroendocrine neoplasm of the digestive tract to indicate the "sort of cancer" morphology of such rare epithelial neoplasms.[7] This "sort of" concept applies for the clinical behavior of carcinoids too, in the sense that such patients may show a slow, deceptive pace, resulting in multisite deposits and unexpectedly long survival in spite of the diffuse cancer burden. Indeed, the definition of "quiet cancer" effectively describes the clinical behavior of carcinoids.[8]

CLASSIFICATION TOOLS

The World Health Organization (WHO) set order into the neuroendocrine cancer world of the digestive system with the classifications devised in 2000 and 2004.[4,5] Such classifications introduced the differentiation status of cancer cells (as defined by traditional morphology) as the main tool for the diagnosis of 2 separate neuroendocrine cancer entities with significantly different behaviors, well differentiated versus poorly differentiated (**Fig. 1**). In addition, the WHO 2000/2004 classification introduced multiparametric clinical-pathological correlations utilizing grading and staging variables to predict the survival of neuroendocrine cancer patients.[4] In particular, the presence of metastases was defined as the only parameter capable of defining as malignant the well-differentiated neuroendocrine neoplasm, associated with a change of neoplasm definition from tumor to carcinoma. Such classifications were broadly effective in predicting patients' survival, but would work only once the neuroendocrine neoplasm's malignant pace was overt, a condition rarely seen at many anatomic sites such as the stomach, the pancreas, and the large intestine, for which an early diagnosis is frequent.

In 2010, under the auspices of the European Neuroendocrine Tumor Society (ENETS) proposals,[9,10] the WHO introduced both grading and staging tools for the stratification of patients with digestive neuroendocrine cancer.[11,12] The American Joint Cancer Committee (AJCC) staging manual, seventh edition rapidly followed.[13] The 2010 WHO/AJCC classifications introduced several principles:

> The term neoplasm was adopted as a unifying concept definition embracing both low- and high-grade neuroendocrine cancer.
> The neuroendocrine neoplasm was by default considered malignant
> A three-tier grading tool was devised based on proliferation markers (either mitotic count or Ki-67).

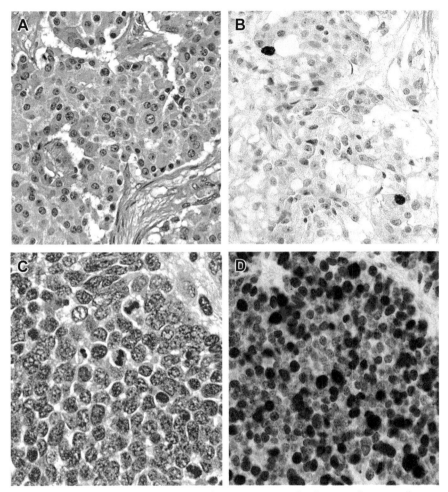

Fig. 1. Morphology and Ki67 labeling in digestive neuroendocrine neoplasms, well versus poorly differentiated. (*A*, *B*) Pancreas well-differentiated NET showing mild cytologic atypia, abundant cytoplasm and only few nuclei labeled for Ki67 (G1). (*C*, *D*) Stomach poorly differentiated NEC, small cell type showing severe atypia, frequent mitoses (middle of the micrograph), a thin rim of cytoplasm and almost all nuclei labeled for Ki67 (G3). (*A*, *C*) H&E. (*B*, *D*) Immunoperoxidase.

Low-intermediate grade (G1-G2), well-differentiated neoplasms were defined neuroendocrine tumors (NETs).

High-grade (G3), poorly differentiated neoplasms were defined as neuroendocrine carcinoma (NEC).

A staging system based on variable and progressive tumor size/local invasion (T1-T4), nodal involvement (N0-N1), and distant metastases (M0-M1) was devised for all anatomic sites.

Several practical application rules for pathologists were also devised, including the concepts that the higher proliferation parameter dictates the G definition for grading, and the Ki-67 labeling index has to be performed in areas of highest nuclear labeling (the so-called hot spots). WHO 2010 proved practically usable[14–16] and was demonstrated to be effective in predicting patient survival.[17–24] **Fig. 1** illustrates the main features of NET compared with NEC (see **Fig. 1**).

The wide application of WHO 2010 resulted in the isolation of a subset of neuroendocrine cancers that are actually well differentiated according to standard morphology but belong to high grade (G3) according to the currently adopted grading tool. This was initiated by the observation of the low response rate to platinum-based chemotherapy in patients with neuroendocrine neoplasm of high grade (G3), although more well than poorly differentiated in morphology.[25] On the same line, different response rates were observed in a large series of NEC patients based on different threshold of Ki-67 index, with relatively better survival for patients with Ki-67 less than 55%.[26] In the pancreas, discrepancies in grading neoplasms (G2 for mitotic count but G3 for Ki67) were noted, with different clinical-pathological profiles and better survival.[27,28] A proposal for NET G3 type was made for high grade neuroendocrine neoplasms displaying high grade Ki-67 index but with a well differentiated morphology.[29] A large, multisite series confirmed its potential clinical efficacy.[30] Finally, it was clarified that such a diagnosis, although rare, can also be extremely challenging even for the expert pathologist; clinical and molecular information, however, could be of help.[31,32]

THE 2017 WORLD HEALTH ORGANIZATION PANCREATIC NEUROENDOCRINE NEOPLASMS CLASSIFICATION

The current WHO classification for endocrine organs (WHO 2017) was devised for neuroendocrine neoplasms of the pancreas (PanNEN) alone (**Table 1**).[33,34] This classification endorses the WHO 2010 principles, introducing however the definition of NET G3 for neoplasms that are well differentiated in morphology but display a proliferation index in the G3 range (**Fig. 2**). This entails the use of the full 3-tier grading

Table 1
The World Health Organization 2017 classification of the neuroendocrine neoplasm of the pancreas

		Neoplasm		Proliferation	
Type	Differentiation Status	Definition	Grade	Ki67 (% of ≥500 cells)	Mitotic Count (2 mm^2)
NEN	Well differentiated	NET	G1	<3	<2
			G2	3–20	2–20
			G3	>20	>20
	Poorly differentiated	NEC Small cell type Large cell type	(default G3)	>20	>20
MiNEN[a]	Well/poorly differentiated	*NET or NEC*	G1-G3	See above	See above
		ADC[b] or SCC	G1-G3	See Ref.[11]	See Ref.[11]

Abbreviations: ADC, adenocarcinoma; MiNEN, mixed non-neuroendocrine-neuroendocrine neoplasm (ie, a neoplasm made by neuroendocrine and non-neuroendocrine [adeno or squamous] tumor cells, either of which accounting for at least 30% of tumor cell population); NEC, neuroendocrine carcinoma; NEN, neuroendocrine neoplasm (ie, a neoplasm uniformly composed by neuroendocrine tumor cells); NET, neuroendocrine tumor; SCC, squamous cell carcinoma.
[a] The features of MiNEN are not detailed in the WHO 2017 classification.
[b] Ductal adenocarcinoma or acinar cell carcinoma for pancreas.
Data from Klöppel G, Couvelard A, Hruban RH, et al. Neoplasms of the neuroendocrine pancreas. Introduction. In: Klöppel G, Osamura RY, Lloyd RV, et al, editors. WHO classification of tumours of the endocrine organs. Lyon (France): IARC; 2017. p. 211–4; with permission.

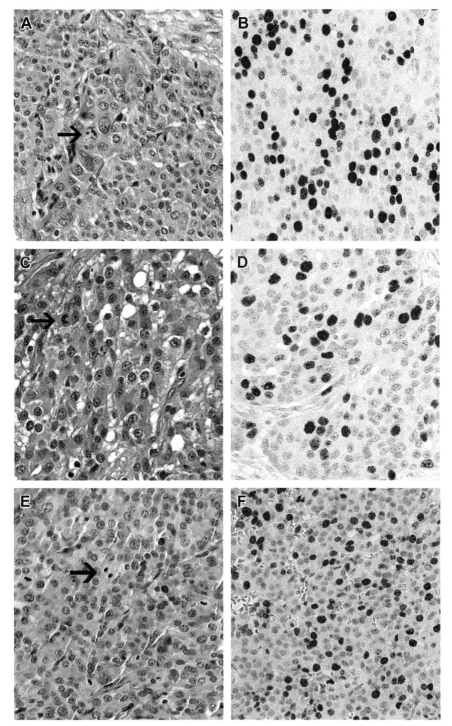

Fig. 2. Morphology and Ki67 labeling in digestive well differentiated high grade (NET G3) neuroendocrine neoplasms. (*A, B*) Stomach. (*C, D*) Pancreas and (*E, F*) colon; at all sites NET G3 display moderate to severe atypia with abundant cytoplasm, mitoses often atypical (*arrows*) and Ki67 labeling well above 20% of tumor cells. (*A, C, E*) H&E; (*B, D, F*) Immunoperoxidase.

definition devised in WHO 2010 for the NET class. The NEC class is by default G3 as defined in WHO 2010. The WHO 2017 classification strongly emphasizes the association of well-differentiated morphology with the NET definition, and the poorly differentiated morphology with the NEC definition. Such marked phenotypic differences likely reflect significantly different genetic backgrounds. Indeed, current molecular evidence points to different molecular pathways for well-differentiated versus poorly differentiated neuroendocrine cancers, with frequent abnormalities of *MEN1, DAXX,* and *ATRX* genes observed in NET but not in NEC and, vice versa, frequent *Tp53* and *RB* gene alterations in NEC but not in NET.[35–37] It is considered possible, although rare, that there is evolution with time of a well-differentiated neuroendocrine neoplasm of low G1-G2 grade to a higher G3 grade[31,36] and, even more rarely, toward a poorly differentiated NEC. In addition, the WHO 2017 PanNEN classification abolishes the preneoplastic class for the pancreas in the light of its rarity and vague definition. Finally, WHO 2017 introduces the concept of non-neuroendocrine neuroendocrine neoplasm (MiNEN) to stress that mixed cancers may contain different types of non-neuroendocrine neoplasm (eg, adeno or squamous) with different grades, as well as different types and grades of neuroendocrine neoplasms (either NET and NEC).

SUMMARY

Based on published data, WHO 2017 introduces the concept of high-grade well-differentiated NET. The new WHO 2017 classification actually recognizes the limits observed following the wide application WHO 2010 in clinical practice, although it is only meant to apply to panNENs; as such it should be utilized only for this group. Although less frequent, NET G3 may occur not only in pancreas but also at other digestive sites (see **Fig. 2**).[30] It is highly likely and indeed desirable that such an improved classification scheme be adopted by WHO for the remaining digestive anatomic sites. This will necessarily require the formal revision of the current digestive WHO classification for the tubular digestive tract, likely to be scheduled in the near future. Conversely, this classification system is currently adopted by the AJCC 2017 for all anatomic sites of the digestive system.[38] Unfortunately, the apparent contradiction between WHO and AJCC may generate some confusion in clinical practice. For the present time, in the rare event of a NET G3 observed outside the pancreas (and most often in the stomach and colon), a reasonable practical approach for pathologists would be to provide in the report both the current WHO 2010 and the AJCC 2017 definitions. An explanatory note should also be added to avoid possible misinterpretation and confusion.

REFERENCES

1. Dasari A, Shen C, Halperin D, et al. Trends in the incidence, prevalence, and survival outcomes in patients with neuroendocrine tumors in the United States. JAMA Oncol 2017;3(10):1335–42.
2. Leoncini E, Boffetta P, Shafir M, et al. Increased incidence trend of low-grade and high-grade neuroendocrine neoplasms. Endocrine 2017;58(2):368–79.
3. Rindi G, Wiedenmann B. Neuroendocrine neoplasms of the gut and pancreas: new insights. Nat Rev Endocrinol 2012;8(1):54–64.
4. Solcia E, Klöppel G, Sobin LH. Histological typing of endocrine tumours. 2nd edition. New York: Springer-Verlag; 2000.
5. DeLellis RA, Lloyd RV, Heitz PU, et al. 3rd edition. Pathology and genetics of tumours of endocrine organs, vol. 8. Lyon (France): IARC Press; 2004.

6. Travis WD, Brambilla E, Burke AP, et al. 4th edition. Pathology and genetics of tumours of the lung, pleura, thymus and heart, vol. 7. Lyon (France): IARC Press; 2015.
7. Oberndorfer S. Karzinoide Tumoren des Dünndarms. Frankf Z Pathol Int 1907;1: 425–32.
8. Harding N. Living with the quiet cancer. The Independent 2009.
9. Rindi G, Kloppel G, Alhman H, et al. TNM staging of foregut (neuro)endocrine tumors: a consensus proposal including a grading system. Virchows Arch 2006; 449(4):395–401.
10. Rindi G, Kloppel G, Couvelard A, et al. TNM staging of midgut and hindgut (neuro) endocrine tumors: a consensus proposal including a grading system. Virchows Arch 2007;451(4):757–62.
11. Bosman F, Carneiro F, Hruban RH, et al. 4th edition. Pathology and genetics of tumours of the digestive system, vol. 3. Lyon (France): IARC Press; 2010.
12. Rindi G, Arnold R, Capella C, et al. Nomenclature and classification of digestive neuroendocrine tumours. In: Bosman F, Carneiro F, editors. World Health Organization classification of tumours, pathology and genetics of tumours of the digestive system. Lyon (France): IARC Press; 2010. p. 10–2.
13. Edge SB, Byrd DR, Compton CC, et al. AJCC cancer staging manual. New York: Springer; 2010.
14. Couvelard A, Deschamps L, Ravaud P, et al. Heterogeneity of tumor prognostic markers: a reproducibility study applied to liver metastases of pancreatic endocrine tumors. Mod Pathol 2009;22(2):273–81.
15. Tang LH, Gonen M, Hedvat C, et al. Objective quantification of the Ki67 proliferative index in neuroendocrine tumors of the gastroenteropancreatic system: a comparison of digital image analysis with manual methods. Am J Surg Pathol 2012;36(12):1761–70.
16. Larghi A, Capurso G, Carnuccio A, et al. Ki-67 grading of nonfunctioning pancreatic neuroendocrine tumors on histologic samples obtained by EUS-guided fine-needle tissue acquisition: a prospective study. Gastrointest Endosc 2012;76(3): 570–7.
17. Pape UF, Jann H, Muller-Nordhorn J, et al. Prognostic relevance of a novel TNM classification system for upper gastroenteropancreatic neuroendocrine tumors. Cancer 2008;113(2):256–65.
18. La Rosa S, Inzani F, Vanoli A, et al. Histologic characterization and improved prognostic evaluation of 209 gastric neuroendocrine neoplasms. Hum Pathol 2011;42(10):1373–84.
19. Jann H, Roll S, Couvelard A, et al. Neuroendocrine tumors of midgut and hindgut origin: tumor-node-metastasis classification determines clinical outcome. Cancer 2011;117(15):3332–41.
20. Norlen O, Stalberg P, Oberg K, et al. Long-term results of surgery for small intestinal neuroendocrine tumors at a tertiary referral center. World J Surg 2012;36(6): 1419–31.
21. Rindi G, Falconi M, Klersy C, et al. TNM staging of neoplasms of the endocrine pancreas: results from a large international cohort study. J Natl Cancer Inst 2012;104(10):764–77.
22. McCall CM, Shi C, Cornish TC, et al. Grading of well-differentiated pancreatic neuroendocrine tumors is improved by the inclusion of both Ki67 proliferative index and mitotic rate. Am J Surg Pathol 2013;37(11):1671–7.
23. Weinstock B, Ward SC, Harpaz N, et al. Clinical and prognostic features of rectal neuroendocrine tumors. Neuroendocrinology 2013;98(3):180–7.

24. Vanoli A, La Rosa S, Klersy C, et al. Four neuroendocrine tumor types and neuro-endocrine carcinoma of the duodenum: analysis of 203 cases. Neuroendocrinology 2017;104(2):112–25.

25. Velayoudom-Cephise FL, Duvillard P, Foucan L, et al. Are G3 ENETS neuroendocrine neoplasms heterogeneous? Endocr Relat Cancer 2013;20(5):649–57.

26. Sorbye H, Welin S, Langer SW, et al. Predictive and prognostic factors for treatment and survival in 305 patients with advanced gastrointestinal neuroendocrine carcinoma (WHO G3): the NORDIC NEC study. Ann Oncol 2013;24(1):152–60.

27. Hijioka S, Hosoda W, Mizuno N, et al. Does the WHO 2010 classification of pancreatic neuroendocrine neoplasms accurately characterize pancreatic neuro-endocrine carcinomas? J Gastroenterol 2015;50(5):564–72.

28. Basturk O, Yang Z, Tang LH, et al. The high-grade (WHO G3) pancreatic neuroendocrine tumor category is morphologically and biologically heterogenous and includes both well differentiated and poorly differentiated neoplasms. Am J Surg Pathol 2015;39(5):683–90.

29. Sorbye H, Strosberg J, Baudin E, et al. Gastroenteropancreatic high-grade neuroendocrine carcinoma. Cancer 2014;120(18):2814–23.

30. Heetfeld M, Chougnet CN, Olsen IH, et al. Characteristics and treatment of patients with G3 gastroenteropancreatic neuroendocrine neoplasms. Endocrine-related cancer 2015;22(4):657–64.

31. Tang LH, Basturk O, Sue JJ, et al. A practical approach to the classification of WHO grade 3 (G3) well-differentiated neuroendocrine tumor (WD-NET) and poorly differentiated neuroendocrine carcinoma (PD-NEC) of the pancreas. Am J Surg Pathol 2016;40(9):1192–202.

32. Konukiewitz B, Schlitter AM, Jesinghaus M, et al. Somatostatin receptor expression related to TP53 and RB1 alterations in pancreatic and extrapancreatic neuro-endocrine neoplasms with a Ki67-index above 20. Mod Pathol 2017;30(4):587–98.

33. Lloyd RV, Osamura R, Kloppel G, et al. 4th edition. WHO classification of tumours of endocrine organs, vol. 10. Lyon (France): IARC Press; 2017.

34. Kloppel G, Couvelard A, Hruban RH, et al. Introduction. In: Lloyd RV, Osamura R, Kloppel G, et al, editors. WHO classification of tumours of endocrine organs. Lyon (France): IARC; 2017. p. 211–4.

35. Basturk O, Tang L, Hruban RH, et al. Poorly differentiated neuroendocrine carcinomas of the pancreas: a clinicopathologic analysis of 44 cases. Am J Surg Pathol 2014;38(4):437–47.

36. Tang LH, Untch BR, Reidy DL, et al. Well-differentiated neuroendocrine tumors with a morphologically apparent high-grade component: a pathway distinct from poorly differentiated neuroendocrine carcinomas. Clin Cancer Res 2016;22(4):1011–7.

37. Scarpa A, Chang DK, Nones K, et al. Whole-genome landscape of pancreatic neuroendocrine tumours. Nature 2017;543(7643):65–71.

38. Amin MB. AJCC cancer staging manual. 8th edition. Boston (NY): Springer-Verlag; 2017.

Liquid Biopsies for Neuroendocrine Tumors: Circulating Tumor Cells, DNA, and MicroRNAs

Francesca Maria Rizzo, MD, Tim Meyer, MD, PhD*

KEYWORDS

- Neuroendocrine • CTCs • ctDNA • miRNAs

KEY POINTS

- Although there have been significant improvements in neuroendocrine tumors treatment over the last years, novel biomarkers are needed to help clinicians in the management of neuroendocrine tumors.
- Liquid biopsies are faster, more economical, and less invasive than tissue biopsies, and have the potential to monitor therapeutic response and to predict recurrences through serial sampling.
- Circulating tumor cells, circulating tumor DNA, and microRNAs have recently emerged as prognostic and predictive novel biomarkers in neuroendocrine tumors.
- Larger, prospective studies are required to fully understand the role of these biomarkers in neuroendocrine tumorigenesis and to incorporate them into routine clinical practice.

INTRODUCTION

Neuroendocrine tumors (NETs) are a heterogeneous group of malignancies, with a variable prognosis and behavior, that to date have been mainly defined by tissue-based characteristics such as Ki67 index, grade, and morphology. Although there have been significant improvements in NET treatment over the last years,[1] challenges still exist with regard to patient stratification and in monitoring treatment. Novel biomarkers are, therefore, needed to aid in clinical decision making and ultimately improve patient outcomes.[2] Biomarkers can be divided into 3 main subgroups: diagnostic if they help to determine the presence and type of cancer, prognostic if they provide information on the patient's overall cancer outcome, or predictive if they

Disclosure Statement: The authors have nothing to disclose.
Department of Oncology, UCL Cancer Institute, University College London, 72 Huntley Street, London WC1E 6DD, UK
* Corresponding author.
E-mail address: t.meyer@ucl.ac.uk

Endocrinol Metab Clin N Am 47 (2018) 471–483
https://doi.org/10.1016/j.ecl.2018.04.002
0889-8529/18/© 2018 Elsevier Inc. All rights reserved.

give information about which particular treatment the patient is most likely to respond to. In the last case, they may be used as a target for therapy.[3]

The identification of robust biomarkers in NETs has proved challenging. Among circulating biomarkers, chromogranin A (CgA) has been considered the most useful and widely used diagnostic and prognostic marker in the past decades.[4] However, the CgA assay has limitations, including low reproducibility, poor sensitivity, and modest specificity, and its overexpression in other diseases have led to diminished enthusiasm in its clinical usefulness.[5] Other monoanalyte biomarkers have also shown poor sensitivity, specificity, and predictive ability, as summarized by Oberg and colleagues.[2] Recently, on the basis of studies performed in a range of other cancers, there has been increasing interest in circulating tumor cells (CTCs), circulating tumor DNA (ctDNA), and microRNAs (miRNAs). Compared with traditional tissue biopsies, liquid biopsies are faster, less invasive, have the potential to reflect all metastatic sites, and can indicate therapeutic response or progression through serial sampling. Moreover, if we consider the potential of the genomic analysis, they offer an alternative means of detecting genomic alterations and their evolution over time in a manner that is not feasible with invasive biopsy.

The aim of this article is to review the current knowledge about 3 new putative prognostic and predictive biomarkers for NETs: CTCs, ctDNA, and miRNAs.

CIRCULATING TUMOR CELLS

CTCs are released into the bloodstream from both primary tumor and secondary sites of disease, and are considered metastatic precursors.[6] CTCs were first detected in patients with NET in 2011.[7] Khan and colleagues[8] demonstrated epithelial cell adhesion molecule (EpCAM) expression in NET by immunohistochemistry suggesting that NET CTCs might be detectable using the *CellSearch* platform for which EpCAM expression is a requirement. In 79 patients with metastatic NETs, CTCs were detected in midgut (43%), pancreatic (21%), and bronchopulmonary NETs (31%). Importantly, it was noted that the presence of CTCs was associated with disease progression and their absence was strongly associated with stable disease. In a subsequent study, the same group defined the prognostic relevance of CTCs in a larger population of 175 patients with NET. The presence of CTCs was associated with increased burden, increased tumor grade, and elevated CgA. There was a highly significant association between presence of CTCs and worse progression-free survival and overall survival (OS). According to multivariate analysis, CTCs were demonstrated to be an independent prognostic factor for survival (hazard ratio, 3.7; $P = .003$) in contrast with CgA (hazard ratio, 1.5; $P = .4$). Subsequently, the predictive role of CTCs was explored in 138 patients with metastatic NETs, in which CTCs were enumerated at baseline, 3 to 5 weeks, and 10 to 15 weeks after commencing treatment.[9] The most commonly used therapies were somatostatin analogues, chemotherapy, peptide receptor radionuclide therapy, and transarterial embolization. Early post-treatment dynamic changes in CTC count were significantly associated with radiologic response and OS. Remarkably, patients who maintained undetectable CTCs after therapy or had a 50% or greater decrease had a lesser chance of progression and superior survival compared with those that had a less than 50% decrease or an increase in CTC count. The authors also compared early and late post-treatment points and did not find any clear advantage for the later time point, consistent with similar studies in prostate and colorectal cancers. CTCs have also been evaluated for the expression of therapeutic targets. For example, somatostatin receptor (SSTR) expression has been measured on CTCs isolated from metastatic patients with gastroenteropancreatic NET.[10] In clinical practice, expression of SSTR2/5 is measured by nuclear medicine imaging, but the resolution of these modalities is insufficient to define intratumoral heterogeneity of SSTR expression, nor is imaging the optimal method to track changes in expression that may arise during therapy. The authors showed that SSTR detection on CTCs is feasible and may provide insights into tumor heterogeneity as well as a means of tracking expression over time and during therapy, as compared with tissue expression. Finally, preliminary results from the same group show that the presence of CTCs is associated with skeletal involvement and that the CXCR4/SDF-1 axis may be a potential mechanism of osteotropism for CTCs in patients with NET (Rizzo and colleagues, unpublished data, 2018).

The usefulness of the CTC count has also been explored in patients with Merkel cell carcinoma. Despite some technical limitations of these studies, CTCs were found to reflect the burden of disease and their presence showed a significant association with survival in 34 patients.[11] Gaiser and colleagues[12] detected EpCAM-positive CTCs in 97% of 30 patients with Merkel cell carcinoma by the Maintrac system and found that the CTC count was elevated in patients with active disease.

Several albeit small trials explored the prognostic and predictive value of CTCs in small cell lung cancer (SCLC). After the first evidence of CTCs in the blood of a patient with SCLC in 2009,[13] several studies have shown that pretreatment CTC number and change in CTC number after chemotherapy or at relapse are independent prognostic factors for patients with SCLC.[14–20] Along this line, a recent report highlighted that copy number alterations in CTCs of SCLC patients could correctly identify patients as chemorefractory or chemosensitive, indicating that CTC copy number alteration may represent a further predictive and prognostic marker in these settings.[21] The most relevant findings on CTCs in NETs are summarized in **Table 1**.

CIRCULATING TUMOR DNA

ctDNA is composed of short nucleic fragments ($\sim$166 bp) released in the blood from apoptotic or necrotic cells.[22] Since the first report in 1977,[23] several studies have investigated its prognostic significance in cancer.[24–27] ctDNA analyses can reveal important information about genomic aberrations relevant to the efficacy of targeted drugs, including epidermal growth factor receptor mutations in non-SCLC,[28] KRAS mutations in colorectal cancer,[29] TP53 and PIK3CA mutations in breast cancer[30,31] and AR mutations in prostate cancer.[32] Consequently, ctDNA has clear applications for monitoring response to therapy in these patients.

A potential challenge with the application of ctDNA to the NET field is the relative lack of recurrent mutations in comparison with other tumors. Molecular profiling of small bowel NETs (SBNETs) revealed the most common recurrent mutations was in cyclin-dependent kinase inhibitor CDKN1B occurring in only 8% of cases.[33] Pancreatic NETs (pNETs) are also characterized by recurrent mutations in a relatively limited number of genes, which include the tumor suppressor gene MEN1, as well as ATRX and DAXX, genes implicated in chromatin remodeling.[34] An abstract presented by Pipinikas and colleagues at ENETS Conference in 2016 demonstrated that ctDNA can be detected in the blood of patients with pNET with a variable concordance between tissue and ctDNA somatic variants, using whole exome sequencing (WES).[35] A subsequent abstract presented by Beltran and colleagues[36] at the American Society of Clinical Oncology Conference in 2017 focused on WES of ctDNA in patients with neuroendocrine prostate cancer (NEPC) to develop a noninvasive tool to assess progression from adenocarcinomas to an NEPC phenotype. WES of ctDNA and matched

Table 1
Prognostic and predictive role of CTCs in NETs

Patients and Primary Site	Findings	Reference
79 metastatic NETs • 19 Pancreatic • 42 Midgut • 13 Bronchopulmonary • 5 Unknown primary	• Significant association between CTC levels and burden of liver metastases ($P<.001$) • Moderate correlation between CTC levels and urinary 5-hydroxyindole acetic acid ($P = .007$) • No correlation between CTCs levels and Ki67 ($P = .59$) and low correlation between CTCs levels and CgA ($P = .03$) • Absence of CTCs associated with stable disease ($P<.001$)	Khan et al,[7] 2011
175 metastatic NETs • 42 Pancreatic • 101 Midgut • 17 Bronchopulmonary • 12 Unknown primary • 3 hindgut	• Significant association between CTC presence and grade ($P = .036$), tumor burden >25% ($P<.001$), and CgA >120 pmol/L ($P<.001$) • Presence of ≥ 1 CTC associated with worse PFS and OS ($P<.001$) • Within grades, the presence of CTCs able to define a poor prognostic subgroup	Khan et al,[8] 2013
138 metastatic NETs • 31 Pancreatic • 81 Midgut • 12 Bronchopulmonary • 11 Unknown primary • 3 Hindgut	• Significant association between the first post-treatment (after 3–5 wk) CTC count and PD ($P<.001$): PD in 8% of patients with favorable CTC response (0 CTCs at baseline and after treatment, or $\geq 50\%$ reduction from baseline) vs 60% in unfavorable group (<50% reduction or increase) • Strong association between changes in CTCs and OS ($P<.001$), the best prognostic group being patients with 0 CTCs before and after therapy, followed by those with $\geq 50\%$ reduction in CTCs, with those with a <50% reduction or increase in CTCs having the worst outcome • In multivariate analysis, changes in CTCs strongly associated with OS ($P<.001$)	Khan et al,[9] 2016
31 metastatic GEP-NETs • 12 Pancreatic • 19 Nonpancreatic	• Detection of CTCs in 68% of patients, of which 33% had evidence of heterogeneous expression of either SSTR2 or SSTR5 • In patients with SSTR$^+$ CTCs, fraction of SSTR2$^+$ or SSTR5$^+$ CTCs variable from 10% to 100% and 50%–100%, respectively, indicating intrapatient heterogeneity of SSTR expression • Variable concordance between the IHC and CTC staining for SSTR 2 and 5	Childs et al,[10] 2016
34 MCC	• Correlation between CTC presence and extent of disease ($P = .004$) • Significant difference in median OS between CTC-positive and CTC-negative samples ($P = .0003$)	Blom et al,[11] 2014

(continued on next page)

Table 1
(*continued*)

Patients and Primary Site	Findings	Reference
30 MCC	• Significantly higher CTC count in patients with active disease ($P<.05$) • Increasing CTC count associated with development of new metastases	Gaiser et al,[12] 2015
50 SCLC	• Longer median survival for patients with <2 CTCs compared with patients with >300 CTCs ($P<.005$) • Persistently increased CTC number at day 22 was an adverse prognostic factors in univariate analysis ($P<.01$)	Hou et al,[14] 2009
97 SCLC	• Significantly shorter PFS and OS for patients with ≥50 CTCs compared with patients with <50 CTCs/7.5 mL of blood ($P<.001$) • A favorable CTC number (<50) after 1 chemotherapy cycle was associated with significantly longer PFS and OS compared with an unfavorable CTC number (≥50; $P<.001$) • Patients with <50 CTCs at both baseline and post-treatment time points had significantly better survival compared with other patients	Hou et al,[15] 2012
59 SCLC	• Association between lack of measurable CTCs and prolonged survival ($P≤.001$) • CTCs count decrease after the first cycle of therapy correlated with longer OS and PFS ($P≤.001$) • CTCs count decrease after 4 cycles of therapy correlated with longer OS ($P = .05$) and PFS ($P = .007$) • CTCs count <2 after the first cycle of therapy was an independent prognostic factor for OS in multivariate analysis ($P = .09$)	Hiltermann et al,[16] 2012
60 SCLC	• Association between a reduction of CTC count >89% after chemotherapy and a lower risk of death (HR, 0.24; 95% CI, 0.09–0.61)	Normanno et al,[17] 2014
30 SCLC	• Significantly longer median survival time for patients with a CTC count of <2 cells/7.5 mL compared with patients with a CTC count of ≥2 cells/7.5 mL before treatment ($P = .007$). Baseline CTC count was an independent prognostic factor for survival time in multivariate analysis ($P = .026$) • Longer median PFS for patients with a CTC count of <2 cells/7.5 mL after 2 cycles of chemotherapy compared with patients who had a CTC count of ≥2 cell/7.5 mL ($P = .07$)	Igawa et al,[18] 2014

(*continued on next page*)

Table 1 (continued)		
Patients and Primary Site	**Findings**	**Reference**
89 SCLC	• Shorter OS in patients with ≥10 CTCs per 7.5 mL compared with patients with <10 CTCs per 7.5 mL (P<.0001) • After the second cycle of chemotherapy, worse OS and PFS in the group with ≥10 CTCs per 7.5 mL (P<.0001 and P = .0002, respectively) • On disease progression, shorter median OS in patients with ≥10 CTCs per 7.5 mL (P = .0053) • Both PFS and OS of patients with a CTC count <10 per 7.5 mL at baseline or a drop in CTCs to <10 per 7.5 mL after the second cycle of chemotherapy longer than in patients with a CTC count ≥10 per 7.5 mL after the second cycle of chemotherapy or patients in whom the CTC count increased to 10 per 7.5 mL after treatment	Cheng et al,[19] 2016
50 SCLC	• Longer PFS in patients with <5 CTCs at baseline (P = .0259) • Significant correlation with both OS (P = .0116) and PFS (P = .0002) if a higher cutoff (CTC <50 or CTC ≥50) was used • Longer PFS and OS in patients with <5 CTC on day 1 of the second cycle of chemotherapy (P = .0001)	Aggarwal et al,[20] 2017
31 SCLC	• Identification of chemosensitive and chemorefractory patients by CTCs copy number aberrations profile and observation of significant difference (P = .0166) in PFS between the 2 groups • Difference in CTCs copy number aberrations profile between initial and acquired chemoresistance	Carter et al,[21] 2017

Abbreviations: CgA, chromogranin A; CI, confidence interval; CTCs, circulating tumor cells; GEP-NETs, gastroenteropancreatic NETs; HR, hazard ratio; IHC, immunohistochemistry; MCC, Merkel cell carcinoma; NET, neuroendocrine tumors; OS, overall survival; PD, progressive disease; PFS, progression-free survival; SCLC, small cell lung cancer; SSTR, somatostatin receptor.

metastatic biopsies showed approximately 80% of shared mutations with a higher similarity of copy number alterations in NEPC compared with adenocarcinomas, suggesting less heterogeneity in NEPC. NEPC alterations were detectable in the circulation before the development of the clinical features of NEPC and, when different metastatic sites were compared with ctDNA, the contribution of tumor alterations in ctDNA was greatest for the liver metastasis versus other sites of disease, with obvious implications for the interpretation of single site biopsies. The authors concluded that WES of ctDNA can be used to better understand intratumoral heterogeneity and to identify patients with a predisposition toward NEPC transformation before clinical progression.

Very few case reports have been published so far on the possible use of ctDNA for personalized medicine in NETs. Recently, Wang and colleagues[37] first reported an

ALK translocation revealed by ctDNA analysis in a patient with a metastatic atypical carcinoid tumor. The *ALK* rearrangement occurred at the canonical intron 19 breakpoint and contained the intact kinase domain of *ALK*. The patient was started on the second-generation ALK inhibitor alectinib with rapid and lasting shrinkage of his disease, supporting the hypothesis that the *ALK* translocation was the driver mutation. In another case report, a woman with a high-grade, large cell neuroendocrine cervical carcinoma was successfully started on nivolumab combined with stereotactic body radiation therapy, based on blood ctDNA results showing alterations suspicious for high tumor mutational burden.[38] Tissue genomic results, available after initiating treatment, confirmed the ctDNA results.

Blood ctDNA can be excreted into urine, where it can be detectable.[39] Patient-matched tissue, plasma, and urine studies indicate concordance of DNA mutation status and comparable sensitivities across the 3 biospecimens.[40] Klempner and colleagues[41] described a patient case with treatment-refractory metastatic high-grade rectal NET harboring a BRAF^{V600E} substitution who achieved a rapid and dramatic response to combination BRAF/MEK-directed therapy and a concurrent decrease in urinary BRAF^{V600E} ctDNA. The correlation between clinical improvement and BRAF^{V600E} urinary ctDNA detection provides evidence for the clinical usefulness of urine ctDNA in the monitoring of tumor dynamics.

MicroRNAs

The miRNAs are a family of 21- to 25-nucleotide small RNAs that regulate gene expression at the post-transcriptional level by binding to target RNAs, resulting in RNA degradation and inhibition of translation.[42] More than 1900 human miRNAs have been discovered since 1993, when the first miRNA was identified,[43] and are annotated in the miRNA registry (http://mirbase.org). miRNAs are relatively stable in human tumor samples and can also be released into blood specimens by passive[44] or active secretion.[45,46] Several studies have recently profiled the expression of miRNAs in pulmonary carcinoids, reporting differences between normal lung tissue and tumor, low- and high-grade bronchial NETs, as well as localized and metastatic disease.[47–49] Ranade and colleagues[50] examined the prognostic role of 880 mature miRNAs and 473 pre-miRNAs in 31 SCLC samples, and found that miR-92a2* levels inversely correlated with survival. The authors also showed that expression levels of miR-92a-2*, miR-147, and miR-574-5p were significantly associated with chemoresistance. Downregulated miR-886-3p, which potentially repress cell proliferation, migration and invasion, correlated with shorter survival in 42 patients with SCLC by Cao and colleagues.[51] This result was subsequently confirmed in a study on 924 miRNAs from 42 patients with SCLC where the authors found that miR-150/miR-886-3p signature significantly correlated with OS and progression-free survival.[52] A prognostic role has also been described for miR-7, which targets the gene MRP1/ABCC1 involved in chemoresistance. A low expression level of miR-7 was significantly associated with drug responsiveness and OS in 44 patients with SCLC.[53] More recently, cytologic samples from 50 patients with SCLC were analyzed for the expression of a 3-miRNA panel (miR-192, miR-200c, and miR-205) and a better OS was described for patients with a low expression level of the 3-miRNA panel.[54] Lee and colleagues[49] evaluated the expression pattern of 3 miRNAs (miR-21, miR-155, and miR let-7a) in a series of 63 lung NETs: the expression level of miR-21 in carcinoid tumors with lymph node metastases was significantly higher than in carcinoid tumors without lymph node metastases. Mairinger and colleagues[55] screened 763 miRNAs known to be involved in pulmonary carcinogenesis in 12 lung NETs and found that 8 miRNAs showed a negative (miR-22, miR-29a, miR-29b, miR-29c, miR-367*; miR-504, miR-513C, and miR-1200) and 4 miRNAs a positive (miR-18a, miR-15b*, miR-335*, and miR-1201) correlation with tumor grade. Moreover, miRNAs let-7d, miR-19, miR-576-5p, miR-340*, and miR-1286 were significantly associated with survival. In contrast, no association between miRNAs expression levels and survival was described in other studies.[47,56] Rapa and colleagues[48] evaluated 56 cases of lung NETs for the expression of 11 miRNAs (miR-15a, miR-22, miR-141, miR-497, miR-503, miR-129-5p, miR-185, miR-409-3p, miR-409-5p, miR-431-5p, and miR-129*), selected on the basis of the results obtained in a previous pilot series. They found 4 miRNAs (miR-129-5p, miR-129*, miR-22, and miR-141) downmodulated in carcinoid cases with high pT3-4 stages and 4 (miR-129-5p, miR-409-3p, miR-409-5p, and miR-431-5p) downmodulated in carcinoid cases with vascular invasion as compared with cases without. Finally, the association with nodal status was statistically confirmed in the whole series for 3 miRNAs (miR-409-3p, miR-409-5p, and miR-431-5p).

Studies on miRNAs in pNETs are scares. miR-21 levels were strongly associated with the Ki-67 index and liver metastases in a series of 40 pNENs.[57] Thorns and colleagues[58] investigated the expression levels of 754 miRNAs in tissue samples of 37 patients with pNET. They found that miR-642 and miR-210 correlated with the Ki-67 index and with metastatic spread, respectively, but could not provide information concerning survival. Lee and colleagues[59] evaluated the expression levels of 8 miRNAs (miRNA-27b, 122, 142-5p, 196a, 223, 590-5p, 630, and 944) in 37 pNENs; only miR-196a level was significantly associated with stage and mitotic count. When pNETs were stratified into high and low miRNA-196a expression groups, miRNA-196a–high pNETs were significantly associated with advanced pathologic stage, higher mitotic counts and Ki-67 index. In addition, high miRNA-196a expression was significantly associated with decreased OS and disease-free survival.

SBNET progression is also characterized by a differential pattern of miRNA expression. Upregulation of miR-183 and downregulation of miR-133a were reported during tumor progression in 2 separate studies[60,61] on 8 and 24 SBNET respectively, making these miRNAs appealing targets for future investigations. Other evidence suggests that miR-129-5p may have an antiproliferative and antimetastatic effect in midgut carcinoid tumors, and that its downregulation during tumor progression might affect factors involved in RNA binding and nucleotide metabolism such as EGR1 and G3BP1.[62] Mandal and colleagues[63] examined miR-96 and miR-133a expression in 51 gastrointestinal NETs and found increased expression of miR-96 and decreased expression of miR-133a during progression from primary to metastatic NETs, suggesting that a combination of both may serve as useful diagnostic and prognostic markers. Miller and colleagues[64] performed miRNA profiling experiments in 90 patient samples and discovered 39 miRNAs significantly deregulated in SBNETs compared with adjacent normal bowel. Moreover, miR-1 and miR-143, which directly regulate *FOSB* and *NUAK2* oncogenes, were found significantly downregulated in metastases compared with primary tumors.

Despite the evidence that tissue miRNAs can be detected in serum samples and that serum levels may correlate with tumor stage and treatment status,[65] few data are available on circulating miRNAs. Bowden and colleagues[66] undertook a multistage study in patients with SBNET. They first developed a panel of 31 candidate miRNAs detectable in patient plasma, based on the evaluation of SBNET samples and matched plasma samples. They refined the panel in an independent cohort of 40 cases and 40 controls and, among the 31 candidate miRNAs, they identified 4 miRNAs (miR-22-3p, miR-21-5p, miR-29b-3p, and miR-150-5p) that were differently expressed between the patient and control groups. In particular, levels of

Table 2
Prognostic miRNAs in NETs

miRNA	NET Histology	Source	Deregulation	References
miR-92a2*	SCLC	Tissue	Upregulated	Ranade et al,[50] 2010
miR-886-3p	SCLC	Tissue	Downregulated	Cao et al,[51] 2013
miR-150 and miR-886-3p	SCLC	Tissue	Downregulated	Bi et al,[52] 2014
miR-7	SCLC	Tissue	Upregulated	Liu et al,[53] 2015
miR-192, miR-200c, miR-205	SCLC	Tissue	Upregulated	Mancuso et al,[54] 2016
miR-21	Lung NETs	Tissue	Upregulated	Lee et al,[49] 2012
let-7d, miR-19, miR576-5p, miR-340ᴬ, miR-1286	Lung NETs	Tissue	Upregulated	Mairinger et al,[55] 2014
miR-409-3p, miR-409-5p, miR-431-5p, miR-129-5p, miR-129*, miR-22, miR-141, miR-431-5p	Lung NETs	Tissue	Downregulated	Rapa et al,[48] 2015
miR-21	pNETs	Tissue	Upregulated	Roldo et al,[57] 2006
miR-642, miR-210	pNETs	Tissue	Upregulated	Thorns et al,[58] 2014
miR-196a	pNETs	Tissue	Upregulated	Lee et al,[59] 2015
miR-183 miR-133a	SBNETs	Tissue	Upregulated Downregulated	Ruebel et al,[60] 2010; Li et al,[61] 2013
miR-129-5p	SBNETs	Tissue	Downregulated	Dossing et al,[62] 2014
miR-96 miR-133a	GI-NETs	Tissue	Upregulated Downregulated	Mandal et al,[63] 2017
miR-1, miR-143	SBNETs	Tissue	Downregulated	Miller et al,[64] 2016
miR-200a	SBNETs	Blood	Upregulated	Li et al,[65] 2015
miR-21-5p, miR-22-3p miR-150-5p	SBNETs	Blood	Upregulated Downregulated	Bowden et al,[66] 2017

Abbreviations: GI-NETs, gastrointestinal NETs; miRNA, microRNA; NET, neuroendocrine tumors; pNETs, pancreatic NETs; SBNETs, small bowel NETs; SCLC, small cell lung cancer.

miR-21-5p and miR-22-3p were higher, and miR-29b-3p and miR-150-5p were lower in the plasma of the 40 patients compared with the 40 healthy controls. They then validated this panel in a second, large cohort of 120 patients and 120 matched independent controls and, as in the previous cohort, they observed upregulation of miR-21-5p and miR-22-3p and downregulation of miR-150-5p in patients with metastatic SBNETs. Moreover, low plasma expression of miR-21-5p and miR-22-3p and high expression of miR-150-5p were significantly associated with prolonged OS. Finally, they generated a high-/low-risk index to combine miR-21-5p, miR-22-3p and miR-150-5p, which was associated with shorter survival. The most relevant findings on prognostic miRNA in NETs are summarized in **Table 2**.

SUMMARY

Despite the identification of CTCs, ctDNA and miRNAs as circulating biomarkers capable of providing prognostic and predictive information in patients with NET, they have not been incorporated into routine clinical practice. This is due in part to technological limitations hampering routine analysis, as well as limited data regarding the implications of clinical decision making based on these biomarkers. Therefore, more prospective evaluations are required to better understand the role of these biomarkers in neuroendocrine tumorigenesis. Incorporation of CTCs, ctDNA, and miRNA analysis into clinical trials is highly recommended to allow greater generalizability and more impactful results, as has already happened for CTCs (NCT02075606) and ctDNA (NCT02973204). The potential to interrogate the tumor genome sequentially using liquid biopsies promises to provide unique insights into tumor heterogeneity, cancer evolution, and the emergence of tumor resistance in the coming years.

REFERENCES

1. Cives M, Strosberg J. Treatment strategies for metastatic neuroendocrine tumors of the gastrointestinal tract. Curr Treat Options Oncol 2017;18(3):14.
2. Oberg K, Modlin IM, De Herder W, et al. Consensus on biomarkers for neuroendocrine tumour disease. Lancet Oncol 2015;16(9):e435–46.
3. Shaw A, Bradley MD, Elyan S, et al. Tumour biomarkers: diagnostic, prognostic, and predictive. BMJ 2015;351:h3449.
4. O'Connor DT, Deftos LJ. Secretion of chromogranin A by peptide-producing endocrine neoplasms. N Engl J Med 1986;314(18):1145–51.
5. Kidd M, Bodei L, Modlin IM. Chromogranin A: any relevance in neuroendocrine tumors? Curr Opin Endocrinol Diabetes Obes 2016;23(1):28–37.
6. Giuliano M, Giordano A, Jackson S, et al. Circulating tumor cells as early predictors of metastatic spread in breast cancer patients with limited metastatic dissemination. Breast Cancer Res 2014;16(5):440.
7. Khan MS, Tsigani T, Rashid M, et al. Circulating tumor cells and EpCAM expression in neuroendocrine tumors. Clin Cancer Res 2011;17(2):337–45.
8. Khan MS, Kirkwood A, Tsigani T, et al. Circulating tumor cells as prognostic markers in neuroendocrine tumors. J Clin Oncol 2013;31(3):365–72.
9. Khan MS, Kirkwood AA, Tsigani T, et al. Early changes in circulating tumor cells are associated with response and survival following treatment of metastatic neuroendocrine neoplasms. Clin Cancer Res 2016;22(1):79–85.
10. Childs A, Vesely C, Ensell L, et al. Expression of somatostatin receptors 2 and 5 in circulating tumour cells from patients with neuroendocrine tumours. Br J Cancer 2016;115(12):1540–7.
11. Blom A, Bhatia S, Pietromonaco S, et al. Clinical utility of a circulating tumor cell assay in Merkel cell carcinoma. J Am Acad Dermatol 2014;70(3):449–55.
12. Gaiser MR, Daily K, Hoffmann J, et al. Evaluating blood levels of neuron specific enolase, chromogranin A, and circulating tumor cells as Merkel cell carcinoma biomarkers. Oncotarget 2015;6(28):26472–82.
13. Bevilacqua S, Gallo M, Franco R, et al. A "live" biopsy in a small-cell lung cancer patient by detection of circulating tumor cells. Lung Cancer 2009;65(1):123–5.
14. Hou JM, Greystoke A, Lancashire L, et al. Evaluation of circulating tumor cells and serological cell death biomarkers in small cell lung cancer patients undergoing chemotherapy. Am J Pathol 2009;175(2):808–16.
15. Hou JM, Krebs MG, Lancashire L, et al. Clinical significance and molecular characteristics of circulating tumor cells and circulating tumor microemboli in patients with small-cell lung cancer. J Clin Oncol 2012;30(5):525–32.
16. Hiltermann TJ, Pore MM, van den Berg A, et al. Circulating tumor cells in small-cell lung cancer: a predictive and prognostic factor. Ann Oncol 2012;23(11):2937–42.

17. Normanno N, Rossi A, Morabito A, et al. Prognostic value of circulating tumor cells' reduction in patients with extensive small-cell lung cancer. Lung Cancer 2014;85(2):314–9.

18. Igawa S, Gohda K, Fukui T, et al. Circulating tumor cells as a prognostic factor in patients with small cell lung cancer. Oncol Lett 2014;7(5):1469–73.

19. Cheng Y, Liu XQ, Fan Y, et al. Circulating tumor cell counts/change for outcome prediction in patients with extensive-stage small-cell lung cancer. Future Oncol 2016;12(6):789–99.

20. Aggarwal C, Wang X, Ranganathan A, et al. Circulating tumor cells as a predictive biomarker in patients with small cell lung cancer undergoing chemotherapy. Lung Cancer 2017;112:118–25.

21. Carter L, Rothwell DG, Mesquita B, et al. Molecular analysis of circulating tumor cells identifies distinct copy number profiles in patients with chemosensitive and chemorefractory small-cell lung cancer. Nat Med 2017;23(1):114–9.

22. Diaz LA Jr, Bardelli A. Liquid biopsies: genotyping circulating tumor DNA. J Clin Oncol 2014;32(6):579–86.

23. Leon SA, Shapiro B, Sklaroff DM, et al. Free DNA in the serum of cancer patients and the effect of therapy. Cancer Res 1977;37(3):646–50.

24. Shaw JA, Page K, Blighe K, et al. Genomic analysis of circulating cell-free DNA infers breast cancer dormancy. Genome Res 2012;22(2):220–31.

25. Oshiro C, Kagara N, Naoi Y, et al. PIK3CA mutations in serum DNA are predictive of recurrence in primary breast cancer patients. Breast Cancer Res Treat 2015; 150(2):299–307.

26. Reinert T, Scholer LV, Thomsen R, et al. Analysis of circulating tumour DNA to monitor disease burden following colorectal cancer surgery. Gut 2016;65(4): 625–34.

27. Tie J, Kinde I, Wang Y, et al. Circulating tumor DNA as an early marker of therapeutic response in patients with metastatic colorectal cancer. Ann Oncol 2015; 26(8):1715–22.

28. Wang W, Song Z, Zhang Y. A comparison of ddPCR and ARMS for detecting EGFR T790M status in ctDNA from advanced NSCLC patients with acquired EGFR-TKI resistance. Cancer Med 2017;6(1):154–62.

29. Mohan S, Heitzer E, Ulz P, et al. Changes in colorectal carcinoma genomes under anti-EGFR therapy identified by whole-genome plasma DNA sequencing. PLoS Genet 2014;10(3):e1004271.

30. Madic J, Kiialainen A, Bidard FC, et al. Circulating tumor DNA and circulating tumor cells in metastatic triple negative breast cancer patients. Int J Cancer 2015; 136(9):2158–65.

31. Murtaza M, Dawson SJ, Tsui DW, et al. Non-invasive analysis of acquired resistance to cancer therapy by sequencing of plasma DNA. Nature 2013; 497(7447):108–12.

32. Romanel A, Gasi Tandefelt D, Conteduca V, et al. Plasma AR and abiraterone-resistant prostate cancer. Sci Transl Med 2015;7(312):312re310.

33. Francis JM, Kiezun A, Ramos AH, et al. Somatic mutation of CDKN1B in small intestine neuroendocrine tumors. Nat Genet 2013;45(12):1483–6.

34. Jiao Y, Shi C, Edil BH, et al. DAXX/ATRX, MEN1, and mTOR pathway genes are frequently altered in pancreatic neuroendocrine tumors. Science 2011; 331(6021):1199–203.

35. Abstracts of the 13th Annual ENETS Conference for the diagnosis and treatment of neuroendocrine tumor disease. March 9-11, 2016, Barcelona, Spain: Abstracts. Neuroendocrinology 2016;103(Suppl 1):1–128.

36. Beltran H, Romanel A, Casiraghi N, et al. Whole exome sequencing (WES) of circulating tumor DNA (ctDNA) in patients with neuroendocrine prostate cancer (NEPC) informs tumor heterogeneity. J Clin Oncol 2017;35(15_suppl):5011.

37. Wang VE, Young L, Ali S, et al. A case of metastatic atypical neuroendocrine tumor with ALK translocation and diffuse brain metastases. Oncologist 2017;22(7): 768–73.

38. Sharabi A, Kim SS, Kato S, et al. Exceptional response to nivolumab and stereotactic body radiation therapy (SBRT) in neuroendocrine cervical carcinoma with high tumor mutational burden: management considerations from the center for personalized cancer therapy at UC San Diego Moores Cancer Center. Oncologist 2017;22(6):631–7.

39. Husain H, Melnikova VO, Kosco K, et al. Monitoring daily dynamics of early tumor response to targeted therapy by detecting circulating tumor DNA in urine. Clin Cancer Res 2017;23(16):4716–23.

40. Reckamp KL, Melnikova VO, Karlovich C, et al. A highly sensitive and quantitative test platform for detection of NSCLC EGFR mutations in urine and plasma. J Thorac Oncol 2016;11(10):1690–700.

41. Klempner SJ, Gershenhorn B, Tran P, et al. BRAFV600E mutations in high-grade colorectal neuroendocrine tumors may predict responsiveness to BRAF-MEK combination therapy. Cancer Discov 2016;6(6):594–600.

42. He L, Hannon GJ. MicroRNAs: small RNAs with a big role in gene regulation. Nat Rev Genet 2004;5(7):522–31.

43. Lee RC, Feinbaum RL, Ambros V. The C. elegans heterochronic gene lin-4 encodes small RNAs with antisense complementarity to lin-14. Cell 1993;75(5): 843–54.

44. Laterza OF, Lim L, Garrett-Engele PW, et al. Plasma MicroRNAs as sensitive and specific biomarkers of tissue injury. Clin Chem 2009;55(11):1977–83.

45. Valadi H, Ekstrom K, Bossios A, et al. Exosome-mediated transfer of mRNAs and microRNAs is a novel mechanism of genetic exchange between cells. Nat Cell Biol 2007;9(6):654–9.

46. Vickers KC, Palmisano BT, Shoucri BM, et al. MicroRNAs are transported in plasma and delivered to recipient cells by high-density lipoproteins. Nat Cell Biol 2011;13(4):423–33.

47. Deng B, Molina J, Aubry MC, et al. Clinical biomarkers of pulmonary carcinoid tumors in never smokers via profiling miRNA and target mRNA. Cell Biosci 2014;4:35.

48. Rapa I, Votta A, Felice B, et al. Identification of microRNAs differentially expressed in lung carcinoid subtypes and progression. Neuroendocrinology 2015;101(3):246–55.

49. Lee HW, Lee EH, Ha SY, et al. Altered expression of microRNA miR-21, miR-155, and let-7a and their roles in pulmonary neuroendocrine tumors. Pathol Int 2012; 62(9):583–91.

50. Ranade AR, Cherba D, Sridhar S, et al. MicroRNA 92a-2*: a biomarker predictive for chemoresistance and prognostic for survival in patients with small cell lung cancer. J Thorac Oncol 2010;5(8):1273–8.

51. Cao J, Song Y, Bi N, et al. DNA methylation-mediated repression of miR-886-3p predicts poor outcome of human small cell lung cancer. Cancer Res 2013;73(11): 3326–35.

52. Bi N, Cao J, Song Y, et al. A microRNA signature predicts survival in early stage small-cell lung cancer treated with surgery and adjuvant chemotherapy. PLoS One 2014;9(3):e91388.

53. Liu H, Wu X, Huang J, et al. miR-7 modulates chemoresistance of small cell lung cancer by repressing MRP1/ABCC1. Int J Exp Pathol 2015;96(4):240–7.

54. Mancuso G, Bovio E, Rena O, et al. Prognostic impact of a 3-microRNA signature in cytological samples of small cell lung cancer. Cancer Cytopathol 2016;124(9): 621–9.

55. Mairinger FD, Ting S, Werner R, et al. Different micro-RNA expression profiles distinguish subtypes of neuroendocrine tumors of the lung: results of a profiling study. Mod Pathol 2014;27(12):1632–40.

56. Lee JH, Voortman J, Dingemans AM, et al. MicroRNA expression and clinical outcome of small cell lung cancer. PLoS One 2011;6(6):e21300.

57. Roldo C, Missiaglia E, Hagan JP, et al. MicroRNA expression abnormalities in pancreatic endocrine and acinar tumors are associated with distinctive patho-logic features and clinical behavior. J Clin Oncol 2006;24(29):4677–84.

58. Thorns C, Schurmann C, Gebauer N, et al. Global microRNA profiling of pancre-atic neuroendocrine neoplasias. Anticancer Res 2014;34(5):2249–54.

59. Lee YS, Kim H, Kim HW, et al. High expression of microRNA-196a indicates poor prognosis in resected pancreatic neuroendocrine tumor. Medicine (Baltimore) 2015;94(50):e2224.

60. Ruebel K, Leontovich AA, Stilling GA, et al. MicroRNA expression in ileal carci-noid tumors: downregulation of microRNA-133a with tumor progression. Mod Pathol 2010;23(3):367–75.

61. Li SC, Essaghir A, Martijn C, et al. Global microRNA profiling of well-differentiated small intestinal neuroendocrine tumors. Mod Pathol 2013;26(5):685–96.

62. Dossing KB, Binderup T, Kaczkowski B, et al. Down-regulation of miR-129-5p and the let-7 family in neuroendocrine tumors and metastases leads to up-regulation of their targets Egr1, G3bp1, Hmga2 and Bach1. Genes (Basel) 2014;6(1):1–21.

63. Mandal R, Hardin H, Baus R, et al. Analysis of miR-96 and miR-133a expression in gastrointestinal neuroendocrine neoplasms. Endocr Pathol 2017;28(4):345–50.

64. Miller HC, Frampton AE, Malczewska A, et al. MicroRNAs associated with small bowel neuroendocrine tumours and their metastases. Endocr Relat Cancer 2016; 23(9):711–26.

65. Li SC, Khan M, Caplin M, et al. Somatostatin analogs treated small intestinal neuroendocrine tumor patients circulating MicroRNAs. PLoS One 2015;10(5): e0125553.

66. Bowden M, Zhou CW, Zhang S, et al. Profiling of metastatic small intestine neuro-endocrine tumors reveals characteristic miRNAs detectable in plasma. Oncotar-get 2017;8(33):54331–44.

The NETest

The Clinical Utility of Multigene Blood Analysis in the Diagnosis and Management of Neuroendocrine Tumors

Irvin M. Modlin, MB ChB, PhD, DSc, FRCS (Ed), FRCS (Eng), FCS (RSA)[a],*,
Mark Kidd, PhD[b], Anna Malczewska, MD[c],
Ignat Drozdov, MD, PhD[b], Lisa Bodei, MD, PhD[d], Somer Matar, BS[b],
Kyung-Min Chung, PhD[b]

KEYWORDS

- NETest • Multigene blood analysis • Neuroendocrine tumors
- Peptide receptor radionuclide therapy • Bronchopulomary carcinoid • Transcript
- Progression • PCR • Blood • Biomarker

KEY POINTS

- The NETest is a blood biomarker test for diagnosis and management of gastroentero-pancreatic and bronchopulmonary neuroendocrine neoplasia.
- The test measures 51 individual circulating genes in 1 mL of blood and algorithmic analysis provides a numeric score of disease status.
- The sensitivity and specificity of the test are respectively >95% and >90%.
- In head-to-head comparisons, the test is ~4-fold more precise than CgA and for monitoring disease progress, it is ~10-fold more accurate.
- Clinically, the test can define the completeness of surgical resection, identify residual disease, monitor disease progression and determine efficacy of treatment.
- PRRT efficacy can be accurately (~95%) predicted using a Predictor Quotient gene set and Ki67 (PPQ).
- Neuroendocrine disease status (stable/progressive) can be assessed by regular monitoring of blood NETest levels.

Disclosure: The authors have nothing to disclose.
[a] Gastroenterological and Endoscopic Surgery, Yale University School of Medicine, 310 Cedar Street, New Haven, CT 06520-8062, USA; [b] Wren Laboratories, 35 NE Industrial Road, Branford, CT 06405, USA; [c] Department of Endocrinology and Neuroendocrine Tumors, Medical University of Silesia, ul. Ceglana 35, Katowice 40-514, Poland; [d] Memorial Sloan Kettering Cancer Center, 1275 York Avenue, Box 77, New York, NY 10065, USA
* Corresponding author. Gastroenterological and Endoscopic Surgery, Yale University School of Medicine, 310 Cedar Street, New Haven, CT 06520-8062.
E-mail address: imodlin@optonline.net

Endocrinol Metab Clin N Am 47 (2018) 485–504
https://doi.org/10.1016/j.ecl.2018.05.002
0889-8529/18/© 2018 Elsevier Inc. All rights reserved.

THE CURRENT CLINICAL STATUS OF NEUROENDOCRINE TUMOR DISEASE

Neuroendocrine neoplasms (NENs), also called neuroendocrine tumors (NETs), and generically referred to as "carcinoids," represent a spectrum of tumors with a diverse range of molecular abnormalities that share a common neuroendocrine cell origin (**Table 1**).[1–9] Anatomically, lesions arise from the diffuse neuroendocrine system of the lungs, gastrointestinal tract, and pancreas as well as discrete organs sites, such as the thymus, pituitary, and adrenal. Functionally, they produce a wide variety of biologically active amines and peptides. As might be predicted, given the diverse cell and tumor types involved, their 5-year survival rates diverge as widely (15%–95%) as their clinical presentations. Overall, this reflects the biological heterogeneity (diverse cell types, disparate molecular regulatory mechanisms, and ill-understood oncogenic drivers) of the tumors and, in reality, suggests that these tumors often bear little relation to each other than their putative common cell of origin.[10,11]

Their management reflects varied approaches often based on local practical experience, eminence-based medicine, or the availability of certain therapies or drug studies. Despite the repetitive development of classification systems and wearisome guidelines (eg, World Health Organization[12] and European Neuroendocrine Tumor Society),[13] there are few evidence-based standardized approaches, particularly for indolent disease or for appropriate sequencing of therapy. Most studies are retrospective, are underpowered, and exhibit significant design flaws. Apart from early identified (usually serendipitous) appendiceal, rectal, or gastric NETs, cure is uncommon and the overwhelming majority of management approaches reflect diverse combinations of strategies in an attempt to delay local or metastatic disease progression and

---

Table 1
Biological and clinical utility of neuroendocrine tumor biomarkers

Detection Indices	Monoanalyte	Circulating Tumor Cells	MicroRNA	mRNA
Pathobiology				
Mutations	No	No	No	Yes
Proliferation	No	No	No	Yes
Secretion	Yes	No	No	Yes
Metabolism	No	No	No	Yes
Epigenetic remodeling	No	No	No	Yes
Apoptosis	No	No	No	Yes
Signaling pathway activity	No	No	No	Yes
Cell of origin	Yes	No[c]	No	Yes
Clinical utility				
Diagnosis	Yes	No	No	Yes
NET disease identification	Yes	No	No	Yes
Somatostatin receptor expression quantification	No	No	No	Yes
Prediction of therapy efficacy	No	Minimal data	No	Yes
Measurement of treatment response	No[a]	Minimal data	No	Yes
Identification of a residual disease	No[b]	Minimal data	No	Yes

[a] Only symptomatic therapy.
[b] Only in specific cases, for example, gastrinoma/insulinoma.
[c] Detection technique identifies EPCAM (Epithelial Cell Adhesion Molecule).

subdue clinical symptomatology.[14] In those with indolent tumor behavior or evidence of stable disease, a watch-and-wait-strategy is considered appropriate by some physicians.[15] Current therapeutic strategies include somatostatin receptor agonists and antagonists, targeted agents (mammalian target of rapamycin inhibitors and vascular endothelial growth factor antagonists), immunotherapy (interferon), cytotoxic chemotherapy, peptide receptor radionuclide therapy (PRRT), external radiation, and interventional radiological or probe-directed ablation.[16] Management choice is often based on local experience, current ongoing pharmaceutical trials, and the composition of the multidisciplinary tumor board rather than a delineation of the molecular biology of the tumor. Relatively simplistic grading and staging classifications tend to drive most decision making in the absence of state-of-the-art assessment of the genomic basis of the individual tumor and the application of system biology techniques to advancing knowledge of the disease.[17]

LIMITATIONS IN THE DELINEATION OF DISEASE STATUS

The continual assessment by imaging, biomarker levels, symptomatology, and evaluation of progression-free survival (PFS) represents the fundamental basis on which NEN management strategies are based. Typically, disease recurrence, progression, or deficits in therapeutic efficacy are defined using an amalgamation of anatomic/morphologic and functional imaging interpolated with alterations in symptomatology and perturbations in biomarkers. Anatomic imaging using the Response Evaluation Criteria in Solid Tumors (RECIST) has well-documented limitations that include suboptimal reproducibility, insensitivity in the interpretation of disease responsiveness to targeted therapies, and relatively low discriminant indices in the identification of metastatic disease.[18–20] Functional imaging with somatostatin receptor–based strategies, for example, ^{68}Ga–somatostatin analog (SSA) PET/CT, has considerable value[21] but limited spatial resolution (several millimeters for PET scanners), and partial volume effects constrain the ability to delineate small lesions. Although the development of new lesions is probably the most powerful indicator of disease progression, the monitoring of therapeutic efficacy and the early detection of residual or progressive disease using imaging remain challenging and are suboptimal.[22–24] Current biomarkers in use are secretory monoanalytes (gastrin and insulin), protein cosecretory products (chromogranin A [CgA]), and urinary degradatory amines (5-hydroxyindoleacetic acid [5-HIAA]) which, in general, have limited predictive or prognostic value.[25]

LIMITATIONS OF CURRENT BIOMARKERS

Biomarkers are tools that diagnose a disease and monitor or predict the outcome of treatment of disease. They are cellular, biochemical, or molecular alterations measurable in biological media, such as tissues, cells, or fluids.[26] NENs secrete bioactive products, including amines and peptides, into the circulation, which are detectable and quantifiable. These include analytes specific to an individual cell type, for example, gastrin (gastrinomas), as well as cosecreted products common to all NENs, for example, CgA or neuron-specific enolase.

CgA is a constitutive product of the neuroendocrine cell secretory granule and is measurable in serum or plasma. It may correlate with tumor mass and seems to function as a prognostic agent.[27,28] Small tumors, however, may be hypersecretory whereas large tumors can exhibit low secretion. Specific receptor targeting agents, for example, SSAs, decrease CgA secretion through inhibition of synthesis and the secretory machinery. The sensitivity of CgA ranges from 60% to 90% with a specificity less than 50% (depending on the population studied).[29] CgA does not correlate with imaging, in particular ^{68}Ga-SSA and fludeoxyglucose F 18 imaging, and its utility with CT or MRI remains to be determined. Biochemical responses to therapy, as measured by changes in circulating CgA levels also generally are nonconcordant with image-based assessments.[25] Poor laboratory metrics, nonspecificity, and diagnostic inaccuracy further contribute to the low enthusiasm for its clinical utility.[25]

Such limitations emphasize the need for alternative tools, such as microRNA (miRNA) or circulating tumor cells (CTCs), or informative molecular tools, such as multianalyte biomarkers that delineate significant biological characteristics of the disease state. Currently, the measurement of miRNA remains complex and is not adequately standardized for clinical usage.[30] CTCs, although intuitively attractive as a direct measurement of tumor cell-related events, have to date failed to provide evidence of broad clinical utility.[25] Dynamic characterization of tumor behavior based on blood-derived genomic information can only be derived from assessment of circulating real-time multianalyte genetic information (NETest, Clifton Life Sciences, Nevis) (see **Table 1**). Blood-based transcriptome analysis and interrogation of the specific genomic drivers of a tumor provide a liquid biopsy, which is an optimal platform to assess tumor status on a real-time basis.[31]

RATIONALE FOR MOLECULAR BIOMARKERS

The complexity and diversity in cancer biological behavior and responses to therapy cannot be adequately defined through measurements of secretory products.[32,33] Measurements of exocytotic and secreted proteins do not adequately capture the biological activity of an active tumor cell, which includes proliferation, metabolic activity, growth factor signaling, and so forth.[33] Clinical scientists in diverse oncological disciplines have, therefore, concluded that a dynamic and panoramic delineation of the molecular biological topography of an evolving neoplasm, that is, the hallmarks of cancer, is best assessed through a multidimensional appraisal of the molecular genomic machinery of the tumor cell. This includes the measurement of mRNA and DNA as well as the delineation of mutational status, and the application of systems biology to the identification of master regulators and oncogenic checkpoints.[10] There is, thus, a focus on the application of molecular technologies to better define a cancer cell state focusing both on detection of mutations (typically in circulating tumor DNA [ctDNA] or transcriptional profiles, including mRNA and signal pathway analyses).[34,35]

Examples of the utility of tumor tissue–based mRNA approaches include MammaPrint (Agendia, Irvine, California), which is a 70-gene assay for predicting the risk of recurrence in an early stage breast cancer while considering adjuvant treatment.[36] Other genomic tests to stratify the risk of cancer recurrence while considering adjuvant treatment are for example, Oncotype DX (Genomic Health, Redwood City, California), used in breast, colon, prostate cancer, or MammoStrat (Clarient Diagnostic Services, Aliso Viejo, California), used in early-stage, hormone receptor–positive breast cancer. The clinical utility of these approaches is highlighted by the recent endorsement of MammaPrint by the American Society for Clinical Oncology, to guide treatment decisions on adjuvant systemic therapy in women with early-stage invasive breast cancer.[37] Although this information underscores the importance and usefulness of gene expression tests, such technology is currently limited to tissue-based testing and would require repetitive biopsy to provide real-time clinical information.

LIQUID BIOPSY STRATEGIES IN OTHER NEOPLASIA

The evolution of strategies to evaluate circulating molecular information from neoplasia, however, has advanced to the point that blood sampling can provide considerable oncological information.[34,35] There is significant interest in the identification and application of such strategies, or liquid biopsies, in the field of oncology (**Fig. 1**).[38,39] In this respect, a circulating neoplastic molecular signature, that is, a circulating Mammaprint-like signature, would have clinical utility to limit invasive biopsies, define therapeutic targets, and provide a real-time monitoring tool to evaluate disease status.[40]

Given the invasive nature and the technical limitations of tissue biopsy, there is added enthusiasm for the development of surrogate markers that can be quantified in blood on a real-time basis.[31] Research has focused on measurement of circulating genetic information, for example, ctDNA, RNA, or tumor cells, or the identification of actionable mutation events, for example, *BRAF* mutations in ctDNA. As such, the use of liquid biopsy allows for patient stratification (eg, as a companion diagnostic) for screening and for monitoring treatment responses. Examples include identification of mutation T790M in ctDNA, which allows for monitoring of treatment responses to EFGR inhibitors in lung cancer.[41,42] Measurements of ctDNA levels have been used for the detection of minimal residual disease after surgery/recurrence for example, in colon cancer.[43]

Unlike a majority of cancers, however, activating mutations are infrequent if not largely unknown in NENs,[10] and most tumors exhibit somatic mutations (when identified) in tumor suppressor genes, for example, *MEN-1,* the predominant pancreatic mutation.[44] The clinical usefulness of other alterations for example, in *ATRX,* *DAXX,*[45] or *YY1*[46] (all identified as sporadic mutations in pancreatic NEN) remains to be proved. In addition, the clinical usefulness of copy number and chromosomal imbalances as well as chemical-based DNA modifications, for example, methylation, requires elucidation.[10] To date, the clinical utility of the measurement of molecular signals, such as ctDNA, methylated gene targets, or CTCs have, therefore, been limited in NENs.[44]

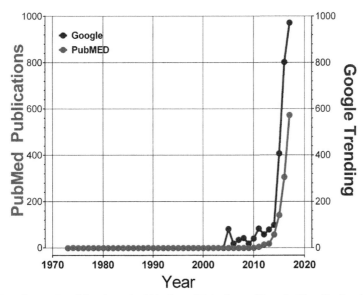

Fig. 1. Numbers of publications (PubMed) or Web focus (Google Trending) relating to "liquid biopsy". Significant public interest was initially noted in 2004 and has escalated since 2012. Academic interest initially lagged but has subsequently escalated from 2012. There has been an exponential explosion in interest in both domains though the medical scientific community appear to be less receptive than the public.

The focus in NENs has thus switched to mRNA-based liquid biopsy approaches, which have been demonstrated to have utility in other diseases. For example, FibroSure/FibroTest (BioPredictive S.A.S., Paris, France) is a blood-based, biochemical, algorithmic test for liver damage used to detect hepatitis C.[47] The FibroSure is a repeatable, noninvasive test that is considered to have high accuracy with the added value of reducing the discomfort or complications related to a liver biopsy.

SCIENTIFIC BASIS OF THE NETest

Transcriptome-based evaluations have proved useful in identifying and differentiating the different subtypes of NEN (based on origin [eg, pancreatic vs small intestinal] and aggressiveness [eg, nonprogressive vs malignant/metastatic]).[48,49] These mRNA-based evaluations also have demonstrable predictive utility at a tissue level.[50]

Transcriptional profiling of tumor tissue has identified a series of neuroendocrine transcripts that are detectable in the circulation[51] and can be used clinically to evaluate gastrointestinal, pancreatic, and bronchopulmonary (BP) NENs.[52-59] This strategy has also been used to define tumors originating in the nervous system, including paragangliomas and adrenal glands, that is, pheochromocytomas.[60] This blood-based multianalyte transcript analysis is the most extensively investigated liquid biopsy tool for this class of tumor.

Individual genes were selected by analyzing microarray data sets of cellular profiles from fresh frozen tumors as well as from whole blood (3 microarray data sets: tumor tissue [n = 15], peripheral blood [n = 7], and adenocarcinoma [n = 363 tumors]) to identify similarities in expression patterns (**Fig. 2**).[51] Once defined, coexpression network inference against normal tissue gene expression was undertaken to eliminate genes that were unlikely to be neoplasia relevant.[51] Tumor-associated genes from other tumor types for example, breast, colon, and so forth, were similarly excluded; 51 candidate marker genes, detectable in the peripheral circulation, were identified to encompass the hallmarks of a NEN. The candidate gene signature was then examined in a training set of 130 blood samples (NEN: n = 63) and validated in 2 independent sets (set 1 [NENs: n = 72] and set 2 [NENs: n = 58]). Correlation analysis of matched blood/tumor identified this as highly significant (R^2 = 0.62–0.91; $P<.0001$), indicating the blood-based measurements were directly attributable to a tumor gene expression signature.

The signature—the NETest—can identify all types NEN, including small nonmetastatic tumors. The sensitivity is such that image-negative lesions in the liver can be identified and subsequently confirmed by histologic demonstration of microscopic tumor deposits. Comparison assessment with other NET biomarkers identifies it to significantly out-perform single analyte-based assays for detection.[51,57] In addition, levels correlate with clinical status, for example, stable or progressive disease.[61] Mathematical analyses have demonstrated that this technique is superior to single analyte assays in the diagnosis of NEN.[11] For example, the area under the curve (AUC) for the NEN gene-based classifier was 0.95 to 0.98 compared with 0.64 for CgA (Z-statistic 6.97–11.42; $P<.0001$).[51] In comparisons with other commonly used biomarkers, like pancreastatin and neurokinin A (AUC: 0.58–0.63), the NETest AUC was 0.98 (area differences: 0.284–0.403, Z statistic 4.85–5.9; $P<.0001$).[57] The utility of the NETest was mathematically confirmed by the use of predictive feature analysis, which established that measuring multiple genes in the circulation exhibited the highest value (69%) for NEN diagnosis compared with measurement of single secreted products (CgA: 13%; pancreastatin: 9%; and neurokinin A: 9%).[57]

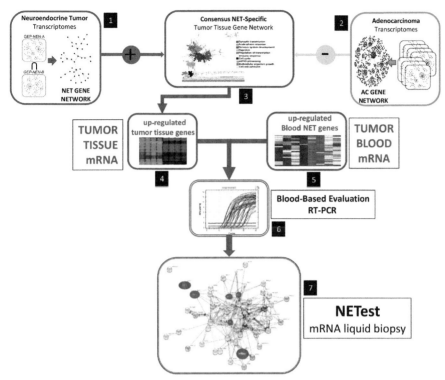

Fig. 2. Computational pipeline used to derive a set of marker genes, the NET Marker Panel that identifies GEP-NEN/NET disease in the blood. Step 1: gene coexpression networks inferred from 2 independent data sets (GEP-NEN-A and GEP-NEN-B) are intersected to produce the GEP-NEN network. Step 2: coexpression networks from neoplastic and normal tissue microarray data sets are combined to produce the normal and neoplastic networks. Step 3: links present in normal and neoplastic networks are subtracted from the GEP-NEN network. Step 4: up-regulated genes in both the GEP-NEN-A and GEP-NEN-B data sets (n = 21) are mapped to the consensus GEP-NEN network. Step 5: identification of consistently up-regulated genes in GEP-NEN blood transcriptome and GEP-NEN-A and GEP-NEN-B data sets, provided 32 putative genes. Step 6: literature curation and cancer mutation database search yielded an additional panel of 22 putative marker genes. A total of 75 marker genes was analyzed prior to delineation of the final NET marker panel. Step 7: the final NETest liquid biopsy includes 51 marker genes that were validated in 3 independent cohorts totaling 193 NETs and 172 controls. RT-PCR, reverse transcription PCR. (*Modified from* Modlin I, Drozdov I, Kidd M. The identification of gut neuroendocrine tumor disease by multiple synchronous transcript analysis in blood. PLoS One 2013;8:e63364; with permission.)

MATHEMATICAL BASIS OF THE NETest

The test uses a 2-step protocol (mRNA isolation, cDNA production, and polymerase chain reaction [PCR])[51,62] from EDTA-collected whole blood (**Fig. 3**).[51,62] Blood gene expression of the 51 markers is normalized to housekeepers and quantified versus a population control.[51] Gene expression levels are related to an outcome using supervised machine learning algorithms, including support vector machines and linear discriminant analyses, both of which have been applied extensively in clinical medicine.[63–68] These algorithms use gene expression levels to learn whether a sample

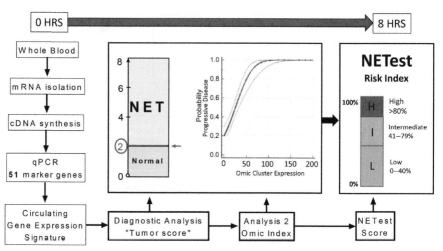

Fig. 3. The multistep protocol used to provide a multianalyte gene expression panel for GEP-NETs. A 2-step protocol (mRNA isolation and cDNA synthesis) is undertaken prior to quantitative PCR gene expression. mRNA levels are normalized using house-keeping gene expression. The normalized 51-marker signature is then interrogated using 2 separate mathematical algorithmic analyses. This provides two readouts. The first generates a score that identifies whether the sample is a NET or non-NET (score 0–8). Samples scored 0 to 2 are classified as normals and levels of 3 to 8 are categorized as NETs. The second analysis evaluates expression of defined clusters of genes involved in the biologically relevant NET pathways. Omic values greater than or equal to 50 have a greater than 75% probability of identifying progressive disease. These 2 information sets are condensed to a single score, which is scaled 0% to 100% (the NETest score). Scaling is undertaken based on weighting the classification score (analysis 1), with the biological gene expression linked to disease status (analysis 2). The NETest delineates in a specific patient whether the tumor falls into a category of low risk (<40%), moderate risk (40%–79%), or high risk (≥80%) for disease activity. HRS, hours; qPCR, quantitative PCR.

should be categorized as either, for example, tumor or control. Algorithm performance is subsequently validated using an independent test set.

The NETest uses 4 different mathematical tools: support vector machine, linear discriminant analysis, k-nearest neighbors, and the naïve Bayes algorithm. These were taught (or trained) using a training set of 130 blood samples (NENs: n = 63 and controls: n = 67) and validated (or tested) in 2 independent sets (set 1 [NENs: n = 72, controls: n = 43] and set 2 [NENs: n = 58; controls: n = 62]). All algorithms were designed to differentiate controls from tumors and stable disease from progressive disease. First, each algorithm labels an unknown sample as either 0 or 1, which corresponds to a prediction of control or tumor, respectively. Then, prediction is applied to tumor samples, labeling them as either 0 (stable) or 1 (progressive). This categorization results in a 0 to 8 score.[51,62] Scores greater than 2 are considered tumor. In the test sets, the AUC values were 0.98 and 0.95, respectively. The test exhibited a high sensitivity (85%–98%), specificity (93%–97%), positive predictive value (95%–96%), and negative predictive value (87%–98%).[51,62] These data confirm that learning algorithms can successfully classify (and, therefore, diagnose) NETs in blood.

To expand the utility of the test from a pure diagnostic to a tool that could capture the biology of neuroendocrine neoplasia, the authors subsequently undertook regulatory network analysis. Briefly, this approach involves mapping NET-specific genes to a database of human protein-protein interactions, thus visualizing marker genes in the context of their respective biological function. This strategy identified 8 biologically relevant gene "omic" clusters (SSTRome, proliferome, signalome, metabolome, secretome, epigenome, plurome, and apoptome), which define the NEN fingerprint and constitute the oncobiome of the NET cell.[31] Differential analysis of gene expression in 6 of the clusters (SSTRome, proliferome, metabolome, secretome, epigenome, and plurome) can then be mathematically analyzed to deduce stable from progressive disease.[31] These constitute a molecular representation of the biological signature of an individual tumor. Overall, this strategy captures the biology of a specific NEN and defines the molecular status of an individual tumor.[31]

To facilitate the clinical interpretation of this information, the diagnostic score is represented as a clinical activity score ranging from 0% (low activity) to 100% (high activity).[31] Thus, a high score, for example, 8, with elevated expression of genes in omic clusters is scaled to 100% (high activity). In contrast, the same score (8) in which a low expression of omic gene clusters is identified is weighted to 53% (see **Fig. 3**). In both examples, the samples are tumor (a score of 8 is equivalent to all 4 algorithms [discussed previously], classifying the sample as a tumor). The difference between the 2 samples reflects differential tumor biology, as captured by omic gene clusters. For example, a score of 100% identifies a more aggressive tumor phenotype than a score of 53%. Using Kaplan-Meier analyses (n = 63, time period 60 months), the authors correlated clinical determinants with gene expression levels. These are low biological activity, less than or equal to 40%; intermediate biological activity, 41% to 79%; and high (biologically aggressive) activity, 80% to 100%.[31,55,56] A similar spectrum of ranges has been identified in BP tumors.[59]

LABORATORY METRICS OF THE NETest

The multianalyte algorithmic analysis procedure has been validated[62] and is undertaken in a Clinical Laboratory Improvement Amendments–certified clinical laboratory (State of Connecticut: 07D2081388). The interassay variability is 2.14% ± 1.14% and the intra-assay variability is 1.02% ± 0.74%.[62] In clinical studies, the intra-assay reproducibility ranges 0.4% to 1% for individual gene expression. Assessment of PCR cycle times, normalized gene expression, and scoring demonstrates high correlation levels (Spearman >0.90). Consecutive daily analysis of NEN samples had a Spearman correlation for scored expression of 0.96 ($P<.001$; coefficient of variation <5%). The summated NETest data assessed in approximately 5500 patient samples from approximately 100 different institutions and approximately 150 physicians indicate that the day-to-day variability for the test is extremely low (<2%) and the test is highly reproducible (sample concordance >95%).

Measurement of the NETest signature in blood is robust and not affected by food intake.[62] Assessment of the gene expression measurements using unsupervised hierarchical clustering failed to identify intrinsic relationships between feeding and gene expression, and the NETest was not altered over a 4-hour period after a test meal.[62] No relationship between age, gender, ethnicity, and proton pump inhibitor (PPI) usage was identifiable.[62] The latter is a particular issue in the measurement of CgA because PPIs significantly increase CgA levels.[69] NETest scores are not affected by long-term PPI treatment (>1 year). Overall, the test has been demonstrated to exhibit a reliably high level of sensitivity and specificity (both >95%),[51] to be standardized and reproducible (interassay and intra-assay coefficient of variation <2%)[62] and not to be affected by age, gender, ethnicity, fasting, or PPI medication.[52,62]

CLINICAL APPLICATIONS OF THE NETest
Diagnosis

Small bowel neuroendocrine neoplasm
The NETest accurately identifies small bowel NENs and differentiates these from other small and large bowel cancers (**Fig. 4**). In 1 prospective study, the accuracy for detecting small bowel NEN was 93% (all NETs positive and 3 [12%] colorectal tumors were positive).[54] CgA was positive in 80%, but 29% (n = 7) of colorectal cancers also exhibited elevated circulating CgA levels. Gene expression scores were elevated ($P<.05$) in subjects with metastatic disease and were more accurate (76%–80%) than CgA levels (20%–32%) for detecting NEN disease.[54] Overall, as a diagnostic test, the NETest was significantly more sensitive than CgA for small bowel NEN.

Pancreatic neuroendocrine neoplasm
The NETest is also useful for accurately confirming neuroendocrine disease (compared with other cancers and non-neoplastic diseases [eg, chronic pancreatitis]) in blood samples from pancreatic disease patients.[54] In 1 study, the accuracy was 94%[54]; 6% (2/31) of intraductal papillary mucinous neoplasms were positive, consistent with the reported coexistence of NEN and these lesions.[70] Only 29% of pancreatic NETs were CgA positive in blood; the overall accuracy of CgA was 56%[54] (**Fig. 5**).

Bronchopulmonary neuroendocrine neoplasm
Detectable mRNA was identified in blood from lung tumors with a neuroendocrine phenotype in greater than 90%.[59] A receiver operating characteristic (ROC) analysis AUC was 0.99 for differentiating lung carcinoids (typical or atypical) versus controls. The sensitivity and specificity ranged from 93% to 95% and from 82% to 93%, respectively.[58] In individuals with RECIST-defined progressive disease, NETest levels were significantly increased (72% ± 23%) irrespective of histology compared with stable disease (33% ± 17%) or those considered surgical cures (10% ± 5%). Levels were

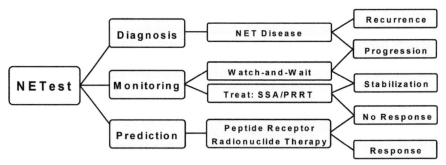

Fig. 4. Clinical utility of a multianalyte assay (NETest) for NET diagnosis and management. The NETest identifies disease status, detects disease progression, is prognostic, and can be used to predict PRRT efficacy. Diagnosis: the NETest can detect BP NET, pancreatic, and gastrointestinal tract NET with greater than or equal to 95% accuracy. In addition, it is effective in the diagnosis of PPGLs (≥95%). Management: NETest has clinical utility in 3 areas: (1) evaluate the effectiveness of a surgical procedure; this allows for a prediction/identification of disease recurrence; (2) evaluate treatment response to SSA or PRRT; and (3) predict treatment failure/disease progression; response to PRRT can be predicted using the NETest and subsequent measurement of transcript levels over time monitor treatment response.

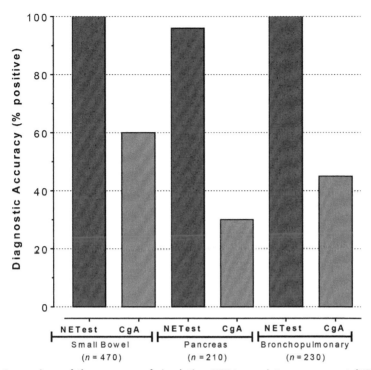

Fig. 5. Comparison of the accuracy of circulating NET transcript measurement (NETest) to CgA. The MAAA (multianalyte algorithm analysis) (NETest) is positive in 96% to 100% of bronchopulmonary, pancreatic, and small bowel NET. CgA in contrast is significantly less accurate. It is positive (elevated) in only approximately 30% to 60%. In pNETs, CgA is elevated in only 30% of tumors. Overall, CgA levels are normal in 40% to 70%, significantly limiting its clinical utility as a biomarker.

greater in metastatic disease (63% ± 26%) in comparison to localized disease (45% ± 21%). As a comparator, blood CgA was elevated in less than 50%. Decision curve analysis demonstrated a greater than 75% standardized clinical net benefit up to a risk threshold of 90% for gene expression analysis compared with CgA. Thus, the use of CgA as a biomarker exhibited a net clinical benefit in less than 30% of patients.

Paragangliomas and pheochromocytomas

The neural-derived lesions, paragangliomas and pheochromocytomas (PPGLs), are NETest-positive in 100% of cases.[60] An ROC analysis AUC was 0.98 for differentiating PPGLs versus controls. Although mutation status was not directly linked to blood gene expression levels, metastatic (80% ± 9%) and multicentric (64% ± 9%) disease had significantly (P<.04) higher scores than localized disease (43% ± 7%). Progressive disease had the highest scores (86% ± 2% vs stable 41% ± 2%; P<.0001).[60] Overall, the NETest was highly sensitive (>95%) as a diagnostic test for PPGLs.

Assessment of the Effectiveness of Surgery for Gastroenteropancreatic and Bronchopulmonary Neuroendocrine Neoplasia

Gastroenteropancreatic neuroendocrine neoplasia

In a prospective GEP-NEN study,[53] the score was elevated in all 35 patients (100%) preoperatively. In comparison, only 14 (40%) had elevated CgA. Resection reduced the NETest from 80% ± 5% to 29% ± 5 (P<.0001). NETest decreases correlated with diminished tumor volume (R^2 = 0.29; P = .03). CgA decrease was insignificant and did not correlate with the extent of tumor resection. The assessment of R0 resections was of particular interest in that 4 (36%) of 11 resections reported as complete had an elevated NETest at 1 month. All 4 subsequently developed positive tumor imaging within 6 months of surgery.

Bronchopulmonary neuroendocrine neoplasm

A prospective BP-NEN study was undertaken in 21 patients.[58] At 6 months after surgery 9 (43%) had evidence of disease (residual/recurrence) and 12 (57%) were disease-free. In the recurrent group, levels were unchanged from before (71% ± 11%) to after surgery (66% ± 8%; P = not significant). In the disease-free group, presurgery gene expression levels (70% ± 7%) were significantly reduced by surgery to 23% ± 3% (P = .0005).

These results demonstrate that blood NET transcripts delineate surgical resection/cytoreduction and facilitate early identification of residual disease in GEP-NEN and BP-NEN.

Monitoring Therapeutic Efficacy

Somatostatin analog

Efficacy was evaluated in a prospective, blinded study.[56] The utility of the NETest was evaluated compared with CgA for the ability to predict treatment failure. In 28 patients receiving SSAs (octreotide [n = 14] and lanreotide [n = 14]), univariate analysis identified that the NETest (P = .002) and tumor grade (P = .054) were associated with therapy responses. Multiple regression analysis identified that only the NETest predicted disease progression during SSA usage (P = .0002). NETest changes occurred significantly earlier than image changes (approximately 5 months prior to image-defined progression). It also was 100% effective in identifying patients who progressed. Multiple regression analysis did not identify CgA as predictive of SSA therapy. This study[56] identified that the NETest exhibited utility in predicting SSA treatment response.

Because biomarker assays that exhibit utility in clinical academic trials do not always effectively translate to real world settings,[71,72] a US registry study (NCT02270567) was undertaken to confirm the clinical utility of the assay in a prospective observational investigation. A study of 51 SSA-treated patients in the United States identified that all patients (n = 37) with a low score (NETest ≤40%) were able to continue without any modification in therapy (type or dose). In contrast, all those with a high score (NETest ≥80%) (n = 24) either underwent a treatment modification (86%) or remained on the current treatment regimen. All (n = 24) exhibited disease progression consistent with failure to respond to SSA. In 21 of these patients, appropriate treatment modifications (dose increases, changing type of SSA, or introduction of selective internal radiation therapy or PRRT) were undertaken. All (n = 21) exhibited disease stabilization at follow-up (6 months: image-based confirmation). The median PFS (mPFS) was not reached for those with low scores. A high score was associated with a mPFS of 5 months (χ^2 = 27.7; hazard ratio [HR] 60.2 (18–201); P<.0001) (Fig. 6).

Peptide radioreceptor therapy

Although previously regarded as an experimental or Hail Mary therapeutic strategy, PRRT is an effective and well-established NET therapy.[73] In principle, selection is based on image-based assessment of somatostatin receptor uptake, although not all patients respond.[74] To better predict efficacy, a combination of tumor grade and a specific omic analysis variant of the NETest gene signature (encompassing growth

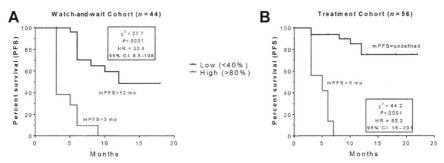

Fig. 6. Relationship between NETest score and PFS in a prospective observational registry cohort. (*A*) Watch-and-wait cohort: a low NETest score was associated with mPFS of 12 months, and a high score was associated with an mPFS of 3 months. This difference was significant (HR 30.4; *P*<.0001). (*B*) Treatment cohort: a low score was associated with an mPFS that was not reached at 12-months, and a high score was associated with an mPFS of 5 months; this difference was significant (HR 60.2; *P*<.0001).

factor signaling and metabolomic gene expression) was developed as a predictive quotient.[75] This was evaluated in 3 prospective studies (n = 158) prior to PRRT therapy.[76] This predictor signature has 2 outputs—positive (predicts response to therapy) and negative (nonresponders). Mathematical assessment using decision curve analysis exhibited greater than 90% standardized predictive benefit up to a risk threshold of 80% for the predictor biomarker analysis. The benefit of a CgA value or grade stratification was equivalent to not using a biomarker (<10% across comparable risk thresholds). Overall, the biomarker was 94% to 97% accurate for predicting a tumor response to PRRT. The mPFS was never reached in those predicted to respond to PRRT (up to 31 months after treatment initiation). For nonresponders, mPFS ranged from 8 months to 14 months. The overall HR for the PRRT predictive biomarker was 47.

As a monitor, measurement of all 51 marker genes identified that the NETest correlated accurately (94%) with PRRT responders (97%) versus nonresponders (91%). Moreover, during therapy, changes in gene expression scores accurately (89%, $P<10^{-6}$) correlated with treatment response assessment (RECIST). In contrast, changes in CgA were only 24% accurate. Overall, the NETest and the predictor analysis (PRRT predictive quotient) identified that PRRT efficacy could be accurately predicted and monitored in greater than 90% of individuals.[75]

Assessment of Long-term Management

Retrospective cohort analysis

A long-term (5-year) study in 34 patients identified that the NETest has predictive and prognostic utility for GEP-NETs. Blood measurement of transcript levels identified clinically actionable alterations approximately 1 year before image-based evidence of progression.[55] Cox modeling identified that the only factor associated with PFS was the NETest. A baseline NETest greater than 80% was significantly associated with disease progression (mPFS: 0.68 years vs 2.78 years, with <40% levels). In contrast, baseline NETest levels greater than 40% in those defined as clinically stable were 100% prognostic of disease progression. Baseline NETest values less than 40% accurately (100%) predicted stability over 5 years. A χ^2 analysis that compared alterations in NETest values to CgA levels demonstrated the NETest 96% more informative than CgA (*P*<.001) in predicting disease status alteration.[55]

Prospective observational study

In a registry study (NCT02270567) (n = 100), a low NETest score was associated with conservative management and maintenance in a watch-and-wait program (n = 28). At follow-up (12 months), all remained stable. All patients (n = 12) with a high score (NETest ≥80%) required treatment interventions and at follow-up (12 months) had disease stabilization (imaging or symptom diminution). A low score was associated with mPFS of 12 months. A high score was associated with an mPFS of 3 months. This difference was significant (χ^2 = 27.7; HR 30.4 [95% CI, 8.5–108]; P<.0001). Comparison of the NETest with CgA using the McNemar test (evaluates 2 biomarkers in paired sample sets) demonstrated CgA of no clinical value in decision making. Overall, a low NETest score reduced imaging approximately 40% (**Fig. 7**).

THE FUTURE

An optimal biomarker needs to have 3 capabilities, namely diagnostic, predictive, and prognostic. Thus, a disease can be identified early, the effect of therapy predicted, and the status of disease monitored. A liquid biopsy fulfills the criteria for real-time disease management and avoids the negative invasive implications and single time-point

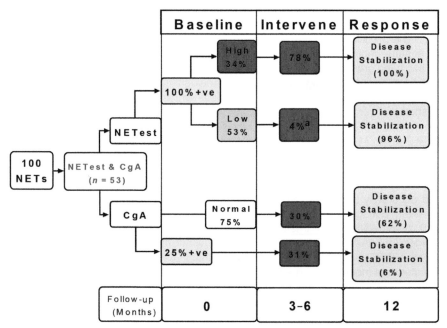

Fig. 7. Comparative clinical utility for CgA and NETest; 100 patients were studied, of whom 53 had both a NETest and CgA. NETest was positive in all 53 samples. CgA levels were elevated in 13 (25%) and were normal in 40 (75%). High NETest scores were noted in 18 (34%) of the 53 patients. Alterations in clinical management (intervene) were made in 78%. All demonstrated disease stabilization at subsequent follow-up (12 months). Low scores were associated with a management change in 1 patient (4%). This patient progressed on everolimus. All other patients (96%) exhibited disease stabilization. CgA was associated with alterations in clinical management in approximately 30% of patients, irrespective of whether the CgA level was elevated. Disease stabilization ranged from 6% to 62% based on intervention and score. CgA levels, therefore, are unable to effectively guide disease management. [a] P<.0001 versus high score. F/Up, Follow-up; Mo, months; +ve, positive.

limitations of tissue biopsy. In addition, it provides information that is of adjunctive value to imaging but is easier to repeat and does not have any of the radiation-related concerns. More recently it has become apparent that a critical requirement is the development of a liquid biopsy that can better identify an appropriate drug target in a particular NEN and, thereafter, define treatment response. This is critical because many therapeutic strategies have limited efficacy, exhibit significant adverse events, and are expensive. In this respect, the PRRT predictive signature demonstrates the utility of circulating RNA as a biomarker (**Fig. 8**). Both the growth factor and the metabolomic genes captured by the signature are specifically related to oxidative stress, metabolism, and hypoxic signaling.[77–79] It is likely that elevated expression of these genes in blood identifies tumors that are more radiosensitive given the role of hypoxia, oxidative stress, and loss of DNA repair associated with radiation responsivity.[80] The specificity of PRRT efficacy prediction, therefore, reflects the identification of molecular mechanisms related to radiation response–associated genes, which modulate tumor response to PRRT.[81]

Given the recent demonstration of the efficacy of PRRT, a predictive strategy is of special relevance. Although PRRT is extremely well tolerated, there is evidence of modest toxicity to the kidney and bone marrow. These are largely unpredictable, because their pathogenesis is poorly understood and, in some cases, apparently idiosyncratic.[16] Irrespective of the etiology, the need to predict or accurately assess the risk of such events is crucial. Blood-based gene expression measurements, therefore, provide an opportunity to identify transcripts relevant to either nephron or myelotoxicity. The development of such a test would provide a complement to the current PRRT predictive quotient and provide a molecular assessment of the risk-benefit ratio for a specific patient.

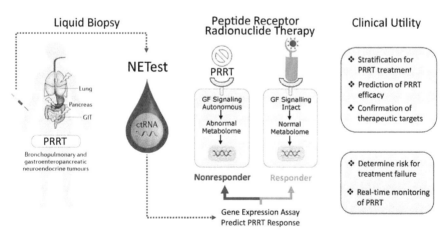

Fig. 8. Cartoon of tumor cell response to ^{177}Lu-octreotate therapy. Tumors (*blue*) responsive to PRRT exhibit a circulating gene fingerprint that has intact, regulated growth factor signaling pathways and normal metabolic pathways. These tumors are predicted to undergo significant DNA damage and tumor apoptosis leading to regression or disease stabilization. Tumors (*orange*) that are autonomous of growth factor modulation and exhibit abnormal metabolome (highly metabolically active) have variable responses to PRRT. Clinical progression is identified after PRRT in the majority (85%–100%) of tumors with predicted nonresponse gene signature. Evaluating blood NET gene expression prior to PRRT facilitates the precise identification of PRRT-responsive tumors. (*Modified from* Kidd M, Modlin IM. Therapy: the role of liquid biopsies to manage and predict PRRT for NETs. Nat Rev Gastroenterol Hepatol 2017;14:6:331–2; with permission.)

CODA

The NETest has been evaluated in more than 5500 NEN patients and identified to exhibit clinical utility in several different areas. These include the assessment of the effectiveness of curative surgery, assessment of the efficacy of SSA therapy, prediction of disease stability/progression, and identification of response to PRRT. The signature was decreased by surgery and values corresponded to the completeness of tumor removal.[53,58] In addition, elevated levels afer R0 resection accurately predicted subsequent disease recurrence. In a separate study, elevated transcript levels were prognostic of SSA failure/disease progression.[56] Alterations in transcript levels occurred significantly earlier than RECIST-based or somatostatin receptor imaging-based measures of disease progression.[56] Finally, levels were prognostic for PRRT efficacy and could be used to evaluate therapeutic efficacy and correlated with image-based assessment.[75]

Current data identify the value of transcript analysis in the monitoring of a variety of therapeutic modalities, particularly in conjunction with other clinical and imaging parameters to monitor disease progression. The authors predict that future strategies for refining and improving the evaluation of therapy will be provided by incorporating imaging modalities and the blood-based molecular information provided by tumor transcriptome analysis.

REFERENCES

1. de Mestier L, Dromain C, d'Assignies G, et al. Evaluating digestive neuroendocrine tumor progression and therapeutic responses in the era of targeted therapies: state of the art. Endocr Relat Cancer 2014;21(3):R105–20. Print 2014.
2. Bergsland EK. The evolving landscape of neuroendocrine tumors. Semin Oncol 2013;40(1):4–22.
3. Wang H, Chen Y, Fernandez-Del Castillo C, et al. Heterogeneity in signaling pathways of gastroenteropancreatic neuroendocrine tumors: a critical look at notch signaling pathway. Mod Pathol 2012;24(10):143.
4. Sundin A, Rockall A. Therapeutic monitoring of gastroenteropancreatic neuroendocrine tumors: the challenges ahead. Neuroendocrinology 2012;96(4):261–71.
5. Kidd M, Schimmack S, Lawrence B, et al. EGFR/TGFalpha and TGFbeta/CTGF signaling in neuroendocrine neoplasia: theoretical therapeutic targets. Neuroendocrinology 2012;15:15.
6. Chan JA, Kulke MH. New treatment options for patients with advanced neuroendocrine tumors. Curr Treat Options Oncol 2011;12(2):136–48.
7. Oberg K. Pancreatic endocrine tumors. Semin Oncol 2010;37(6):594–618.
8. Garcia-Carbonero R, Capdevila J, Crespo-Herrero G, et al. Incidence, patterns of care and prognostic factors for outcome of gastroenteropancreatic neuroendocrine tumors (GEP-NETs): results from the National Cancer Registry of Spain (RGETNE). Ann Oncol 2010;21(9):1794–803.
9. Strosberg J, Gardner N, Kvols L. Survival and prognostic factor analysis of 146 metastatic neuroendocrine tumors of the mid-gut. Neuroendocrinology 2009; 89(4):471–6.
10. Kidd M, Modlin I, Bodei L, et al. Decoding the molecular and mutational ambiguities of gastroenteropancreatic neuroendocrine neoplasm pathobiology. Cell Mol Gastroenterol Hepatol 2015;1:131–53.
11. Lewis MA, Yao JC. Molecular pathology and genetics of gastrointestinal neuroendocrine tumours. Curr Opin Endocrinol Diabetes Obes 2013;4:4.

12. Bosman FT. 4th edition. WHO classification of tumours of the digestive system, volume 3. Lyon (France): World Health Organization; International Agency for Research on Cancer; 2010.

13. Salazar R, Wiedenmann B, Rindi G, et al. ENETS 2011 consensus guidelines for the management of patients with digestive neuroendocrine tumors: an update. Neuroendocrinology 2012;95(2):71–3.

14. Pavel M. Translation of molecular pathways into clinical trials of neuroendocrine tumors. Neuroendocrinology 2013;97(1):99–112.

15. Alexandraki KI, Kaltsas GA, Grozinsky-Glasberg S, et al. Appendiceal neuroendocrine neoplasms: diagnosis and management. Endocr Relat Cancer 2016; 23(1):R27–41.

16. Frilling A, Modlin I, Kidd M, et al. Recommendations for management of patients with neuroendocrine liver metastases. Lancet Oncol 2014;15(1):e8–21.

17. Alvarez MA, Subramaniam PS, Grunn A, et al. Pharmacological targeting of master regulator proteins in neuroendocrine tumors: a novel strategy for precision cancer medicine applications. Nat Genet, in press.

18. Eisenhauer EA, Therasse P, Bogaerts J, et al. New response evaluation criteria in solid tumours: revised RECIST guideline (version 1.1). Eur J Cancer 2009;45(2): 228–47.

19. Neperud J, Mahvash A, Garg N, et al. Can imaging patterns of neuroendocrine hepatic metastases predict response yttruim-90 radioembolotherapy? World J Radiol 2013;5(6):241–7.

20. Denecke T, Baur AD, Ihm C, et al. Evaluation of radiological prognostic factors of hepatic metastases in patients with non-functional pancreatic neuroendocrine tumors. Eur J Radiol 2013;82(10):e550–5.

21. Toumpanakis C, Kim MK, Rinke A, et al. Combination of cross-sectional and molecular imaging studies in the localization of gastroenteropancreatic neuroendocrine tumors. Neuroendocrinology 2014;21:21.

22. Binderup T, Knigge U, Loft A, et al. 18F-fluorodeoxyglucose positron emission tomography predicts survival of patients with neuroendocrine tumors. Clin Cancer Res 2010;16(3):978–85.

23. Castano JP, Sundin A, Maecke HR, et al. Gastrointestinal neuroendocrine tumors (NETs): new diagnostic and therapeutic challenges. Cancer Metastasis Rev 2014;5:5.

24. Faivre S, Ronot M, Dreyer C, et al. Imaging response in neuroendocrine tumors treated with targeted therapies: the experience of sunitinib. Target Oncol 2012; 7(2):127–33.

25. Oberg K, Modlin I, DeHerder W, et al. Biomarkers for neuroendocrine tumor disease: a delphic consensus assessment of multianalytes, genomics, circulating cells and monoanalytes. Lancet Oncol 2015;16:e435046.

26. Hulka B. Overview of biological markers. In: Hulka B, Griffith J, Wilcosky T, editors. Biological markers in epidemiology. New York: Oxford University Press; 1990. p. 3–15.

27. Modlin IM, Gustafsson BI, Moss SF, et al. Chromogranin A–biological function and clinical utility in neuro endocrine tumor disease. Ann Surg Oncol 2010; 17(9):2427–43.

28. Yao JC, Pavel M, Phan AT, et al. Chromogranin A and neuron-specific enolase as prognostic markers in patients with advanced pNET treated with everolimus. J Clin Endocrinol Metab 2011;96(12):3741–9.

29. Lawrence B, Gustafsson BI, Kidd M, et al. The clinical relevance of chromogranin A as a biomarker for gastroenteropancreatic neuroendocrine tumors. Endocrinol Metab Clin North Am 2011;40(1):111–34, viii.

30. Malczewska A, Kidd M, Matar S, et al. A comprehensive assessment of the role of miRNAs as biomarkers in gastroenteropancreatic neuroendocrine tumors. Neuroendocrinology 2018;107(1):73–90.

31. Kidd M, Drozdov I, Modlin I. Blood and tissue neuroendocrine tumor gene cluster analysis correlate, define hallmarks and predict disease status. Endocr Relat Cancer 2015;22(4):561–75.

32. Hanahan D, Weinberg RA. The hallmarks of cancer. Cell 2000;100(1):57–70.

33. Hanahan D, Weinberg RA. Hallmarks of cancer: the next generation. Cell 2011; 144(5):646–74.

34. Walenkamp A, Crespo G, Fierro Maya F, et al. Hallmarks of gastrointestinal neuroendocrine tumours: implications for treatment. Endocr Relat Cancer 2014;21(6): R445–60.

35. Wang E, Zaman N, McGee S, et al. Predictive genomics: a cancer hallmark network framework for predicting tumor clinical phenotypes using genome sequencing data. Semin Cancer Biol 2014;18(14):00050–9.

36. Cardoso F, van't Veer LJ, Bogaerts J, et al. 70-gene signature as an aid to treatment decisions in early-stage breast cancer. N Engl J Med 2016;375(8):717–29.

37. Krop I, Ismaila N, Andre F, et al. Use of biomarkers to guide decisions on adjuvant systemic therapy for women with early-stage invasive breast cancer: american society of clinical oncology clinical practice guideline focused update. J Clin Oncol 2017;35(24):2838–47.

38. Curtis C. Genomic profiling of breast cancers. Curr Opin Obstet Gynecol 2015; 27(1):34–9.

39. Diaz LA Jr, Bardelli A. Liquid biopsies: genotyping circulating tumor DNA. J Clin Oncol 2014;32(6):579–86.

40. Siravegna G, Marsoni S, Siena S, et al. Integrating liquid biopsies into the management of cancer. Nat Rev Clin Oncol 2017;2(10):14.

41. Oxnard GR, Paweletz CP, Kuang Y, et al. Noninvasive detection of response and resistance in EGFR-mutant lung cancer using quantitative next-generation genotyping of cell-free plasma DNA. Clin Cancer Res 2014;20(6):1698–705.

42. Remon J, Caramella C, Jovelet C, et al. Osimertinib benefit in EGFR-mutant NSCLC patients with T790M-mutation detected by circulating tumour DNA. Ann Oncol 2017;28(4):784–90.

43. Reinert T, Scholer LV, Thomsen R, et al. Analysis of circulating tumour DNA to monitor disease burden following colorectal cancer surgery. Gut 2015; 4(308859):625–34.

44. Kidd M, Modlin I, Oberg K. Towards a new classification of gastroenteropancreatic neuroendocrine neoplasms. Nat Rev Clin Oncol 2016;13(11):691–705.

45. Jiao Y, Shi C, Edil BH, et al. DAXX/ATRX, MEN1, and mTOR pathway genes are frequently altered in pancreatic neuroendocrine tumors. Science 2011; 331(6021):1199–203.

46. Shay JW, Reddel RR, Wright WE. Cancer. Cancer and telomeres–an ALTernative to telomerase. Science 2012;336(6087):1388–90.

47. Patel K, Friedrich-Rust M, Lurie Y, et al. FibroSURE and FibroScan in relation to treatment response in chronic hepatitis C virus. World J Gastroenterol 2011; 17(41):4581–9.

48. Kidd M, Modlin IM, Drozdov I. Gene network-based analysis identifies two potential subtypes of small intestinal neuroendocrine tumors. BMC Genomics 2014;15: 595.

49. Duerr EM, Mizukami Y, Ng A, et al. Defining molecular classifications and targets in gastroenteropancreatic neuroendocrine tumors through DNA microarray analysis. Endocr Relat Cancer 2008;15(1):243–56.

50. Drozdov I, Kidd M, Nadler B, et al. Predicting neuroendocrine tumor (carcinoid) neoplasia using gene expression profiling and supervised machine learning. Cancer 2009;115(8):1638–50.

51. Modlin I, Drozdov I, Kidd M. The Identification of gut neuroendocrine tumor disease by multiple synchronous transcript analysis in blood. PLoS One 2013;8: e63364.

52. Modlin IM, Aslanian H, Bodei L, et al. A PCR blood test outperforms chromogranin A in carcinoid detection and is unaffected by PPIs. Endocr Connect 2014;14: 14–0100.

53. Modlin IM, Frilling A, Salem RR, et al. Blood measurement of neuroendocrine gene transcripts defines the effectiveness of operative resection and ablation strategies. Surgery 2016;159(1):336–47.

54. Modlin IM, Kidd M, Bodei L, et al. The clinical utility of a novel blood-based multi-transcriptome assay for the diagnosis of neuroendocrine tumors of the gastrointestinal tract. Am J Gastroenterol 2015;110(8):1223–32.

55. Pavel M, Jann H, Prasad V, et al. NET blood transcript analysis defines the crossing of the clinical rubicon: when stable disease becomes progressive. Neuroendocrinology 2017;104(2):170–82.

56. Cwikla JB, Bodei L, Kolasinska-Cwikla A, et al. Circulating transcript analysis (NETest) in GEP-NETs treated with somatostatin analogs defines therapy. J Clin Endocrinol Metab 2015;100(11):E1437–45.

57. Modlin IM, Drozdov I, Alaimo D, et al. A multianalyte PCR blood test outperforms single analyte ELISAs (chromogranin A, pancreastatin, neurokinin A) for neuroendocrine tumor detection. Endocr Relat Cancer 2014;21(4):615–28.

58. Filosso PL, Kidd M, Roffinella M, et al. The utility of blood neuroendocrine gene transcript measurement in the diagnosis of bronchopulmonary neuroendocrine tumors (BPNET) and as a tool to evaluate surgical resection and disease progression. Eur J Cardiothorac Surg 2017;53(3):631–9.

59. Kidd M, Modlin I, Drozdov I, et al. A liquid biopsy for bronchopulmonary/lung carcinoid diagnosis. Oncotarget 2017;9(6):7182–96.

60. Peczkowska M, Cwikla J, Kidd M, et al. The clinical utility of circulating neuroendocrine gene transcript analysis in well-differentiated paragangliomas and pheochromocytomas. Eur J Endocrinol 2017;176(2):143–57.

61. Modlin I, Drozdov I, Kidd M. A multitranscript blood neuroendocrine tumor molecular signature to identify treatment efficacy and disease progress. J Clin Oncol 2013;31(Suppl):A4137.

62. Modlin I, Drozdov I, Kidd M. Gut neuroendocrine Tumor Blood qPCR fingerprint assay: characteristics and reproducibility. Clin Chem 2014;52(3):419–29.

63. Kononenko I. Machine learning for medical diagnosis: history, state of the art and perspective. Artif Intell Med 2001;23(1):89–109.

64. Darcy AM, Louie AK, Roberts LW. Machine learning and the profession of medicine. JAMA 2016;315(6):551–2.

65. Bustin SA. Absolute quantification of mRNA using real-time reverse transcription polymerase chain reaction assays. J Mol Endocrinol 2000;25(2):169–93.

66. Jia X, Ju H, Yang L, et al. A novel multiplex polymerase chain reaction assay for profile analyses of gene expression in peripheral blood. BMC Cardiovasc Disord 2012;12:51.

67. Schmittgen TD, Zakrajsek BA, Mills AG, et al. Quantitative reverse transcription-polymerase chain reaction to study mRNA decay: comparison of endpoint and real-time methods. Anal Biochem 2000;285(2):194–204.

68. Ding C, Cantor CR. A high-throughput gene expression analysis technique using competitive PCR and matrix-assisted laser desorption ionization time-of-flight MS. Proc Natl Acad Sci U S A 2003;100(6):3059–64.

69. Giusti M, Sidoti M, Augeri C, et al. Effect of short-term treatment with low dosages of the proton-pump inhibitor omeprazole on serum chromogranin A levels in man. Eur J Endocrinol 2004;150(3):299–303.

70. Ishida M, Shiomi H, Naka S, et al. Concomitant intraductal papillary mucinous neoplasm and neuroendocrine tumor of the pancreas. Oncol Lett 2013;5(1):63–7.

71. Ginsburg GS, Kuderer NM. Comparative effectiveness research, genomics-enabled personalized medicine, and rapid learning health care: a common bond. J Clin Oncol 2012;30(34):4233–42.

72. Malik SM, Pazdur R, Abrams JS, et al. Consensus report of a joint NCI thoracic malignancies steering committee: FDA workshop on strategies for integrating biomarkers into clinical development of new therapies for lung cancer leading to the inception of "master protocols" in lung cancer. J Thorac Oncol 2014; 9(10):1443–8.

73. Strosberg J, El-Haddad G, Wolin E, et al. Phase 3 Trial of 177Lu-Dotatate for midgut neuroendocrine tumors. N Engl J Med 2017;376(2):125–35.

74. Bodei L, Kidd M, Paganelli G, et al. Clinical features are not reliable in predicting long-term toxicity after PRRT - Evidence from >800 patients to support genetic screen development. Paper presented at: ENETS Conference. Barcelona (Spain), March 6–8, 2014.

75. Bodei L, Kidd M, Modlin IM, et al. Measurement of circulating transcripts and gene cluster analysis predicts and defines therapeutic efficacy of peptide receptor radionuclide therapy (PRRT) in neuroendocrine tumors. Eur J Nucl Med Mol Imaging 2016;43(5):839–51.

76. Bodei L, Kidd MS, Singh A, et al. PRRT genomic signature in blood for prediction of 177Lu-octreotate efficacy. Eur J Nucl Med Mol Imaging 2018;45(7):1155–69.

77. Valli A, Rodriguez M, Moutsianas L, et al. Hypoxia induces a lipogenic cancer cell phenotype via HIF1alpha-dependent and -independent pathways. Oncotarget 2015;6(4):1920–41.

78. Olsson AH, Yang BT, Hall E, et al. Decreased expression of genes involved in oxidative phosphorylation in human pancreatic islets from patients with type 2 diabetes. Eur J Endocrinol 2011;165(4):589–95.

79. Day TF, Mewani RR, Starr J, et al. Transcriptome and proteome analyses of TNFAIP8 knockdown cancer cells reveal new insights into molecular determinants of cell survival and tumor progression. Methods Mol Biol 2017;1513: 83–100.

80. Hill RP. The changing paradigm of tumour response to irradiation. Br J Radiol 2017;90(1069):20160474.

81. Kidd M, Modlin IM. Therapy: the role of liquid biopsies to manage and predict PRRT for NETs. Nat Rev Gastroenterol Hepatol 2017;14(6):331–2.

Novel Functional Imaging of Neuroendocrine Tumors

Anders Sundin, MD, PhD

KEYWORDS

- ^{68}Ga-Dota-toc ● ^{68}Ga-Dota-tate ● ^{68}Ga-Dota-noc,^{18}FDG ● ^{18}F-Dopa
- ^{11}C-5-hydroxy-tryptophan

KEY POINTS

- ^{68}Ga-DOTA-somatostatin analogue-PET/computed tomography constitutes an integral part in neuroendocrine tumor visualization and is especially advantageous to detect metastases to lymph nodes, bone, liver, peritoneum, and brain.
- PET/computed tomography should be performed together with diagnostic intravenous contrast-enhanced computed tomography to take full advantage of the technique.
- Similarly, MRI with PET/MRI should use dynamic intravenous contrast enhancement of the liver and pancreas and whole-body diffusion-weighted imaging.
- MRI is superior to computed tomography for neuroendocrine tumor imaging of liver, pancreas, brain, and bone, but may miss small lung metastases, which are best visualized by computed tomography.

INTRODUCTION

Imaging of neuroendocrine tumors (NETs) is based on the combination of morphologic (radiologic) and functional (nuclear medicine) techniques because they provide complementary information (**Box 1**). Functional imaging with modern scanners can currently be performed as hybrid imaging procedures, whereby PET and single photon emission computed tomography (SPECT) are performed together with computed tomography (CT) scan as PET/CT scan and SPECT/CT scanning, and in recent years also PET/MRI. Hybrid procedures generally achieve a better imaging yield, as compared with separate interpretation of morphologic and functional imaging, and additionally improve reader confidence. Because conventional radiologic cross-sectional methods (CT scanning and MRI) constitute the basis for NET imaging and because the quality of both components is crucial for the result of hybrid imaging (PET/CT scanning and PET/MRI), this article concentrates on the functional

Disclosure: The author has nothing to disclose.

Department of Radiology, Molecular Imaging, Institution of Surgical Sciences, Uppsala University, Uppsala University Hospital, Uppsala SE-751 85, Sweden

E-mail address: anders.sundin@radiol.uu.se

Endocrinol Metab Clin N Am 47 (2018) 505–523
https://doi.org/10.1016/j.ecl.2018.04.003
0889-8529/18/© 2018 Elsevier Inc. All rights reserved.

Box 1
Points of interest

- NET imaging should always use a combination of morphologic and functional whole-body imaging.

- In low grade NETs, somatostatin receptor imaging with ^{68}Ga-DOTA-somatostatin analogue-PET/CT is preferred to scintigraphy because of the vastly superior performance of PET/CT.

- In high-grade NETs, somatostatin receptor expression is usually low or absent and metabolic imaging with ^{18}FDG-PET/CT is, therefore, preferred.

- Above a suggested approximate 15% KI-67 cutoff, metabolic imaging with ^{18}FDG-PET/CT is usually preferred rather than ^{68}Ga-DOTA-somatostatin analogue-PET/CT because of the risk of low or absent somatostatin receptor expression in the NET lesions.

- A combination of ^{68}Ga-DOTA-somatostatin analogue-PET/CT and ^{18}FDG-PET/CT is advantageous because high-grade NETs may show somatostatin receptor expression sufficient for PRRT and low-grade NETs may be ^{18}FDG-avid, which is a negative prognostic indication, although this policy is usually not possible because of financial constraints.

- The most commonly used ^{68}Ga-DOTA-somatostatin analogue preparations are ^{68}Ga-DOTA-TOC (tyrosine octreotide), ^{68}Ga-DOTA-TATE (octreotate) and ^{68}Ga-DOTA-NOC (1-Nal3-octreotide), with no convincingly reported differences in imaging capacity.

- ^{18}F-DOPA is an alternative PET tracer for lesion detection available in some countries.

- ^{11}C-5-hydroxy-tryptophan is yet another PET tracer; however, it has limited availability, which can be used when ^{68}Ga-DOTA-somatostatin analogue-PET/CT fails.

- For CT together with PET/CT, a fully diagnostic examination protocol should be used, including IV contrast-enhanced CT of the liver and pancreas in the late arterial phase and of the whole body in the venous phase.

- Small (<5 mm) NET lesions may be missed by PET because of its limited spatial resolution and concomitant IV contrast-enhanced CT may pick up these lesions.

- Because of the better tissue contrast, MRI is better than CT for imaging of the liver, pancreas, bone and brain, and can be considered in addition to PET/CT.

- Diffusion-weighted imaging and dynamic IV gadolinium contrast-enhanced MRI should be included for optimal NET imaging of the liver and pancreas.

- For MRI of the liver, hepatocyte-specific contrast media are available.

- PET/MRI is so far available for clinical NET imaging in merely a few centers and should use fully diagnostic whole-body MRI protocols.

- The recent development of somatostatin receptor antagonists for clinical applications hold interesting potentials for future NET hybrid imaging.

Abbreviations: CT, computed tomography; IV, intravenous; NET, neuroendocrine tumor; PRRT, peptide receptor radiotherapy.

---

techniques and comments on relevant details related to the concomitant morphologic imaging procedures.

Depending on how the NET patient presents with the disease, the requirements for imaging are very varying. A functioning pancreatic NET may produce pronounced hormonal symptoms and yet be very small, and for its preoperative localization several morphologic and functional imaging techniques and also endoscopy may be required. The other end of the spectrum may be represented by a patient presenting with a disseminated small intestinal NET (SI-NET) and bulky liver metastases for whom the imaging workup by comparison is straightforward and will comprise tumor staging by CT scanning or MRI and somatostatin receptor imaging by PET (or scintigraphy if PET is not available).

Also, these imaging requirements differ depending on the particular application, that is, whether the imaging is performed for primary tumor detection, tumor staging of the primary tumor and regional and distant metastases, surveillance and detection of recurrent disease after surgery with curative intent, or therapeutic monitoring of locoregional and systemic therapies.

SOMATOSTATIN RECEPTOR IMAGING

Somatostatin receptor imaging is performed in patients with NET because several additional metastases are regularly revealed as compared with radiologic cross-sectional imaging (CT scanning and MRI), and the tumor somatostatin receptor status provides information on the patient's eligibility for treatment with somatostatin analogues labeled with therapeutic beta-emitting radionuclides, that is, peptide receptor radiotherapy (PRRT). The previous mainstay for somatostatin receptor imaging, somatostatin receptor scintigraphy (including SPECT) with predominately ^{111}In-pentetreotide (Octreoscan), but also with [99]mTc-labelled octreotide, has during the last decade been replaced in an increasing number of centers by PET/CT scanning with ^{68}Ga-DOTA-somatostatin analogues because of its considerably better imaging yield.[1,2,3,4] An additional advantage is the lower radiation dose to the patient.[5] This considerably better diagnostic performance is explained by the higher spatial resolution of PET as compared with SPECT (approximately 0.5 cm vs 1.0–1.5 cm) and the better tumor-to-normal-tissue contrast. It is, therefore, much more advantageous for the patient to be referred to a nearby center for ^{68}Ga-DOTA-somatostatin analogue-PET/CT scanning rather than to undergo scintigraphy in their local hospital. The description of somatostatin receptor imaging provided herein is concentrated on PET/CT scanning and PET/MRI and not on scintigraphy.

In recent reviews, the reported mean sensitivity and specificity of ^{68}Ga-DOTA-somatostatin analogue-PET/CT scanning for NET diagnoses ranges between 88% and 93%[6,7,8,9] and 88% and 95%, respectively.[6,7] The reported mean sensitivity and specificity for the diagnosis of duodenopancreatic NETs was 92% and 83%, respectively, and for the detection of bone metastases ranges 97% to 100% and 92% to 100%, respectively.[7]"

The sensitivity of ^{68}Ga-DOTA-somatostatin analogue-PET/CT scanning to detect gastrinomas is considerably lower at 68%, and the detection of the primary NET in cancer with an unknown primary is even less, at 52%.[7]

^{68}Ga-DOTA-Somatostatin Analogue Preparations

The most commonly used ^{68}Ga-DOTA-somatostatin analogue preparations are ^{68}Ga-DOTA-TOC (tyrosine octreotide), TATE (octreotate), and NOC (1-Nal3-octreotide), which all closely resemble the original peptide octreotide (used for scintigraphy) but with 1 amino acid (TOC and NOC) or 2 amino acids (TATE) replaced, resulting in very varying affinities of the 3 peptides in vitro for the different somatostatin receptor subtypes. These differences in vitro have, however, been difficult to convincingly show in comparative trials in the clinical setting.[10,11] DOTA (1,4,7,10-tetraazacyclododecane-1,4,7,10-tetraacetic acid) is a chelate that allows for conjugating the radiometal (^{68}Ga) with the peptide.

Generally, 2 MBq of ^{68}Ga-DOTA-somatostatin analogue (TOC/TATE/NOC) per kilogram of body weight is injected intravenously (IV) and the PET/CT examination starts 1 hour after injection, although some centers examine at 30 minutes to achieve faster patient throughput that will allow for examination of more patients per tracer preparation. The highest tumor uptake of ^{68}Ga-DOTATOC has, however, been shown approximately 70 minutes after injection.[1]

PET/Computed Tomography Examination Procedure

Stand-alone PET scanners are currently rare and modern equipment comprise hybrid PET/CT systems with the PET detector rings generally in the back of the scanner and the CT scanner in front. Consequently, the gantry (tunnel) of the PET/CT scanner is somewhat longer than that of a regular CT scanner, but is otherwise very similar, with a bed for the patient. To take full advantage of the PET/CT examination, the CT scanning in conjunction with PET should be performed as a fully diagnostic examination, including IV contrast enhancement and using similar CT examination protocols as in the radiology department. CT scanning should be limited to a non–contrast-enhanced examination when the patient has recently (during the last 3–4 weeks) already undergone a diagnostic CT scan of the thorax–abdomen and pelvis, and when the patient cannot receive IV contrast media because of previous serious adverse effects or impaired kidney function. For filling of the stomach and bowel and to enhance renal excretion of the CT contrast medium, the patient drinks approximately 800 mL over the 1.5 hours before the start of the PET/CT examination.

A standard PET/CT examination protocol generally begins with a frontal (and sometimes also a lateral) CT overview (scout view, scannogram, topogram) extending from the head to the proximal thighs. The fields of view for the CT and PET examinations are indicated on this CT overview. The axial fields of view for both CT scans and PET usually comprise the whole body from the base of the skull to the proximal thighs, but CT examination also includes additional scanning of the liver (described elsewhere in this article). The PET/CT examination sequence usually continues with a very low radiation dose whole body CT scanning, used to later correct the ensuing PET images for attenuation, then the whole body PET acquisition is performed. The PET detector rings in most scanners cover 15 to 20 cm and the patient therefore needs to be moved stepwise through the gantry to perform the PET acquisition 2 to 3 minutes per bed position. The examination sequence usually ends with the diagnostic CT scanning, which includes scanning of the liver in the late arterial contrast enhancement phase and whole body CT scanning in the venous phase. Some protocols also include a precontrast examination of the liver that can be added when required. All CT examinations are performed while the patient continues tidal breathing to allow for coregistration with the PET image volume. In patients who do not undergo a diagnostic CT scan, the initial CT scan for attenuation correction should be performed with a somewhat higher radiation dose to allow also for coregistration and anatomic correlation of the PET findings.

The PET and CT images are reconstructed and reformatted in the transverse, coronal, and sagittal planes, and as corresponding PET/CT fusion images. Also, a 3-dimensional whole body reconstruction of the PET image volume as a maximum intensity projection is supplied to facilitate the image reading. The PET/CT images are reviewed in a computer workstation, usually by using software supplied by the PET/CT vendor, or by using similar functions available in some picture archive and communication system workstation software.

Nonsomatostatin Analogue-PET/Computed Tomography

In some European countries, PET/CT scanning with ^{18}F-DOPA is similarly available as with ^{68}Ga-DOTA-somatostatin analogues. Although ^{18}F-DOPA-PET/CT scanning does not provide information on somatostatin receptor expression, it is useful for tumor visualization and has been shown to be superior to Octreoscan[12] and similar to ^{68}Ga-somatostatin analogue-PET/CT scanning in a patient-based analysis, although fewer tumor lesions were found by ^{18}F-DOPA-PET/CT scanning.[13,14] ^{18}F-DOPA-PET/CT scanning is valuable when ^{68}Ga-somatostatin analogue-PET/CT scanning fails, such as in NETs with low or absent somatostatin receptor expression. Another alternative in these patients, although with availability restricted to 2 European centers, is PET/CT scanning with the serotonin precursor ^{11}C-5-hydroxy-trypto-phan.[15,16,17] Although still investigational for benign insulinoma with frequently low somatostatin receptor expression, high sensitivity has been reported for PET/CT scanning with ^{68}Ga-labelled tracers binding to the glucagon-like peptide receptor-1.[18]

Usually, somatostatin receptor expression in the NETs decreases in parallel with increasing tumor proliferation (KI-67 index), and the ^{68}Ga-DOTA-somatostatin analogue uptake in high grade NETs is consequently low or negative.[19] For metabolic imaging with [^{18}F]fluoro-deoxy-glucose ([18]FDG), the principal tracer for PET/CT scanning in general oncology, the situation is generally the reverse, and in parallel with increasing proliferation the NETs generally become more [18]FDG avid. For lesion detection of higher grade NETs, and especially with neuroendocrine cancers, [18]FDG-PET/CT scanning is therefore preferred. There is, however, a very wide overlap in this respect in the sense that even low G2 NETs can be [18]FDG avid and high G2 and G3 tumors may show high somatostatin receptor expression, rendering the patient eligible for PRRT. Optimally, it is preferable to perform both somatostatin receptor imaging and [18]FDG-PET/CT scanning because the tracers are complementary and increase the sensitivity for lesion detection.[20] In most centers, dual PET/CT scanning is, however, not feasible because of financial constraints, and the choice of PET tracer needs to be based on the NET proliferation. A very approximate KI-67 cutoff of 15% may be applied, above which [8]FDG probably is a more suitable tracer than ^{68}Ga-DOTA-somatostatin analogues for lesion detection.[21] Consequently, the imaging capacity of [18]FDG-PET/CT scanning depends on the proportions of the various NET grades in the group of patients examined, and this is reflected in the wide variations in sensitivities in different reports, ranging from 37% to 72%.[19,20,22,23,24] Interestingly, the presence or absence of [18]FDG avidity has also been shown to predict prognosis.[21,22]

[18]FDG-PET/CT scanning is generally performed 60 minutes after injection of 4 MBq [18]FDG per kilogram body weight and with an examination protocol similar to that for ^{68}Ga-DOTA-somatostatin analogue-PET/CT scanning.

Computed Tomography

CT scanning constitutes the basic NET imaging technique, irrespective of disease presentation and imaging application. Current CT scanners include detectors comprising a large number of parallel rows, at least 64, and in combination with short ($\leq$0.5 seconds) x-ray tube rotation time the whole thorax, abdomen and pelvis examination may be examined during 1 breath hold. The resulting hundreds of transverse 1 mm or less images are generally automatically reformatted by the scanner software to produce image volumes also in the coronal and sagittal planes multiplanar reformatted images to better appreciate anatomy and pathologic findings. To this end, the transverse images may additionally be used to produce 3-dimensional image volumes, typically maximum intensity projection and volume-rendering technique images. Equally important, these modern fast scanners allow for better use of IV iodine-based contrast media, and CT scanning of the liver and pancreas should always be performed during several contrast-enhancement phases (discussed elsewhere in this article).

Spectral CT scanning or dual-energy CT scanning is a recent development that allows for simultaneous detection of x-rays with different energy during the same CT scanning procedure, typically at 80 and 140 kV. The difference in x-ray attenuation in the images achieved by using a high and low tube tension, respectively, is greater for a high-attenuating than for low-attenuating tissues. Consequently, a low x-ray tube tension may be applied to better use iodine-based contrast media (with high attenuation) to achieve better contrast enhancement at a standard contrast medium dose, or to attain the same contrast enhancement at a lower dose of the contrast medium. The iodine content of a tissue may be determined by this technique, and its role in tissue characterization is currently also investigated. Dual-energy CT scanning applications for hybrid imaging of NETs have, however, not yet been established.

^{68}Ga-DOTA-Somatostatin Analogue-PET/Computed Tomography Findings

Characteristic PET/CT findings of various NET lesions are illustrated in the figures. NET liver metastases generally show high ^{68}Ga-DOTA-somatostatin analogue accumulation (**Fig. 1**) and lesions not depicted on CT scans are often seen (**Fig. 2**). Considerably lower tracer accumulation is seen in liver metastases in a patient with a SI-NET with a Ki-67 index of 15% (**Fig. 3**), and is completely absent in the liver metastases in a patient with a high-grade (G3) NET (**Fig. 4**). As pointed out, small lymph node metastases are by morphologic imaging techniques (CT scanning and MRI) often overlooked or, when depicted, cannot be characterized as such because

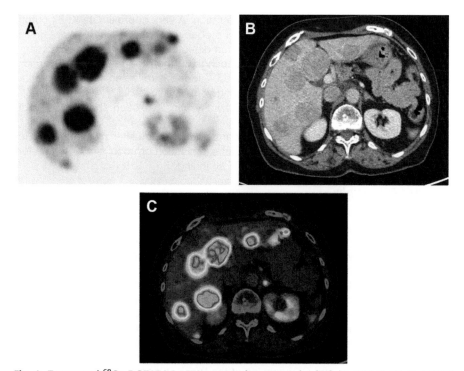

Fig. 1. Transversal ^{68}Ga-DOTATOC-PET/computed tomography (CT) (*A*, PET; *B*, CT; *C*, PET/CT fusion) showing very high tracer uptake in multiple small intestinal neuroendocrine tumor liver metastases.

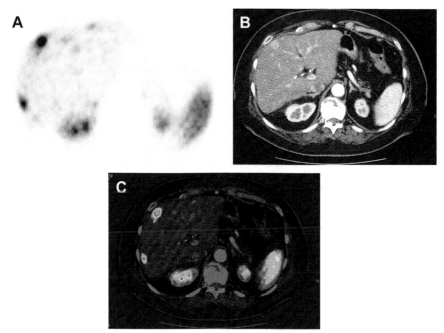

Fig. 2. Transversal ^{68}Ga-DOTATOC-PET/computed tomography (CT) (*A*, PET; *B*, CT; *C*, PET/CT fusion) showing high uptake in 2 neuroendocrine tumor liver metastases, of which the ventrally located lesion on CT corresponds with a hypervascular lesion, whereas the dorsally located liver metastasis is not visualized by CT.

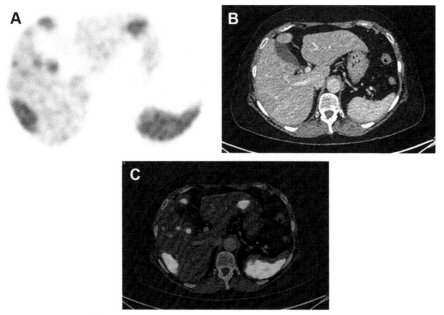

Fig. 3. Transversal ^{68}Ga-DOTATOC-PET/computed tomography (CT) (*A*, PET; *B*, CT; *C*, PET/CT fusion) showing comparably much lower tracer uptake in multiple liver metastases in this patient with a small intestinal neuroendocrine tumor with a ki-67 index of 15%.

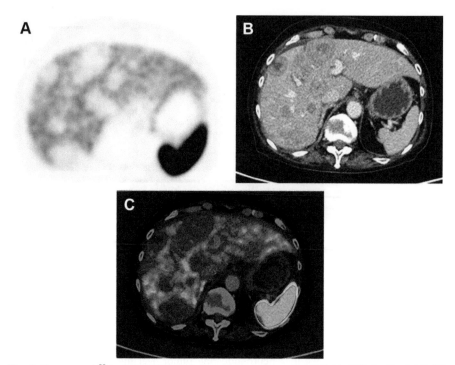

Fig. 4. Transversal ⁶⁸Ga-DOTATOC-PET/computed tomography (CT) (*A*, PET; *B*, CT; *C*, PET/CT fusion) showing PET-negative multiple liver metastases in this patient with a high G2 neuro-endocrine tumor.

lymph nodes with a short axis diameter (≤10 mm) are considered benign. The tracer uptake in small (<10 mm) metastatic lymph nodes is often high, and these lesions are generally easily identified by ⁶⁸Ga-DOTA-somatostatin analogue-PET/CT scanning (**Fig. 5**). This is also illustrated in **Fig. 6**, in which PET/CT scanning with both ⁶⁸Ga-DOTATOC and ¹¹C-5-hydroxy-tryptophan is shown for comparison. Bone metastases are frequently missed by CT scans, but are generally well-shown by ⁶⁸Ga-DOTA-somatostatin analogue-PET/CT scans, as in this patient with a rectal NET (**Fig. 7**) with disseminated bone metastases (**Fig. 8**). Peritoneal metastases are easy to miss with CT scanning. Although their diagnosis generally is facilitated by ⁶⁸Ga-DOTA-somatostatin analogue-PET/CT scans (**Fig. 9**) they may nevertheless be overlooked, as recently reported.[25] The importance of diagnosing the primary SI-NET (or primaries) is under debate. To achieve oncological surgical resection, the whole small intestine needs to be palpated during surgery and all primary SI-NETs removed. In many patients, the primary SI-NET (or SI-NETs) may be visualized by ⁶⁸Ga-DOTA-somatostatin analogue-PET/CT scanning (**Fig. 10**). Endoscopic ultrasound imaging is the optimal technique to detect pancreatic NETs, but because of the limited availability, noninvasive imaging methods are often tried first. In many patients, CT scans and MRI may localize the tumor and in others ⁶⁸Ga-DOTA-so-matostatin analogue-PET/CT scanning may be helpful (**Fig. 11**). The advantage of metabolic imaging with ¹⁸FDG-PET/CT scanning in high-grade tumors is illustrated in this patient with a neuroendocrine cancer of the thymus (**Fig. 12**). A high somato-statin receptor expression in this lung tumor indicates a NET (**Fig. 13**).

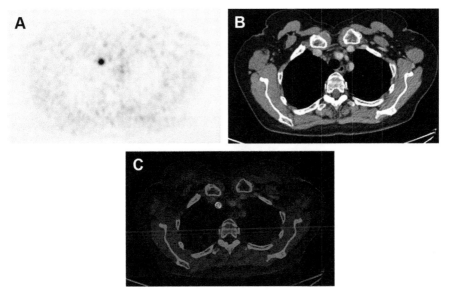

Fig. 5. Transversal ^{68}Ga-DOTATOC-PET/computed tomography (CT) (*A*, PET; *B*, CT; *C*, PET/CT fusion) showing distinct high tracer uptake in a small (7-mm) paratracheal lymph node metastasis, previously overlooked on CT, in this patient with a small-intestinal neuroendocrine tumor.

MRI

The tissue contrast of MRI is better than that of CT scanning. MRI is better than CT scanning for imaging of the liver and pancreas and to detect metastases in bone and brain, and should be favored before CT scanning for these applications. This factor should be considered before hybrid imaging in centers where both PET/CT and PET/MRI scanners are available.

The pharmacokinetics of the gadolinium-based extracellular contrast media for MRI is similar to that of the iodine-based contrast media for CT scanning, and the high temporal resolution of MRI similarly allows for dynamic acquisitions in several contrast enhancement phases.

In addition, hepatocyte-specific MRI contrast media (Gd-DTPA and Gd-EOB-DTPA) are available. Immediately after injection, they act as extracellular contrast agents but are then accumulated in the hepatocytes, which allows for late imaging after several minutes (15–120 minutes depending on the chelate) to achieve maximum signal difference (contrast) between liver metastases: these become low signaling (dark) in relation to the contrast-enhanced high-signaling (bright) normal liver. These liver-specific contrast media are partly excreted into the bile, which may be used for MR cholangiography.

Diffusion-weighted imaging (DWI) is based on the random Brownian movement of water molecules, which is free in cystic structures, but is restricted in highly cellular tissues such as malignant tumors. DWI is performed by using several (usually 3) so-called b values, a factor reflecting the respective strength and timing of the gradient that is used to generate the images. These images are also used and to calculate the degree of restriction of the water molecules in the examined tissues, which is shown in corresponding images of the apparent diffusion coefficient map. DWI is well-established in neurologic imaging and is currently being investigated for lesion

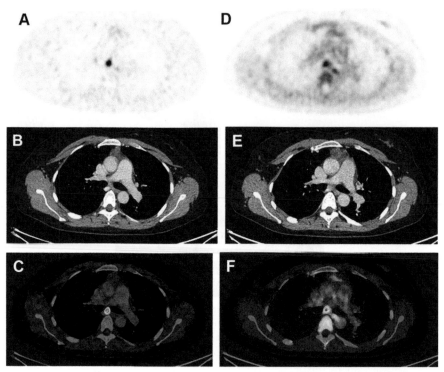

Fig. 6. Transversal ^{68}Ga-DOTATOC-PET/computed tomography (CT) (*A*, PET; *B*, CT; *C*, PET/CT fusion) and ^{11}C-5-hydroxy-tryptophan-PET/CT (*D*, PET; *E*, CT; *F*, PET/CT fusion) showing high focal tracer uptake in a subcarinal lymph node metastasis in this patient with a neuroendocrine tumor with unknown primary tumor (cancer unknown primary).

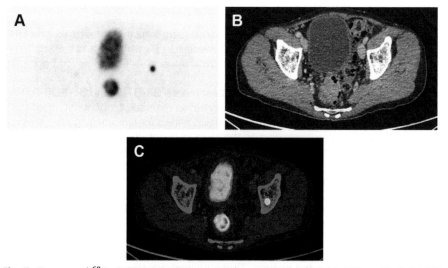

Fig. 7. Transversal ^{68}Ga-DOTATOC-PET/computed tomography (CT) (*A*, PET; *B*, CT; *C*, PET/CT fusion) showing a high tracer uptake in a primary rectal neuroendocrine tumor. A small bone metastasis in the left acetabulum is clearly diagnosed by PET but is not visualized by CT.

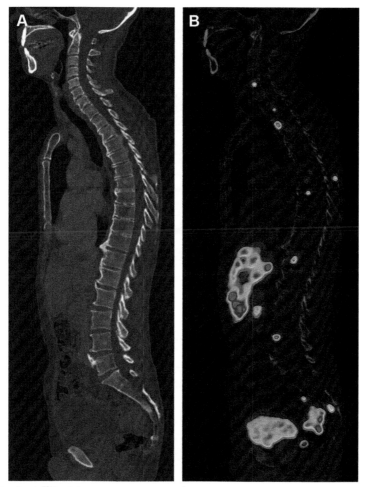

Fig. 8. Sagittal ^{68}Ga-DOTATOC-PET/computed tomography (CT) (*A*, CT; *B*, PET/CT fusion) showing PET-positive multiple bone metastases in the spine that are not visualized on CT. This is the same patient as in **Fig. 7**.

detection and as a means for therapy monitoring in general oncology, and recently also in patients with NET. Because of the advantageous detection of NET lesions, DWI-MRI should be a part of the MRI examination protocol.

PET/MRI Examination

Modern MRI equipment allows for whole body MRI examination protocols (head to proximal thighs) that may be performed either alone or as hybrid imaging procedure in PET/MRI scanners. To not prolong the examination beyond 1 hour, the composition of the MRI protocol needs to be a trade-off between image detail and examination time. The number of MRI sequences and their respective acquisition lengths will both usually need to be decreased, and will typically result in lower spatial resolution than for MRI of a limited part of the body. Similarly to stand alone MRI, whole body MRI may miss small lung metastases, which are best diagnosed by CT scanning.

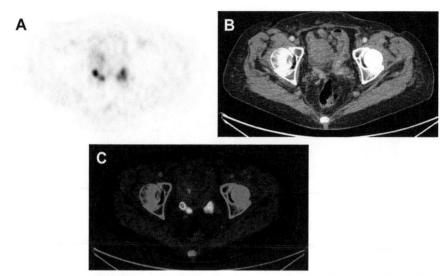

Fig. 9. Transversal ^{68}Ga-DOTATOC-PET/computed tomography (CT) (*A*, PET; *B*, CT; *C*, PET/CT fusion) showing peritoneal metastases in the pelvis in a patient with a small-intestinal neuroendocrine tumor.

In a whole body examination protocol, short acquisitions may be achieved by using, for example, the Dixon technique that will provide 3-dimensional T1-weighted in-phase, out-of-phase, water-only, and fat-only images. Also, whole body coronary T2-weighted sequences, preferably fat suppressed, such as short T1 inversion

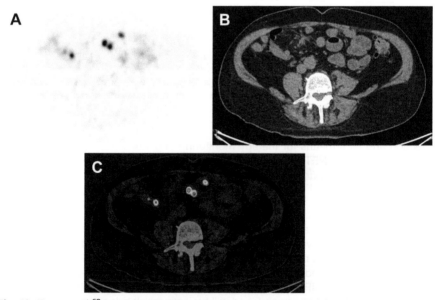

Fig. 10. Transversal ^{68}Ga-DOTATOC-PET/computed tomography (CT) (*A*, PET; *B*, CT; *C*, PET/CT fusion) showing multiple primary small-intestinal neuroendocrine tumors. In this patient, the concomitant CT scan was performed without intravenous contrast enhancement.

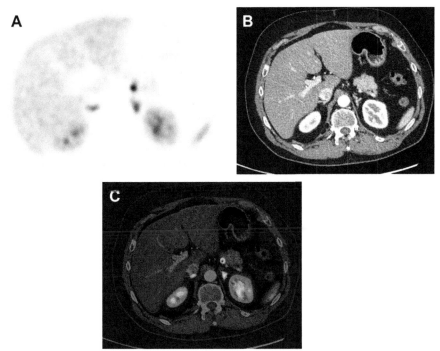

Fig. 11. Transversal ^{68}Ga-DOTATOC-PET/computed tomography (CT) (*A*, PET; *B*, CT; *C*, PET/CT fusion). This patient with multiple neuroendocrine neoplasia type I with a pancreatic neuroendocrine tumor shows a distinctive focal tracer uptake that is not visualized on the CT scan.

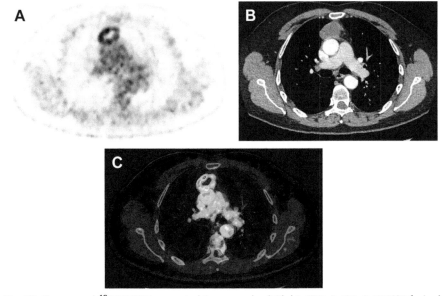

Fig. 12. Transversal ^{18}FDG-PET/computed tomography (CT) (*A*, PET; *B*, CT; *C*, PET/CT fusion) shows a high peripheral ^{18}FDG uptake in this centrally necrotic thymus neuroendocrine cancer.

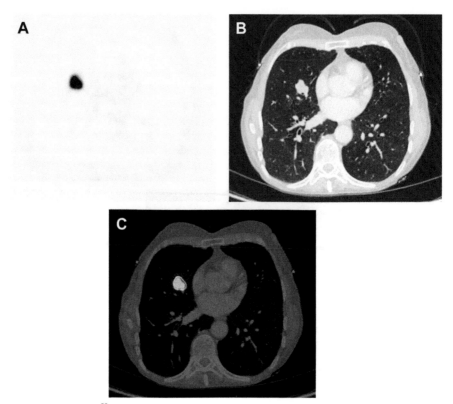

Fig. 13. Transversal ⁶⁸Ga-DOTATOC-PET/computed tomography (CT) (*A*, PET; *B*, CT; *C*, PET/CT. The high somatostatin receptor expression in this lung tumor indicates a neuroendocrine tumor.

recovery, can then be added and, for the spine, sagittal T1-weighted and T2-weighted fat-suppressed (short T1 inversion recovery) sequences. Whole body DWI should always be included, preferably by using 3 b-values (eg, 50, 400, and 900) or to save time 2 b-values (50 and 900). Time consuming, but important, is dynamic IV gadolinium contrast-enhanced examination of the liver and pancreas. Similar to CT scanning, and performed together with PET/CT scanning, which needs to include IV contrast-enhanced examination of the liver and pancreas, also PET/MRI should include dynamic IV contrast-enhanced MRI, because small lesions (≤0.5 cm) in the liver and pancreas otherwise may be missed because of the limited spatial resolution of the PET camera. The MRI acquisitions may be performed during breath-hold or by using techniques to allow for free breathing.

Because PET/MRI scanners regularly are equipped with a 3 T rather than a 1.5 T magnet, the high field strength allows for either better spatial resolution or shorter acquisition time, or a little of both. For example, the high field strength is an advantage for the DWI. By contrast, MRI acquisitions at 3 T are very susceptible to movement-induced image artifacts and it is, therefore, necessary to prepare the patient immediately before PET/MRI by IV injection of an antiperistaltic drug, for example, butylscopolamine 20 mg (or glucagon 1 mg), and this injection may have to be repeated during the examination.

The risk of claustrophobia is more pronounced with PET/MRI than PET/CT because of the longer tunnel (gantry). The patient should, therefore, be informed well in advance regarding the examination procedure and its approximate duration. Diazepam orally 2.5 to 5.0 mg administered one-half of an hour before PET/MRI is usually helpful to prepare patients who have experienced claustrophobia during a previous PET/MRI, MRI, or PET/CT examination. IV administration of diazepam or another an anxiolytic agent during the examination procedure may sometimes be necessary.

As with stand-alone MRI machines, the presence of pacemakers and some types of magnetic metal implants is considered a contraindication for PET/MRI. This factor needs to be clarified well in advance of the examination.

Attenuation correction of the PET images constitutes a problem with PET/MRI. Instead of the low-dose CT scan performed together with PET/CT scans for this purpose, the PET images are corrected for attenuation by using a whole body MRI sequence, which is segmented to represent the attenuation of water, fat, and air. The technical problems in connection with this process and the related issues concerning PET measurements of tracer uptake in tumors and normal tissues lay outside the scope of this article.

PET/MRI is still in many centers investigational, and so far few studies on PET/MRI for NET imaging have been published.[26,27,28,29,30] The advantage of MRI over CT scanning for the detection of hepatic metastases has also been shown also by software fusion of ^{68}Ga-DOTATOC-PET/CT scanning with IV contrast-enhanced MRI of the liver.[31]

SUMMARY

To take full advantage of hybrid techniques for NET imaging, which in the clinical setting currently uses PET/CT scanning, and hitherto in occasional centers PET/MRI, both the functional and morphologic imaging component needs to be optimized.

Modern high-resolution multidetector CT scanning allows for detailed fast imaging of the whole thorax, abdomen, and pelvis during one breath-hold and takes advantage of IV iodine-based contrast media by repeated scanning, including the liver and pancreas in the native (precontrast) and late arterial phases and the thorax–abdomen–pelvis in the venous phase. Also, it is universally available and constitutes the basic radiologic method for NET imaging. Thus, CT scanning provides a means for primary NET tumor diagnosis, assessing its local extent, staging of regional and distant metastases, surveillance after surgery, and locoregional therapies and for therapy monitoring. However, because of inadequate morphologic criteria, based on a short axis diameter of greater than 10 mm, the detection of lymph node metastases by CT scanning is unreliable. Smaller metastatic nodes may, thus, be missed and the detection of enlarged reactive nodes can produce false-positive results. Another important shortcoming of CT scanning is that bone metastases are often not visible or are easily overlooked.

MRI offers vastly better image contrast and is superior to CT scanning for imaging of the liver, pancreas, bone, and brain, and also allows for the use of hepatocyte-specific contrast media. With current scanners, whole body MRI examination protocols can be completed within approximately 1 hour or less and include IV dynamic contrast enhancement of the liver and pancreas and whole-body diffusion-weighted MRI. MRI may, however, miss small lung metastases.

In low-grade NETs (G1 and low G2), complementary somatostatin receptor imaging with ^{68}Ga-DOTA-somatostatin analogue-PET/CT scanning is crucial for the diagnosis of additional NET lesions that have been missed by morphologic imaging, such as small primary tumors, and metastases to bone, liver, peritoneum, and lymph nodes that are too small to be characterized as such by CT/MRI. Information on the overall tumor somatostatin receptor status is also provided to assess the patient's eligibility for PRRT. Alternatively, ^{18}F-DOPA-PET/CT can be used for lesion detection, but obviously the tumor somatostatin receptor expression may not be evaluated. For high-grade NETs, metabolic imaging by [18]FDG-PET/CT is usually preferred for lesion detection. [18]FDG positivity indicates a worse prognosis. Optimally, PET/CT includes a fully diagnostic IV contrast-enhanced CT scan to facilitate image reading and allows for the depiction of small lesions that may be missed by PET because of its limited spatial resolution, such as hypervascular liver metastases. However, PET-negative small hemangiomas should not be confused with hypervascular liver metastases.

PET/MRI remains mainly investigational, but to take full advantage of this hybrid imaging technique, the whole body MRI examination protocol also needs to be optimized and include IV dynamic contrast-enhanced imaging of the liver and pancreas and whole body DWI.

Ultrasound imaging is not a part of hybrid imaging, but its merits should nevertheless be briefly mentioned in a review on NET imaging. Ultrasound imaging often offers the initial diagnosis of liver metastases and constitutes the method of choice to guide the biopsy needle for histopathologic diagnosis of abdominal NET lesions. IV contrast-enhanced ultrasound imaging is an excellent method to detect small liver metastases and to characterize liver lesions that remain equivocal on CT/MRI. Endoscopic ultrasound imaging is the most sensitive method to diagnose pancreatic NETs, and also allows for biopsy. Endoscopic ultrasound imaging is mandatory for surveillance in patients with multiple endocrine neoplasia type 1. Intraoperative ultrasound imaging facilitates lesion detection and localization in the pancreas and liver.

A very intriguing area of research that recently has also been applied in clinical trials is PET/CT scans and PRRT using somatostatin receptor antagonists.[32,33,34,35] In contrast with the agonist-receptor complex, this antagonist-receptor complex is not internalized but nevertheless remains bound to the NET cell membrane, and published reports indicate advantages of using somatostatin receptor antagonists instead of agonists for imaging and PRRT.

To conclude, accurate imaging of NETs is crucial for patient management, and a knowledge of the advantages and shortcomings of the different available methods is important to choose the appropriate techniques that match the relevant clinical questions. Hybrid imaging with PET/CT scanning needs to use fully diagnostic examination protocols for both imaging components to take make optimal use of the technique. This also holds true for PET/MRI, which so far is mainly investigative and clinically available in only a few centers. The recent development of somatostatin receptor antagonists for clinical applications hold interesting potentials for future NET hybrid imaging.

REFERENCES

1. Gabriel M, Decristoforo C, Kendler D, et al. 68Ga-DOTA-Tyr3-octreotide PET in neuroendocrine tumors: comparison with somatostatin receptor scintigraphy and CT. J Nucl Med 2007;48:508–18.

2. Srirajaskanthan R, Kayani I, Quigley AM, et al. The role of 68Ga-DOTATATE PET in patients with neuroendocrine tumors and negative or equivocal findings on 111In-DTPA-octreotide scintigraphy. J Nucl Med 2010;51:875–82.

3. Frilling A, Sotiropoulos GC, Radtke A, et al. The impact of 68Ga-DOTATOC positron emission tomography/computed tomography on the multimodal management of patients with neuroendocrine tumors. Ann Surg 2010;252:850–6.

4. Van Binnebeek S, Vanbilloen B, Baete K, et al. Comparison of diagnostic accuracy of 111In-pentetreotide SPECT and 68Ga-DOTATOC PET/CT: a lesion-by-lesion analysis in patients with metastatic neuroendocrine tumours. Eur Radiol 2016;26:900–9.

5. Sandström M, Velikyan I, Garske-Román U, et al. Comparative biodistribution and radiation dosimetry of 68Ga-DOTATOC and 68Ga-DOTATATE in patients with neuroendocrine tumors. J Nucl Med 2013;54:1755–9.

6. Yang J, Kan Y, Ge BH, et al. Diagnostic role of Gallium-68 DOTATOC and Gallium-68 DOTATATE PET in patients with neuroendocrine tumors: a meta-analysis. Acta Radiol 2014;55:389–98.

7. Johnbeck CB, Knigge U, Kjær A. PET tracers for somatostatin receptor imaging of neuroendocrine tumors: current status and review of the literature. Future Oncol 2014;10:2259–77.

8. Geijer H, Breimer LH. Somatostatin receptor PET/CT in neuroendocrine tumours: update on systematic review and meta-analysis. Eur J Nucl Med Mol Imaging 2013;40:1770–80.

9. Treglia G, Castaldi P, Rindi G, et al. Diagnostic performance of Gallium-68 somatostatin receptor PET and PET/CT in patients with thoracic and gastroenteropancreatic neuroendocrine tumours: a meta-analysis. Endocrine 2012;42:80–7.

10. Poeppel TD, Binse I, Petersenn S, et al. 68Ga-DOTATOC versus 68Ga-DOTATATE PET/CT in functional imaging of neuroendocrine tumors. J Nucl Med 2011;52:1864–70.

11. Velikyan I, Sundin A, Sörensen J, et al. Quantitative and qualitative intrapatient comparison of 68Ga-DOTATOC and 68Ga-DOTATATE: net uptake rate for accurate quantification. J Nucl Med 2014;55:204–10.

12. Balogova S, Talbot JN, Nataf V, et al. 18F-fluorodihydroxyphenylalanine vs other radiopharmaceuticals for imaging neuroendocrine tumours according to their type. Eur J Nucl Med Mol Imaging 2013;40:943–66.

13. Ambrosini V, Tomassetti P, Castellucci P, et al. Comparison between 68Ga-DOTA-NOC and 18F-DOPA PET for the detection of gastro-entero-pancreatic and lung neuro-endocrine tumours. Eur J Nucl Med Mol Imaging 2008;35:1431–8.

14. Putzer D, Gabriel M, Kendler D, et al. Comparison of (68)Ga-DOTA-Tyr(3)-octreotide and (18)F-fluoro-L-dihydroxyphenylalanine positron emission tomography in neuroendocrine tumor patients. Q J Nucl Med Mol Imaging 2010;54:68–75.

15. Orlefors H, Sundin A, Eriksson B, et al. PET-guided surgery - high correlation between positron emission tomography with 11C-5-Hydroxytryptophane (5-HTP) and surgical findings in abdominal neuroendocrine tumours. Cancers 2012;4:100–12.

16. Orlefors H, Sundin A, Garske U, et al. Whole-body (11)C-5-hydroxytryptophan positron emission tomography as a universal imaging technique for neuroendocrine tumors: comparison with somatostatin receptor scintigraphy and computed tomography. J Clin Endocrinol Metab 2005;90:3392–400.

17. Koopmans KP, Neels OC, Kema IP, et al. Improved staging of patients with carcinoid and islet cell tumors with 18F-dihydroxy-phenyl-alanine and 11C-5-hydroxytryptophan positron emission tomography. J Clin Oncol 2008;26:1489–95.

18. Luo Y, Pan Q, Yao S, et al. Glucagon-like peptide-1 receptor PET/CT with 68Ga-NOTA-Exendin-4 for detecting localized insulinoma: a prospective cohort study. J Nucl Med 2016;57:715–20.

19. Binderup T, Knigge U, Loft A, et al. Functional imaging of neuroendocrine tumors: a head-to-head comparison of somatostatin receptor scintigraphy, 123I-MIBG scintigraphy, and 18F-FDG PET. J Nucl Med 2010;51:704–12.

20. Has Simsek D, Kuyumcu S, Turkmen C, et al. Can complementary 68Ga-DOTA-TATE and 18F-FDG PET/CT establish the missing link between histopathology and therapeutic approach in gastroenteropancreatic neuroendocrine tumors? J Nucl Med 2014;55:1811–7.

21. Binderup T, Knigge U, Loft A, et al. 18F-fluorodeoxyglucose positron emission to-mography predicts survival of patients with neuroendocrine tumors. Clin Cancer Res 2010;16:978–85.

22. Bahri H, Laurence L, Edeline J, et al. High prognostic value of 18F-FDG PET for metastatic gastroenteropancreatic neuroendocrine tumors: a long-term evalua-tion. J Nucl Med 2014;55:1786–90.

23. Kayani I, Conry BG, Groves AM, et al. A comparison of 68Ga-DOTATATE and 18F-FDG PET/CT in pulmonary neuroendocrine tumors. J Nucl Med 2009;50: 1927–32.

24. Squires MH 3rd, Volkan Adsay N, Schuster DM, et al. Octreoscan versus FDG-PET for neuroendocrine tumor staging: a biological approach. Ann Surg Oncol 2015;22:2295–301.

25. Norlén O, Montan H, Hellman P, et al. Preoperative 68Ga-DOTA-somatostatin analog-PET/CT hybrid imaging increases detection rate of intra-abdominal small intestinal neuroendocrine tumor lesions. World J Surg 2018;42(2):498–505.

26. Hope TA, Pampaloni MH, Nakakura E, et al. Simultaneous (68)Ga-DOTA-TOC PET/MRI with gadoxetate disodium in patients with neuroendocrine tumor. Ab-dom Imaging 2015;40:1432–40.

27. Beiderwellen KJ, Poeppel TD, Hartung-Knemeyer V, et al. Simultaneous 68Ga-DOTATOC PET/MRI in patients with gastroenteropancreatic neuroendocrine tu-mors: initial results. Invest Radiol 2013;48:273–9.

28. Mayerhoefer ME, Ba-Ssalamah A, Weber M, et al. Gadoxetate-enhanced versus diffusion-weighted MRI for fused Ga-68-DOTANOC PET/MRI in patients with neuroendocrine tumours of the upper abdomen. Eur Radiol 2013;23: 1978–85.

29. Berzaczy D, Giraudo C, Haug AR, et al. Whole-body 68Ga-DOTANOC PET/MRI versus 68Ga-DOTANOC PET/CT in patients with neuroendocrine tumors: a pro-spective study in 28 patients. Clin Nucl Med 2017;42:669–74.

30. Sawicki LM, Deuschl C, Beiderwellen K, et al. Evaluation of 68Ga-DOTATOC PET/MRI for whole-body staging of neuroendocrine tumours in comparison with 68Ga-DOTATOC PET/CT. Eur Radiol 2017;27:4091–9.

31. Schreiter NF, Nogami M, Steffen I, et al. Evaluation of the potential of PET-MRI fusion for detection of liver metastases in patients with neuroendocrine tumours. Eur Radiol 2012;22:458–67.

32. Wild D, Fani M, Fischer R, et al. Comparison of somatostatin receptor agonist and antagonist for peptide receptor radionuclide therapy: a pilot study. J Nucl Med 2014;55:1248–52.

33. Nicolas GP, Beykan S, Bouterfa H, et al. Safety, biodistribution, and radiation dosimetry of 68Ga-OPS202 (68Ga-NODAGA-JR11) in patients with gastroenter-opancreatic neuroendocrine tumors: a prospective phase I imaging study. J Nucl Med 2017. [Epub ahead of print].

34. Nicolas GP, Schreiter N, Kaul F, et al. Comparison of 68Ga-OPS202 (68Ga-NO-DAGA-JR11) and 68Ga-DOTATOC (68Ga-Edotreotide) PET/CT in patients with

gastroenteropancreatic neuroendocrine tumors: evaluation of sensitivity in a pro-spective phase II imaging study. J Nucl Med 2017. [Epub ahead of print].
35. Nicolas GP, Mansi R, McDougall L, et al. Biodistribution, pharmacokinetics, and dosimetry of 177Lu-, 90Y-, and 111In-labeled somatostatin receptor antagonist OPS201 in comparison to the agonist 177Lu-DOTATATE: the mass effect. J Nucl Med 2017;58:1435–41.

Molecular Genetic Studies of Pancreatic Neuroendocrine Tumors: New Therapeutic Approaches

Mark Stevenson, BSc, PhD, Kate E. Lines, BSc, PhD,
Rajesh V. Thakker, MD, ScD, FRCP, FMedSci, FRS*

KEYWORDS

- MEN1 • VHL • PNETs • Menin • mTOR • Epigenetic • SSTRs • RAS

KEY POINTS

- Pancreatic neuroendocrine tumors (PNETs) can occur as sporadic neoplasms or as part of hereditary syndromes such as multiple endocrine neoplasia type 1 (MEN1).
- MEN1, which is an autosomal dominant disorder, is due to loss-of-function mutations of the tumor suppressor *MEN1* gene that encodes menin.
- Approximately 40% of nonfamilial (ie, sporadic) PNETs have *MEN1* mutations, with subsequent loss of menin, which acts as a tumor suppressor.
- Menin is a scaffold protein with roles in transcriptional regulation, genome stability, DNA repair, protein degradation, cell motility and adhesion, microRNA biogenesis, cell division, cell cycle control, epigenetic regulation, and Wnt signaling.
- Emerging therapies targeting the functional roles of menin with *Men1* gene replacement therapy, epigenetic modulators, and antagonists of Wnt-signaling may prove useful for future treatment of PNETs.

INTRODUCTION

Pancreatic neuroendocrine tumors (PNETs), which account for 1% to 2% of all pancreatic neoplasms, are pathologically heterogeneous and consist of epithelial cells with phenotypic and ultrastructural neuroendocrine differentiation.[1,2] PNETs may be classified according to their proliferation, which is assessed by the Ki-67 index or mitotic count. Well-differentiated PNETs grade (G)-1 have a Ki-67 index of less than

Disclosure Statement: This work was funded by the UK Medical Research Council (MRC) program grants G9825289 and G1000467 (M. Stevenson, K.E. Lines, and R.V. Thakker), and UK National Institute for Health Research (NIHR)–Oxford Biomedical Research Centre program. R.V. Thakker is a Wellcome Trust Investigator and NIHR senior investigator.
Radcliffe Department of Medicine, Oxford Centre for Diabetes, Endocrinology and Metabolism (OCDEM), University of Oxford, Churchill Hospital, Headington, Oxford OX3 7LJ, UK
* Corresponding author.
E-mail address: rajesh.thakker@ndm.ox.ac.uk

Endocrinol Metab Clin N Am 47 (2018) 525–548
https://doi.org/10.1016/j.ecl.2018.04.007
0889-8529/18/© 2018 Elsevier Inc. All rights reserved.

endo.theclinics.com

3% or mitotic count of less than 2 mitoses per 10 high-power fields (HPFs). Well-differentiated G2 PNETs have a Ki-67 index of 3% to 20% or 2 to 20 mitoses per 10 HPFs. Well-differentiated G3 PNETs, or poorly differentiated pancreatic neuroendocrine carcinomas (PNECs), have a Ki-67 index of greater than 20% and greater than 20 mitoses per 10 HPFs.[1,3,4] The incidence of PNETs, also known as pancreatic islet cell tumors, has doubled between 1973 and 2004 from 0.16 to 0.33 per 100,000 individuals, and this may in part be due to improvements in diagnostic imaging and detection, whereas autopsy studies have shown that as many as 0.8% to 10% of individuals have PNETs.[2,5–7] PNETs may secrete hormones or vasoactive substances, such as gastrin, insulin, glucagon, or vasoactive intestinal peptide (VIP), and be associated with clinical symptoms due to the hormonal overproduction, or they may be nonsecreting (ie, nonfunctional) and clinically present, often with locally advanced or metastatic disease.[8]

Treatments for primary PNETs include surgery, whereas nonresectable PNETs and metastases are treated with biotherapies that include somatostatin analogues, inhibitors of receptors and monoclonal antibodies, chemotherapy, and radionuclide therapy.[9] The median survival time for patients with PNETs is approximately 3.6 years,[10] whereas the prognosis for patients whose PNETs have metastasized is poor ,with a survival of 1 to 3 years.[5,6,11,12] However, the pathologic molecular state of well-differentiated PNETs is not sufficiently understood for the prediction of the aggressiveness of individual tumors that would reliably identify patients who would benefit from early therapy, or for indolent disease for which the risk-to-benefit ratio of treatment may not be advantageous for patients.[13] Thus, improved understanding of the molecular basis of PNETs, as well as better treatments, is required. Recent preclinical studies have identified new cellular pathways and therapeutic targets for treating PNETs, including epigenetic modification, the β-catenin–Wnt pathway, hedgehog signaling, somatostatin receptors (SSTRs), and *MEN1* gene replacement therapy. This article reviews these advances in the molecular genetics of PNETs that have stemmed from studies of hereditary syndromes associated with PNETs, as well as sporadic PNETs, and the cellular pathways that these studies have identified for therapeutic approaches.

PANCREATIC NEUROENDOCRINE TUMORS IN HEREDITARY SYNDROMES

PNETs most frequently (~90%) arise as a nonfamilial isolated endocrinopathy (ie, sporadically) but they can also occur as part of a complex familial syndrome that includes multiple endocrine neoplasia type 1 (MEN1), von Hippel-Lindau disease (VHL), neurofibromatosis type 1 (NF1), and the tuberous sclerosis complex (TSC).[1,2,9] Indeed, PNETs have been reported to occur in 30% to 80% of MEN1 patients, greater than 15% of VHL patients, less than 10% of NF1 patients, and less than 1% of patients with TSC.[9] These hereditary tumor syndromes are briefly reviewed because they provide molecular insights into PNET development.

Multiple Endocrine Neoplasia Type 1

The most common hereditary syndrome associated with PNETs is MEN1, which is an autosomal dominant disorder characterized by the combined occurrence of 2 or more tumors involving the parathyroids, pancreatic islets, anterior pituitary, and adrenals.[14,15] In MEN1, PNETs are typically multiple, whereas in sporadic cases tumors are generally solitary masses. Patients with the MEN1 syndrome have germline mutations in the *MEN1* tumor suppressor gene, which is located on chromosome 11q13 and encodes a 610 amino acid protein, menin. *MEN1* germline mutations are found in greater than 90% of MEN1 patients and comprise whole or partial gene deletions; frameshift deletions or insertions; in-frame deletions or insertions; and splice site, missense, and nonsense mutations, which result in a functional deficiency of menin.[16,17] MEN1 tumors have somatic mutations, as well as germline mutations consistent with the Knudson 2-hit hypothesis for the role of tumor suppressor genes in oncogenesis, and in most (>90%) MEN1 tumors the somatic abnormality is loss of heterozygosity (LOH), with the remaining 10% having intragenic deletions or point mutations.[17–19]

Menin is a ubiquitously expressed protein that functions as a nuclear scaffold protein that interacts with greater than 40 interacting proteins (**Fig. 1**), thereby enabling it to have multiple roles in pathways of cellular proliferation by influencing transcriptional regulation, genome stability, DNA repair, protein degradation, cell motility and adhesion, microRNA (miRNA) biogenesis, cell division, cell cycle control, and epigenetic regulation.[17,20–25] For example, menin inhibits: (1) wingless integration (Wnt) 1 signaling by transferring β-catenin from the nucleus, which reduces cell proliferation[21,26]; (2) the activity of JunD protooncogene (JunD) by blocking its phosphorylation and, therefore, potentially subsequent interaction with coactivators,[22,27] causing JunD to prevent rather than promote cell growth[28]; and (3) Hedgehog pathway signaling, which influences several functions, including tumorigenesis by recruitment of a protein arginine methyltransferase 5 (PRMT5), which inactivates the Hedgehog pathway promoter growth arrest specific 1 (*Gas1*) gene[29] (**Fig. 2**). In addition, menin interacts with the mixed lineage leukemia (MLL) protein 1 histone methyltransferase complex to methylate histone H3 (lysine 4 [Lys4]), causing chromatin modification and increased transcriptional activity of genes, including those encoding the cyclin-dependent kinase inhibitors p27 and p18, which are involved in cell cycle regulation[30,31] (see **Fig. 2**). Menin also promotes the cytostatic effects of transforming growth factor-beta (TGF-β) by interaction with the small body size mothers against decapentaplegic homolog (Smad) pathway[32–34] (see **Fig. 2**), as well as interacting with nuclear factor kappa B subunit (NF-kB) proteins to modulate NF-kB transactivation.[35] Furthermore, menin can prevent the interaction between the guanine triphosphate (GTP) hydrolase (GTPase) Kirsten rat Sarcoma viral oncogene homolog (K-RAS) and sons of sevenless (SOS) that is essential for K-RAS activation.[36] Moreover, in murine pancreatic β-cells, menin has been shown to activate opposing K-RAS pathways that comprise a proliferative pathway, likely via regulation of mitogen-activated protein kinase (MAPK) and extracellular signal-regulated kinase (ERK) phosphorylation, and an antiproliferative pathway via ras association domain family member 1 (RASSF1A).[37] Thus, menin is considered to interact with K-RAS to block the MAPK-ERK pathway, thereby inhibiting proliferation. In addition, menin loss removes this inhibition and leads to increased cell proliferation.[37] Menin also acts as a suppressor of ERK-dependent phosphorylation of target proteins[38] (see **Fig. 2**). In addition, SSTR modulation of proliferation may also occur through K-RAS signaling, thereby highlighting the importance of K-RAS signaling in PNETs and indicating that menin may play a possible role in SSTR downstream signaling[39] (see **Fig. 2**). Furthermore, menin is an inhibitor of the phosphatidtylinositol-3-kinase (PI3K)–viral oncogene of Akt8 retrovirus (Akt) (ie, protein kinase B [PKB]–mammalian target of rapamycin [mTOR] [PI3K-Akt-mTOR]) signaling pathway, by binding to Akt and preventing its translocation to the plasma membrane[40] (see **Fig. 2**). The mTOR pathway regulates cell proliferation, cell metabolism, survival, motility, and autophagy.[41]

von Hippel-Lindau Disease

PNETs develop in patients with VHL disease, which is an autosomal dominant disorder with an incidence of 1 in 36,000 individuals.[42] The *VHL* gene is located on

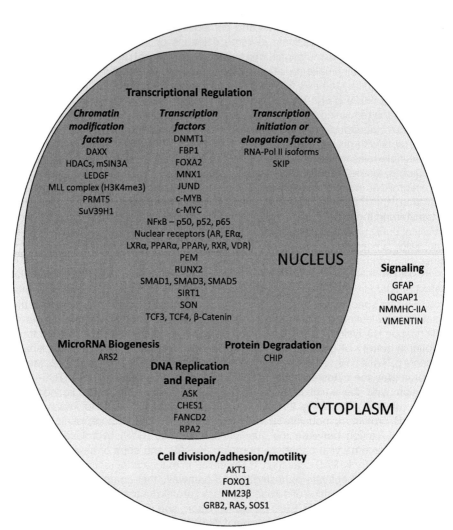

Fig. 1. Menin-interacting proteins. More than 40 different proteins have been reported to interact with menin, which is a multifunctional protein with roles in transcriptional regulation as a corepressor or coactivator (via interactions with chromatin modifying proteins, transcription factors, and transcription initiation or elongation proteins), DNA repair associated with response to DNA damage, cell signaling, cytoskeletal structure, cell division, cell adhesion, or cell motility. AKT1, viral oncogene of Akt8 retrovirus (AKT) serine-threonine kinase 1; FOXO1, forkhead box O1; AR, androgen receptor; ARS2, arsenite-resistance protein 2; ASK, apoptosis signal regulating kinase; CHES1, checkpoint suppressor 1; CHIP, carboxy terminus of hsp70-interacting protein; c-MYB, MYB (myeloblastosis) protooncogene; c-MYC, MYC (myelocytomatosis) protooncogene; DAXX, death domain associated protein; DNMT1, DNA methyltransferase 1; ERα, estrogen receptor alpha; FANCD2, Fanconi anemia complementation group D2; FBP1, fructose bisphosphatase 1; FOXA2, forkhead box A2; GFAP, glial fibrillary acidic protein; GRB2, growth factor receptor-bound protein 2; HDACs, histone deacetylases; IQGAP1, IQ motif containing GTPase activating protein 1; JUND, JunD protooncogene; LEDGF, lens epithelium-derived growth factor; LXRα, liver X receptor alpha; MLL, mixed lineage leukemia; MNX1, motor neuron and pancreas homeobox 1; mSIN3A, SIN3 transcription regulator family member A; NFκB, nuclear factor kappa B; NM23β,

chromosome 3p25 and encodes the protein VHL (pVHL) tumor suppressor, involved in the oxygen-sensing pathway that regulates hypoxia-inducible factors (HIFs).[43] Truncation of the pVHL prevents the ubiquitination of HIF transcription factors, leading to expression of target genes favoring angiogenesis (see **Fig. 2**). Individuals with VHL disease typically inherit a germline *VHL* mutation and those cells that acquire a somatic mutation (ie, the second hit) of the wild-type allele develop tumors. *VHL* germline mutations, which are detected in virtually all VHL patients,[44,45] comprise missense, frameshift, nonsense, in-frame deletions or insertions, large or complete deletions, and splice site abnormalities, with mutations located in exon 3 being associated with an increased risk of malignant PNETs.[45–47] Mouse models of conditional inactivation of *Vhl* in specific pancreatic cell populations have revealed that a lack of pVHL in pancreatic progenitor cells results in significant postnatal death, and the few surviving mice then develop islet hyperplasia and microcystic adenomas, which are also found to occur in 35% to 70% of VHL patients.[48]

Neurofibromatosis Type 1

Patients with NF1, which is an autosomal dominant disorder, may develop PNETs. The *NF1* tumor suppressor gene is located on chromosome 17q11.2 and encodes the cytoplasmic protein neurofibromin that controls cellular proliferation by inactivating the ras signal transduction pathway[49] (see **Fig. 2**). Loss of function *NF1* mutations lead to increased activity of the MAPK and PI3K-Akt-mTOR pathways,[50] and the PNETs that develop have a great potential for malignancy.[51,52]

Tuberous Sclerosis Complex

Patients with TSC may develop PNETs such as gastrinomas, insulinomas, and nonfunctioning tumors. TS is an autosomal dominant disease caused by mutations in *TSC1* located on chromosome 9q34 or *TSC2* located on chromosome 16p13.3, which encode the hamartin and tuberin proteins, respectively. Mutations in *TSC1* and *TSC2* can activate the mTOR pathway to increase cell proliferation[52,53] (see **Fig. 2**).

SPORADIC PANCREATIC NEUROENDOCRINE TUMORS

Most sporadic PNETs are associated with somatic mutations, although some patients with sporadic PNETs may have germline mutations.

Somatic Mutations in Sporadic Pancreatic Neuroendocrine Tumors

The most commonly mutated gene in sporadic PNETs is the *MEN1* gene. Thus, 40% of sporadic PNETs have somatic *MEN1* mutations, indicating that *MEN1* mutations are major drivers in the development of all PNETs (**Table 1**).[13,54] In addition, whole exome

---

NME/NM23 nucleoside diphosphate kinase 2; NMMHC-IIA, nonmuscle myosin heavy chain IIA; PEM, PEM homeobox; PPARα, peroxisome proliferator-activated receptor alpha; PRMT5, protein arginine methyltransferase 5; RAS, KRAS (Kirsten rat sarcoma virus) proto-oncogene; RPA2, replication protein 2; RUNX2, runt-related transcription factor 2; RXR, retinoic X receptor; SIRT, Sirtuin 1; SKIP, SKI interacting protein; SMAD, small body size mothers against decapentaplegic homolog; SON, SON DNA binding protein; SOS1, son of sevenless homolog 1; SUV39H1, suppressor of variegation 3 to 9 homolog 1; TCF, transcription factor; VDR, vitamin D receptor. (*Data from* Thakker RV. Multiple endocrine neoplasia type 1 (MEN1) and type 4 (MEN4). Mol Cell Endocrinol 2014;386(1–2):2–15; and Agarwal SK. The future: genetics advances in MEN1 therapeutic approaches and management strategies. Endocr Relat Cancer 2017;24(10):T119–34.)

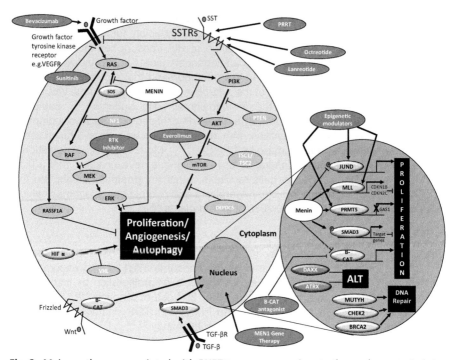

Fig. 2. Major pathways associated with PNET tumor progression. In the nucleus menin interacts with the transcription factor JunD to prevent its phosphorylation and activation of target genes, such as gastrin (*GAST*); β-catenin mediating its export from the nucleus and inhibiting Wnt signaling; PRMT5 to inactivate the Hedgehog pathway promoter *Gas1*; and MLL1 and MLL2, and Smad3, which is a TGF-β signaling component, to promote transcription of target genes that reduce cellular proliferation. DAXX and ATRX are responsible for telomere maintenance with genetic mutations, leading to the Altered Lengthening of Telomere (ALT) phenotype, whereas MUTYH, CHEK2, and BRCA2 are involved in DNA repair. In the cytoplasm menin inhibits the mTOR pathway, which regulates cellular proliferation and autophagy by binding to Akt, which are part of RTK and SSTR signaling pathways; and K-RAS–induced proliferation by both inhibition of ERK-dependent phosphorylation of target proteins and prevention of the SOS–K-RAS interaction. PTEN, TSC1, TSC2, and DEPDC5 are also involved in regulating the mTOR signaling pathway, whereas NF1 regulates RAS signaling via MEK-ERK and mTOR pathways by regulating the conversion of inactive RasGDP to active RasGTP. VHL is part of a multiprotein complex responsible for ubiquitination and degradation of the α subunits of HIF1 and 2; thus *VHL* mutations can lead to stabilization of HIFs, increasing angiogenesis through increased expression of hypoxia-inducible target genes. Targeted therapies (*white text in ovals with solid outlines*) include mTOR inhibitors, such as everolimus; Wnt pathway inhibitors, such as β-catenin antagonists; epigenetic modulators; *MEN1* gene therapy; RTK inhibitors, such as sunitinib; and somatostatin analogues, such as octreotide and lanreotide or PRRT. AKT, AKT serine-threonine kinase 1; ATRX, alpha thalassemia or mental retardation syndrome X-linked; B-cat, β-catenin; BRCA2, breast cancer 2; CDKN1B or 2C, cyclin-dependent kinase inhibitor 1 B or 2C; CHEK2, checkpoint kinase 2; DEPDC5, DEP domain containing protein 5; ERK, extracellular signal-regulated kinase; HIF-α, hypoxia-inducible factor alpha; JUND, JunD protooncogene; MEK, mitogen-activated protein kinase–ERK kinase 1; mTOR, mechanistic target of rapamycin kinase; MUTYH, MutY homolog; PI3K, phosphatidylinositol-4,5-bisphosphate 3 kinase; PRRT, peptide receptor radionuclide therapy; PTEN, phosphatase and tensin homolog; Raf, B-Raf protooncogene; RASSF1A, ras association domain family member 1; RTK, receptor tyrosine kinase; VEGFR, vascular endothelial growth factor receptor.

Table 1
Germline and somatic driver mutations identified in clinically sporadic pancreatic neuroendocrine tumors reported in 2 whole genome sequencing studies

Gene	Pathway, Function	Type	Somatic (%)	Germline (%)	Mutation	Ref.
MEN1	Chromatin remodeling, mTOR, TGF-β	S or G	37–44	6	fs, in, ns, ms, sp	Scarpa et al,[13] 2017; Jiao et al,[54] 2011
DAXX	Chromatin remodeling, ALT	S	22–25	—	fs, in, ns, ms, sp	Scarpa et al,[13] 2017; Jiao et al,[54] 2011
ATRX	Chromatin remodeling, ALT	S	11–17	—	fs, in, ns, sp	Scarpa et al,[13] 2017; Jiao et al,[54] 2011
PTEN	mTOR pathway	S	7–9	—	fs, ns, ms,	Scarpa et al,[13] 2017; Jiao et al,[54] 2011
SETD2	Chromatin remodeling	S	6	—	fs, ns, ms, sp, re	Scarpa et al,[13] 2017
MLL3	Chromatin remodeling	S	3	—	ns, ms, re	Scarpa et al,[13] 2017
TP53	Cell cycle arrest, apoptosis, DNA repair	S	2	—	ns, ms	Scarpa et al,[13] 2017; Jiao et al,[54] 2011
TSC1	mTOR pathway	S	2	—	ms, sp	Scarpa et al,[13] 2017
TSC2	mTOR pathway	S	2	—	fs, ms	Scarpa et al,[13] 2017; Jiao et al,[54] 2011
CDC42BPB	Cytoskeletal reorganization and cell migration	S	2	—	ms	Scarpa et al,[13] 2017
KLF7	Transcriptional activator	S	2	—	ns	Scarpa et al,[13] 2017
BCOR	Transcriptional corepressor	S	2	—	ns	Scarpa et al,[13] 2017
PRRC2A	Inflammation	S	2	—	fs, ns	Scarpa et al,[13] 2017
URGCP	Cell cycle progression	S	2	—	ns	Scarpa et al,[13] 2017
ARID1A	Chromatin remodeling	S	2	—	ns	Scarpa et al,[13] 2017
DIS3L2	mRNA degradation	S	2	—	ms	Scarpa et al,[13] 2017
DEPDC5	mTOR pathway	S	2	—	fs	Scarpa et al,[13] 2017
CDKN2A	Cell cycle progression	S	1	—	CNV/re, meth	Scarpa et al,[13] 2017
EYA1	Transcriptional coactivator, DNA repair	S	1	—	CNV	Scarpa et al,[13] 2017
FMBT1	Chromatin remodeling	S	1	—	CNV	Scarpa et al,[13] 2017

(continued on next page)

Table 1
(continued)

Gene	Pathway, Function	Type	Somatic (%)	Germline (%)	Mutation	Ref.
RABGAP1L	GTPase	S	2	—	CNV	Scarpa et al,[13] 2017
PSPN	mTOR pathway	S	1	—	CNV	Scarpa et al,[13] 2017
ULK1	mTOR pathway	S	1	—	CNV	Scarpa et al,[13] 2017
MTAP	Polyamine metabolism	S	4	—	re	Scarpa et al,[13] 2017
ARID2	Chromatin remodeling	S	5	—	re	Scarpa et al,[13] 2017
SMARCA4	Chromatin remodeling	S	3	—	re	Scarpa et al,[13] 2017
DST	Cell adhesion	S	3	—	ms	Scarpa et al,[13] 2017
ZNF292	Transcriptional regulation	S	2	—	ns	Scarpa et al,[13] 2017
EWSR	mTOR pathway	S	3	—	re	Scarpa et al,[13] 2017
PIK3CA	mTOR pathway	S	1	—	ms	Jiao et al,[54] 2011
VHL	Degradation of HIFs	S or G	1	1	ns	Scarpa et al,[13] 2017
CDKN1B	Cell cycle progression	G	—	1		Scarpa et al,[13] 2017
MUTYH	Base excision repair	G	—	5		Scarpa et al,[13] 2017
BRCA2	DNA damage repair	G	—	1		Scarpa et al,[13] 2017
CHEK2	DNA damage repair	G	—	4		Scarpa et al,[13] 2017

Germline mutations were identified in MEN1, CDKN1B, VHL, BRCA2, and MUTYH and CHEK2.[13] One study reported whole exome sequencing findings from 10 sporadic PNETs and screened the most commonly mutated genes in an additional 58 PNETs, which together comprised 66 nonfunctional tumors and 2 functional PNETs.[54] Another study reported the genomic findings from 98 clinically sporadic PNETs comprising 78 nonfunctional tumors, 8 insulinomas, 1 glucagonoma, 2 gastrinomas, 1 clear cell tumor, 1 PPoma (PNET that secretes pancreatic polypeptide), 1 VIPoma (PNET that secretes vasoactive intestinal peptide), 1 unspecified functional tumor, and 5 well-differentiated or well-differentiated or poorly differentiated neuroendocrine carcinomas.[13] This identified approximately 3100 somatic coding mutations, approximately 2500 of which were non-silent in greater than 2550 genes, and some of these mutations were verified in a further 62 additional PNETs.[13] Sixteen significantly and recurrently mutated genes defined by IntOGen analysis are shown. In addition, recurrent mutations were identified in TSC1 and TSC2,[13,54] which encode negative regulators of the mTOR pathway, and the histone modifier gene SETD2 was reported to have multiple independent mutations in subclones of a tumor. Recurrent regions of gain and loss, as well as chromosomal rearrangements were also identified.[13]

Abbreviations: ALT, altered lengthening of telomere; CNV, copy number variant; fs, frame shift insertion or deletion; G, germline; in, in frame insertion or deletion; meth, hypermethylation of the promoter; ms, missense mutation; ns, nonsense mutation; re, chromosomal rearrangement; S, somatic; sp, splice site mutation.

and whole genome sequencing studies have identified the involvement of other genes and cellular pathways in chromatin modification, telomere length maintenance, growth control, DNA damage, and cell metabolism, as well as alterations in gene copy number, chromosomal rearrangements, gene fusions, telomere integrity, and miRNAs.[13,54]

Mutations in genes involved in chromatin remodeling

Approximately 25% to 45% of sporadic PNETs have somatic mutations in *MEN1* with LOH seen at the *MEN1* locus in 30% to 70% of cases, including those without somatic *MEN1* mutations[13,54–56]; and approximately 45% have inactivating somatic mutations of either the death domain-associated protein (*DAXX*) or α-thalassemia, or mental retardation syndrome X-linked (*ATRX*) genes that are associated with loss of protein expression, detected by immunohistochemical analysis of PNETs.[57–61] Mutations in both *MEN1* and either *ATRX* or *DAXX* occur in 18% to 25% of PNETs, whereas *ATRX* and *DAXX* mutations do not occur concurrently in the same tumor.[13,54] This is consistent with the functional roles of DAXX-encoded and ATRX-encoded proteins being within the same pathway.[62] Indeed, the DAXX and ATRX proteins, which are involved in apoptosis and chromatin remodeling,[13,54,63] are critical for the maintenance of stable telomere length. Thus, both DAXX and ATRX proteins, which form an H3.3 histone chaperone complex, are required to enable incorporation of histone H3.3 at telomeres. ATRX is also required for suppressing the expression of the long noncoding RNA (lncRNA) telomeric repeat-containing RNA (TERRA), which maintains telomeric structure by regulating telomerase activity and heterochromatin formation.[64–68] Thus, DAXX and ATRX are involved in controlling telomere length, and the loss of DAXX or ATRX function due to mutations leads to an increase in telomere length in tumors with *DAXX* or *ATRX* mutations,[13] and these tumors are referred to as having the alternative lengthening of telomeres (ALT) phenotype (see **Fig. 2**).[58,59] Reactivation of telomerase leads to resistance to senescence in tumor cells with *ATRX* mutations, and tumors lacking telomerase activity display telomerase-independent ALT.[69,70] Patients who have PNETs with mutations in *MEN1*, *DAXX*, or *ATRX*, or a combination of both *MEN1* and *DAXX* or *ATRX*, are reported to have a better prognosis when compared with patients who had PNETs that lacked these mutations.[54] Somatic mutations of the set domain-containing 2 (*SETD2*) gene have also been detected in approximately 20% of sporadic PNETs (see **Table 1**).[13,71] Inactivating mutations of *SETD2*, which is involved in chromatin remodeling, have previously been linked with clear cell renal carcinoma.[72] *MEN1*, *DAXX*, and *ATRX* are tightly related to chromatin remodeling, thereby suggesting that PNETs are tightly regulated by epigenetic mechanisms, which are important drivers of tumorigenesis. Other epigenetic alterations found in PNETs include hypermethylation of the promoter region of *RASSF1* and cyclin-dependent kinase inhibitor 2A (*CDKN2A*).[73–75] In addition, insulin-like growth factor 2 (*IGF2*) has a unique hypermethylation signature in insulinomas, and this is of interest in relation to the reported epigenetic changes in insulin-like growth factor and insulinoma.[76] Finally, the pleckstrin homology-like domain family A member 3 (*PHLDA3*) genomic locus, which is a p53-regulated repressor of Akt, has been reported to have LOH and promoter methylation at a high frequency, thereby indicating that PHLDA3 is probably a tumor suppressor in PNETs.[77]

The occurrence of *MEN1* and *DAXX* or *ATRX* mutations in sporadic non-MEN1 insulinomas is reported to be 3% to 8% and 3%, respectively.[78,79] However mutations and differential expression of epigenetic modifying genes and their targets are reported to occur more frequently.[78,79] Thus, the somatic Trp372Arg gain of function mutation of the Ying Yang 1 (*YY1*) transcription factor, which regulates mitochondrial function and insulin or insulin-like growth factor signaling and is a target for mTORC1,[80,81] has been reported to occur in 15% to 30% of sporadic insulinomas.[78,79] The Trp372Arg mutation increased transcriptional activity of YY1, which resulted in greater transcription of target genes isocitrate dehydrogenase 3 (NAD [+]) alpha (*IDH3A*) and uncoupling protein 2 (*UCP2*).[78] Other recurrently mutated genes detected in insulinomas include H3 histone family 3A (*H3F3A*), lysine-specific demethylase 6A (*KDM6A*), and ataxia telangiectasia and Rad3-related protein (ATR) serine-threonine kinase (*ATR*), which are reported in 8%, 8%, and 8% of insulinomas, respectively.[79]

Mutations affecting the mammalian target of rapamycin signaling pathway

Approximately 15% of sporadic PNETs harbor somatic mutations of genes in the mTOR cell signaling pathway, including mutations of phosphatidylinositol-4,5-bisphosphate 3-kinase catalytic subunit alpha (*PIK3CA*); phosphatase and tensin homolog (*PTEN*); *TSC1* and *TSC2*; and disheveled, Egl-10, and Pleckstrin (DEP) domain-containing protein 5 (*DEPDC5*)[13,54] (see **Fig. 2, Table 1**). Mutations in *PTEN*, *TSC2*, and *DEPDC5*, which are mutually exclusive, are typically inactivating mutations, and 75% of sporadic PNETs have decreased expression of PTEN and TSC2,[82] whereas the *PIK3CA* mutation, which involves a hotspot for activation of the kinase domain, has been reported to be oncogenic.[62,83] Moreover, gastroentero-pancreatic neuroendocrine tumors (GEPNETs) with *TSC2*, *KRAS*, and tumor protein p53 (*TP53*) mutations are reported more probably associated with disease progression and reduced survival in patients. These possible aggressive alterations were observed in 6% of patients with PNETs less than 2 cm and limited to the pancreas, which is defined as stage 1 disease by the European Neuroendocrine Tumor Society (ENET) tumor-node-metastasis classification and combined ENET and American Joint Commission on Cancer,[84] thereby identifying a potential group of patients that may benefit from early surgery or systemic therapy.[85] Gene fusion events involving the Ewing sarcoma breakpoint region 1 (*EWSR1*) gene, which can activate mTOR signaling, have also been putatively identified in PNETs.[13]

Copy number changes

Copy number changes, which may reflect chromosomal instability comprising loss and gain, have been reported in PNETs, and these alterations may accumulate during tumor growth and progression with multiple chromosomal abnormalities being associated with a worse prognosis.[1,86] Recurrent regions of chromosomal loss involve the known NET tumor suppressors, including *MEN1*, *CDKN2A*, eyes absent homolog (EYA) transcriptional coactivator and phosphatase 1 (*EYA1*), sex comb on midleg (Scm)-like with 4 malignant brain tumor (Mbt) domains 1 (*SFMBT1*), and RAB GTPase-activating protein 1-like (*RABGAP1L*), which are located on chromosomes 11q13.1, 9q21.3, 8q13.3, 3p21.1, and 1q25.1, respectively.[13] Recurrently amplified regions include persephin (*PSPN*) on chromosome 19p13.3 and Unc-51 (*Caenorhabditis elegans*)-like autophagy-activating kinase 1 (*ULK1*) on chromosome 12q24.33, which are involved in rearranged during transfection (RET)-signaling and mTOR-regulated autophagy, respectively.[13]

MicroRNAs

MiRNAs *miR-103* and *miR-155* are up-regulated and down-regulated in PNETs and pancreatic acinar cancers when compared with normal tissue, respectively.[87] *MiR-204* expression in insulinomas is reported to correlate with insulin expression and mir-21, which represses *PTEN*, is reported to be associated with an increased proliferation index in insulinomas and their hepatic metastases.[87] The miRNA profiles of insulinomas and nonfunctioning PNETs are reported to be indistinguishable, although overexpression of *miR-204* and *miR-211*, which are closely related, have been reported to be restricted to insulinomas.[73,86,88]

Pancreatic neuroendocrine carcinomas

G3 PNETs, or PNECs, have a distinct molecular signature from G1 and G2 PNETs, in having frequent mutations of the *TP53* and retinoblastoma 1 (*RB1*) genes, which are very rare in well-differentiated PNETs.[13,89] The prevalence of *TP53* aberrations is also significantly greater in liver metastases than in primary PNETs.[85] There are also significant differences in the distribution of variants in the *RET*, Harvey rat sarcoma viral oncoprotein (*HRAS*), *MEN1*, *DAXX*, and *ATRX* genes, with *MEN1* variants being more common in early stage disease and *DAXX* and *ATRX* being more frequent in advanced disease.[85]

Germline Mutations In Patients with Sporadic Pancreatic Neuroendocrine Tumors

Germline mutations of the *MEN1*, *CDKN1B*, and *VHL* genes have been reported to occur in approximately 6%, approximately 1%, and approximately 1% of patients with sporadic PNETs, which also had LOH involving these genes in the tumors[13] (see **Table 1**). The identification of germline *MEN1* mutations in patients with apparently sporadic PNETs is important because it indicates that these patients and their children are at greater risk of developing MEN1-associated tumors. This has implications for the clinical management and surveillance of MEN1-associated tumors in the patients and for genetic screening and tumor surveillance in their children and possibly their first-degree relatives. In addition, germline alterations in DNA-repair genes have also been reported to result in characteristic mutational signatures in tumor genomes. Thus, inactivating germline mutations of the base-excision repair gene Mut Y homolog (*MUTYH*), which occurred with somatic LOH in PNETs of approximately 5% of patients[13] (see **Table 1**), had a mutational signature of guanine:cytosine (G:C) to thymine:alanine (A:T) transversions throughout the tumor genome. Germline biallelic inactivation of MUTYH has been also reported to cause autosomal recessive MUTYH-associated colorectal polyposis syndrome, which is also associated with somatic G:C to T:A transversions involving the *APC* gene, which is the driver of colorectal polyps.[13,90] This suggests that MUTYH deficiency likely plays a role in the development of PNETs and that polyadenosine diphosphate (ADP) ribose polymerase (PARP) inhibitors, which are directed at defective DNA-damage repair mechanisms, may represent potential treatments that would require further assessments. In addition, approximately 1% and approximately 4% of patients with sporadic PNETs have been observed to have germline mutations of breast cancer 2 (*BRCA2*) and checkpoint kinase 2 (*CHEK2*) that were associated with reduced kinase activity, respectively[13] (see **Table 1**).

CURRENT THERAPEUTIC APPROACHES FOR PANCREATIC NEUROENDOCRINE TUMORS

Surgical resection with regional lymph node dissection offers the only potentially curative treatment of well-differentiated PNETs (G1 and G2).[9] For advanced PNETs and metastatic disease medical therapies (eg, biotherapies, which target tumor-specific receptors and intracellular pathways, and chemotherapies, which generally target cell division) and radiological treatments (eg, peptide receptor radionuclide therapy [PRRT], radiofrequency ablation, transarterial embolization, and selective internal radiation therapy) are available.[9] Medical chemotherapy is usually reserved for patients with PNET metastases, high tumor burden, high proliferative index (eg, Ki-67 index >5%), rapid tumor progression, or symptoms not controlled by biotherapy.[9] Chemotherapy for such PNET disease usually comprises combined cytotoxic regimes (eg, streptozocin with 5-fluorouracil or doxorubicin[91] or temozolomide with capecitabine[92]), and tumor response rates of 70% have been reported.[92] Medical biotherapies for PNETs, which can be hormonal and based on somatostatin (a peptide hormone that inhibits release of other hormones, cell proliferation, and angiogenesis[93]) or targeted to tumor-specific molecular changes (eg, in receptors and signaling pathways) that help tumors to grow and spread, include mTOR signaling inhibitors, receptor tyrosine kinase (RTK) inhibitors, and antibodies targeting vascular endothelial growth factor (VEGF) or VEGF receptor (VEGFR)[9] (see **Fig. 2**). The recent advances in medical biotherapies are briefly reviewed, followed by a discussion of emerging therapies.

Somatostatin Analogues

Somatostatin analogues (eg, octreotide and lanreotide) have been used to control excessive hormone secretion and for their potential antiproliferative effects in patients with low-grade (Ki-67 index <5%) PNETs that express SSTRs, which are G-protein-coupled receptors (GPCRs).[94–97] There are 5 SSTRs ($SSTR_{1-5}$) and each has specific functions. $SSTR_2$ and $SSTR_5$ predominantly mediate inhibition of hormone secretion. $SSTR_1$, $SSTR_2$, $SSTR_4$, and $SSTR_5$ mediate cell cycle arrest and antiproliferative actions, whereas $SSTR_3$ mediates apoptosis.[98,99] Moreover, the aberrantly truncated variant of $SSTR_5$ (sst5TMD4) is overexpressed in GEPNETs, in which it is associated with increased aggressiveness.[100] In addition, sst5TMD4 disrupts the normal function of $SSTR_2$ and decreases the response of different tumor cells and tissues in response to somatostatin analogues.[101,102] These findings suggest that identification of sst5TMD4 may be a useful biomarker to predict responses to somatostatin analogues and the aggressiveness of PNETs.[86,100] PNETs may express all 5 subtypes, although approximately 80% of PNETs will predominantly express $SSTR_2$, for which octreotide and lanreotide have high affinities (see **Fig. 2**),[94] such that treatment with lanreotide resulted in an approximately 50% reduction in the risk of disease progression and a prolonged progression-free survival (PFS) (median in lanreotide treated group not reached vs median in placebo treated group of 18 months, $P<.001$) in non-MEN1 subjects with treatment-naive well-differentiated G1 and G2 nonfunctioning GEP-NETs,[96,103,104] whereas octreotide resulted in tumor response in 10%, stable disease in 80%, and progression of disease in 10% of MEN1 subjects with duodeno-pancreatic neuroendocrine tumors (NETs) who were treated over 12 to 15 months.[105] In addition PRRT using a somatostatin analogue (eg, octreotide, octreotate, dotatate, and dota-toc) labeled with a β-emitting nuclide in the form of either [177]lutetium or [90]yttrium has been reported to be effective for treating NETs. Thus, treatment with: [177]lutetium-octreotide or [90]yttrium-octreotide in patients with gastrointestinal NETs and metastatic NETs,[106–111] has been reported to result in objective response rates of approximately 20% to 60%,[106,108–110] PFS of 20 to 34 months,[108,110] and an overall survival of 53 months.[108] Combining [177]lutetium and [90]yttrium nuclides has also been reported to increase survival in patients with PNETs[111]; and the combination of [177]luoctreotate, capecitabine, and temozolomide, in a phase 1-2 study has been reported to result in complete or partial response in greater than 50% of the subjects with advanced NETs (including PNETs).[107]

Mammalian Target of Rapamycin Inhibitors

mTOR activation is associated with poor prognosis and there is a significant correlation between a high proliferation index (Ki-67) values and expression of mTOR, PIK3CA, and eukaryotic translation initiation factor 4E binding protein 1 (p-4EBP1).[86,112] Moreover, somatic mutations of genes associated with the mTOR pathway[13,54] are found in approximately 15% of PNETs. The mTOR inhibitor everolimus, which suppresses multiprotein complexes to inhibit downstream signaling (see **Fig. 2**), has been reported to increase PFS from approximately 6 to 11 months in patients with advanced NETs, including PNETs.[113–116] However, a companion diagnostic test that would help to identify patients who could benefit from treatment with mTOR inhibitors is not available,[2] although preclinical data have suggested that aberrations of *PI3KCA* and *PTEN*, and high pAKT levels, may predict sensitivity to rapamycin in NET cell lines and rapalogs in NET patients.[117] However, protein and/or messengerRNA (mRNA) analysis might be a better indicator of mTOR pathway activation than mutational status because it would avoid errors due to epigenetic changes that affect protein expression.[86] Loss of AKT repression, may also occur in patients with PHLDA3 LOH or methylation; therefore, these patients may also potentially respond well to everolimus.[77]

Receptor Tyrosine Kinase Inhibitors

PNETs are highly vascular and frequently express VEGFRs[118,119] and RTK inhibitors (eg, sunitinib, which targets VEGFRs) and platelet-derived growth factor receptors (PDGFRs) (see **Fig. 2**) have been reported to increase PFS from approximately 5.5 to 11.4 months, in subjects with PNETs.[120] In a phase 2 trial, pazopanib, another RTK inhibitor, has also been reported to result in response and disease control rates of approximately 20% and greater than 75%, respectively, of non-MEN1 subjects with metastatic GEPNETs.[121] However, therapeutic resistance to RTK inhibitors may arise through induction of hypoxic stress and upregulation of transcription factors controlling expression of proangiogenic molecules, or through reduced lysosomal stability leading to autophagy.[122,123] Companion diagnostic tests that would help to identify such resistance remain to be developed.

EMERGING THERAPIES FOR PANCREATIC NEUROENDOCRINE TUMORS

MEN1 mutations, which occur in approximately 40% of sporadic PNETs and almost all MEN1 PNETs, represent the major drivers for PNET development, and therapies based on an increased understanding of menin, together with that of receptors and signaling pathways in PNETs, are helping to develop new therapies. Assessment of the efficacy of these therapies have been facilitated by cellular and in vivo models, which include conventional and conditional *Men1* knockout mouse models that develop MEN1-associated tumors, including PNETs,[124–133] and some of these preclinical advances are discussed.

MEN1 Gene Replacement Therapy

Menin acts as a tumor suppressor and, as such, its loss due to *MEN1* mutations leads to tumor development and growth. Thus, *MEN1* gene replacement therapy should be able to suppress tumor proliferation. Indeed, *Men1* gene replacement therapy into pituitary NETs that developed in conventional knockout mice lacking 1 allele of *Men1* (*Men1*[+/−]), using a recombinant nonreplicating adenoviral serotype 5 vector (rAd5), containing *Men1* complementary DNA (cDNA) under the control of a cytomegalovirus promoter (rAd5-MEN1), resulted in increased menin expression with decreased proliferation of the pituitary NETs. The *Men1* gene therapy did not induce an immune T-cell response or increased apoptosis.[134] These findings established proof of principle for the efficacy of *Men1* gene replacement therapy. In addition, use of a hybrid adeno-associated virus and phage (AAVP) vector displaying biologically active octreotide on the viral surface for ligand-directed delivery of the proapoptotic tumor necrosis factor (*TNF*) transgene to PNETs developing in a pancreatic-specific *Men1* knockout mouse model has also been reported to reduce tumor size and improve survival of the mutant mice.[135] These results suggest that systemic, ligand-directed transgene treatment of PNETs could potentially evolve as a novel and effective treatment.

Epigenetic Modulators

Menin interacts with several histone-modifying proteins, including histone methyltransferase (MLL1 and PRMT5) and deacetylase complexes (mSin3A-histone deacetylase)[17] (see **Fig. 1**). The use of epigenetic modulators, which represent a novel class of anticancer drugs[136] to treat PNETs, has been used in in vitro and in vivo studies.[137] These studies used JQ1, an inhibitor of the bromodomain and extraterminal domain (BET) family of proteins that bind to acetylated histone residues to promote gene transcription.[137] In vitro studies revealed that JQ1 decreased proliferation and increased apoptosis of a PNET cell line. In vivo studies, using a pancreatic β-cell–specific conditional *Men1* knockout mouse model, revealed that JQ1 decreased proliferation and increased apoptosis of PNETs.[137] CP103, another BET inhibitor, has also been reported to reduce PNET proliferation in a human PNET cell line xenograft mouse model.[138] Thus, epigenetic modulators; for example, via BET inhibition, may offer potential therapies for PNETs lacking *MEN1* expression.

Wnt Signaling Modulators

Menin inhibits Wnt signaling because it promotes phosphorylation of β-catenin and its transfer from the nucleus via nuclear-cytoplasmic shuttling, which reduces cell proliferation.[21,26] Moreover, the conditional knockout of β-catenin in PNETs of mice with pancreatic β-cell conditional knockout of menin decreased the number and size of PNETs, as well as increased survival, whereas use of a β-catenin antagonist (PKF115–584) decreased PNET cell proliferation in β-cell menin knockout mice.[139] Thus, Wnt-signaling modulators may provide a novel approach for treatment of MEN1-deficient PNETs.

RAS Signaling

Aberrant activation of Ras signaling can occur in NETs due to mutations in Ras or Ras regulatory proteins, such as NF1, or downstream effectors, such as Raf-MEK-ERK. Aberrant activation of Ras depends on absolute dependency on protein kinase C delta (PKCδ)-mediated survival pathways.[140,141] This sensitizes cells to apoptosis induced by suppression of PKCδ activity, which is not toxic to cells with normal Ras activity. The PNET cell line, BON-1, is sensitive to PKCδ inhibition induced by shRNA knockdown or diverse small molecule inhibitors, such as Rottlerin,[142] and such molecules may prove to be useful for treating PNETs that have activated Ras signaling.

Antiangiogenic Compounds

Most antiangiogenic compounds block the activity of the cytokine VEGF, which promotes the growth and survival of blood vessels. Treatment with bevacizumab, which is an anti-VEGF monoclonal antibody, in combination with chemotherapy, has been reported to delay the progression of moderately well-differentiated and advanced gastrointestinal NETs, which included metastatic well-differentiated PNETs.[143–146] However, inhibiting VEGF signaling has been reported to be accompanied by increased invasiveness and metastasis of cancers, possibly due to the upregulation of proangiogenic factors, including fibroblast growth factors (FGFs); therefore, targeting FGFs in addition to VEGF and PDGF may improve the efficacy of treatment.[147–149] Furthermore, the combination of sunitinib, or an anti-VEGF antibody, with inhibitors (eg, PF-04217903 or PF-0241066 [crizotinib]) of hepatocyte growth factor receptor (HGFR) or c-Met, which promotes cell proliferation, invasion, and metastasis, prevented the increased tumor aggressivity without impairment to the activity of restricting tumor growth.[150] Thus, these studies suggest that the increase in invasion and metastasis that are promoted by selective inhibition of VEGF signaling may be reduced by combining the treatment with a c-Met inhibitor. In addition, inhibition of nitric oxide (NO) synthase may have a role because the use of L-arginine methyl ester (L-NAME), an NO synthase inhibitor, in ex vivo treatment of PNETs from conventional $Men1^{+/-}$ knockout mice caused impaired blood perfusion and increased constriction of the tumor-supplying arterioles.[151]

Use of Somatostatin Analogues for Pancreatic Neuroendocrine Tumor Chemoprevention

Somatostatin analogues may have a potential role in chemoprevention of MEN1-associated NETs because they have been shown to have antiproliferative, and anti-secretory effects on NETs.[103,104,152,153] Thus, treatment with pasireotide, which is a multiple-receptor–targeted somatostatin analogue that acts via $SSTR_{1,2,3}$ and $SSTR_5$,[94] decreased proliferation and increased apoptosis of PNETs in conventional $Men1^{+/-}$ and pancreatic-specific conditional Men1 knockout mutant mice, as well as increasing survival of the conventional $Men1^{+/-}$ mutant knockout mice.[154,155] In addition to these antiproliferative and proapoptotic effects, pasireotide was also found to inhibit the development of PNETs in the $Men1^{+/-}$ mutant mice.[154] These findings, which indicate that pasireotide treatment resulted in fewer $Men1^{+/-}$ mice with PNETs that also had fewer PNETs per pancreas when compared with control phosphate buffered saline–treated $Men1^{+/-}$ mice, are consistent with a lower development of new NETs, in pasireotide-treated $Men1^{+/-}$ mice.[154] These findings suggest that somatostatin analogues may play a chemopreventive role in the treatment of MEN1-associated PNETs in patients, and 2 studies in MEN1 subjects have reported such antiproliferative actions of somatostatin analogues. In 1 study, octreotide was given to MEN1 subjects to treat duodeno-pancreatic NETs. Retrospective analysis revealed that 10% of PNETs had tumor response and that 80% had stable disease[105]; whereas, in another study, octreotide was given prospectively to 8 MEN1 subjects with GEPNETs, and was found to be safe and decrease gastrointestinal hormone secretion, and to be associated with stable PNET disease.[156]

SUMMARY

MEN1 mutations are major drivers for development of familial and sporadic forms of PNETs. Additional genetic studies of PNETs have further improved the understanding of the molecular alterations and cellular pathways associated with these tumors, including the roles of genes involved in chromatin remodeling and epigenetic regulation, mTOR signaling, K-RAS signaling, β-catenin–Wnt signaling, and SSTR signaling. This has led to the development of medical biotherapies, which can inhibit SSTR, mTOR, or RTK signaling. In addition, recent preclinical studies have also demonstrated the efficacy of MEN1 gene replacement therapy, epigenetic modulators, Wnt pathway targeting β-catenin antagonists, and multi-SSTR–targeted analogues in treating PNETs. Clinical evaluation of such emerging treatments may help to provide new therapies for improving outcomes and life expectancies in PNET patients.

REFERENCES

1. Reid MD, Saka B, Balci S, et al. Molecular genetics of pancreatic neoplasms and their morphologic correlates an update on recent advances and potential diagnostic applications. Am J Clin Pathol 2014;141(2):168–80.
2. Ohmoto A, Rokutan H, Yachida S. Pancreatic neuroendocrine neoplasms: basic biology, current treatment strategies and prospects for the future. Int J Mol Sci 2017;18(1) [pii:E143].
3. Bosman FT, Carneiro F, Hruban RH, et al. WHO classification of tumours of the digestive system. 4th edition. Lyon (France): International Agency for Research on Cancer (IARC); 2010.
4. Lloyd RV, Osamura RY, Klöppel G, et al. WHO classification of tumours of endocrine organs. 4th edition. Lyon (France): International Agency for Research on Cancer (IARC); 2017.
5. Yao JC, Hassan M, Phan A, et al. One hundred years after "Carcinoid": epidemiology of and prognostic factors for neuroendocrine tumors in 35,825 cases in the United States. J Clin Oncol 2008;26(18):3063–72.
6. Halfdanarson TR, Rabe KG, Rubin J, et al. Pancreatic neuroendocrine tumors (PNETs): incidence, prognosis and recent trend toward improved survival. Ann Oncol 2008;19(10):1727–33.
7. Kimura W, Kuroda A, Morioka Y. Clinical pathology of endocrine tumors of the pancreas. Analysis of autopsy cases. Dig Dis Sci 1991;36(7):933–42.
8. Di Domenico A, Wiedmer T, Marinoni I, et al. Genetic and epigenetic drivers of neuroendocrine tumours (NET). Endocr Relat Cancer 2017;24(9):R315–34.
9. Frost M, Lines KE, Thakker RV. Current and emerging therapies for PNETs in patients with or without MEN1. Nat Rev Endocrinol 2018;14(4):216–27.
10. Dasari A, Shen C, Halperin D, et al. Trends in the incidence, prevalence, and survival outcomes in patients with neuroendocrine tumors in the United States. JAMA Oncol 2017;3(10):1335–42.
11. Yao JC, Eisner MP, Leary C, et al. Population-based study of islet cell carcinoma. Ann Surg Oncol 2007;14(12):3492–500.
12. Zhang J, Francois R, Iyer R, et al. Current understanding of the molecular biology of pancreatic neuroendocrine tumors. J Natl Cancer Inst 2013; 105(14):1005–17.
13. Scarpa A, Chang DK, Nones K, et al. Whole-genome landscape of pancreatic neuroendocrine tumours. Nature 2017;543(7643):65–71.
14. Thakker RV, Newey PJ, Walls GV, et al. Clinical practice guidelines for multiple endocrine neoplasia type 1 (MEN1). J Clin Endocrinol Metab 2012;97(9): 2990–3011.
15. Yates CJ, Newey PJ, Thakker RV. Challenges and controversies in management of pancreatic neuroendocrine tumours in patients with MEN1. Lancet Diabetes Endocrinol 2015;3(11):895–905.
16. Lemos MC, Thakker RV. Multiple endocrine neoplasia type 1 (MEN 1): analysis of 1336 mutations reported in the first decade following identification of the gene. Hum Mutat 2008;29(1):22–32.
17. Thakker RV. Multiple endocrine neoplasia type 1 (MEN1) and type 4 (MEN4). Mol Cell Endocrinol 2014;386(1–2):2–15.
18. Goudet P, Murat A, Binquet C, et al. Risk factors and causes of death in MEN1 disease. A GTE (Groupe d'Etude des tumeurs endocrines) cohort study among 758 patients. World J Surg 2010;34(2):249–55.

19. Ito T, Igarashi H, Uehara H, et al. Causes of death and prognostic factors in multiple endocrine neoplasia type 1: a prospective study comparison of 106 MEN1/Zollinger-Ellison syndrome patients with 1613 literature MEN1 patients with or without pancreatic endocrine tumors. Medicine 2013;92(3):135–81.

20. Agarwal SK. The future: genetics advances in MEN1 therapeutic approaches and management strategies. Endocr Relat Cancer 2017;24(10):T119–34.

21. Cao Y, Liu R, Jiang X, et al. Nuclear-cytoplasmic shuttling of menin regulates nuclear translocation of {beta}-catenin. Mol Cell Biol 2009;29(20):5477–87.

22. Huang J, Gurung B, Wan B, et al. The same pocket in menin binds both MLL and JUND but has opposite effects on transcription. Nature 2012;482(7386): 542–6.

23. Matkar S, Thiel A, Hua X. Menin: a scaffold protein that controls gene expression and cell signaling. Trends Biochem Sci 2013;38(8):394–402.

24. Agarwal SK, Kennedy PA, Scacheri PC, et al. Menin molecular interactions: insights into normal functions and tumorigenesis. Horm Metab Res 2005;37(6): 369–74.

25. Balogh K, Racz K, Patocs A, et al. Menin and its interacting proteins: elucidation of menin function. Trends Endocrinol Metab 2006;17(9):357–64.

26. Klaus A, Birchmeier W. Wnt signalling and its impact on development and cancer. Nat Rev Cancer 2008;8(5):387–98.

27. Agarwal SK, Guru SC, Heppner C, et al. Menin interacts with the AP1 transcription factor JunD and represses JunD-activated transcription. Cell 1999;96(1): 143–52.

28. Agarwal SK, Novotny EA, Crabtree JS, et al. Transcription factor JunD, deprived of menin, switches from growth suppressor to growth promoter. Proc Natl Acad Sci U S A 2003;100(19):10770–5.

29. Gurung B, Feng Z, Iwamoto DV, et al. Menin epigenetically represses Hedgehog signaling in MEN1 tumor syndrome. Cancer Res 2013;73(8):2650–8.

30. Hughes CM, Rozenblatt-Rosen O, Milne TA, et al. Menin associates with a trithorax family histone methyltransferase complex and with the hoxc8 locus. Mol Cell 2004;13(4):587–97.

31. Milne TA, Hughes CM, Lloyd R, et al. Menin and MLL cooperatively regulate expression of cyclin-dependent kinase inhibitors. Proc Natl Acad Sci U S A 2005;102(3):749–54.

32. Attisano L, Wrana JL. Signal transduction by the TGF-beta superfamily. Science 2002;296(5573):1646–7.

33. Hendy GN, Kaji H, Sowa H, et al. Menin and TGF-beta superfamily member signaling via the Smad pathway in pituitary, parathyroid and osteoblast. Horm Metab Res 2005;37(6):375–9.

34. Canaff L, Vanbellinghen JF, Kaji H, et al. Impaired transforming growth factor-beta (TGF-beta) transcriptional activity and cell proliferation control of a menin in-frame deletion mutant associated with multiple endocrine neoplasia type 1 (MEN1). J Biol Chem 2012;287(11):8584–97.

35. Heppner C, Bilimoria KY, Agarwal SK, et al. The tumor suppressor protein menin interacts with NF-kappaB proteins and inhibits NF-kappaB-mediated transactivation. Oncogene 2001;20(36):4917–25.

36. Wu Y, Feng ZJ, Gao SB, et al. Interplay between menin and K-Ras in regulating lung adenocarcinoma. J Biol Chem 2012;287(47):40003–11.

37. Chamberlain CE, Scheel DW, McGlynn K, et al. Menin determines K-RAS proliferative outputs in endocrine cells. J Clin Invest 2014;124(9):4093–101.

38. Gallo A, Cuozzo C, Esposito I, et al. Menin uncouples Elk-1, JunD and c-Jun phosphorylation from MAP kinase activation. Oncogene 2002;21(42):6434–45.

39. Patel YC. Somatostatin and its receptor family. Front Neuroendocrinol 1999; 20(3):157–98.

40. Wang Y, Ozawa A, Zaman S, et al. The tumor suppressor protein menin inhibits AKT activation by regulating its cellular localization. Cancer Res 2011;71(2): 371–82.

41. Laplante M, Sabatini DM. mTOR signaling in growth control and disease. Cell 2012;149(2):274–93.

42. Maher ER, Iselius L, Yates JRW, et al. Von Hippel-Lindau disease - a genetic-study. J Med Genet 1991;28(7):443–7.

43. Maher ER, Neumann HPH, Richard S. Von Hippel-Lindau disease: a clinical and scientific review. Eur J Hum Genet 2011;19(6):617–23.

44. Stolle C, Glenn G, Zbar B, et al. Improved detection of germline mutations in the von Hippel Lindau disease tumor suppressor gene. Hum Mutat 1998;12(6): 417–23.

45. Findels-Hosey JJ, McMahon KQ, Findeis SK. Von Hippel-Lindau disease. J Pediatr Genet 2016;5(2):116–23.

46. Blansfield JA, Choyke L, Morita SY, et al. Clinical, genetic and radiographic analysis of 108 patients with von Hippel-Lindau disease (VHL) manifested by pancreatic neuroendocrine neoplasms (PNETs). Surgery 2007;142(6):814–8 [discussion: 818.e1-2].

47. Nordstrom-O'Brien M, van der Luijt RB, van Rooijen E, et al. Genetic analysis of von Hippel-Lindau disease. Hum Mutat 2010;31(5):521–37.

48. Shen HCJ, Adem A, Ylaya K, et al. Deciphering von Hippel-Lindau (VHL/Vhl)-associated pancreatic manifestations by inactivating VHL in specific pancreatic cell populations. PLoS One 2009;4(4):e4897.

49. Martin GA, Viskochil D, Bollag G, et al. The gap-related domain of the neurofi-bromatosis type-1 gene-product interacts with Ras P21. Cell 1990;63(4):843–9.

50. Brems H, Beert E, de Ravel T, et al. Mechanisms in the pathogenesis of malig-nant tumours in neurofibromatosis type 1. Lancet Oncol 2009;10(5):508–15.

51. Nishi T, Kawabata Y, Hari Y, et al. A case of pancreatic neuroendocrine tumor in a patient with neurofibromatosis-1. World J Surg Oncol 2012;10:153.

52. Minnetti M, Grossman A. Somatic and germline mutations in NETs: implications for their diagnosis and management. Best Pract Res Clin Endocrinol Metab 2016;30(1):115–27.

53. Lebwohl D, Anak O, Sahmoud T, et al. Development of everolimus, a novel oral mTOR inhibitor, across a spectrum of diseases. Ann N Y Acad Sci 2013;1291: 14–32.

54. Jiao Y, Shi C, Edil BH, et al. DAXX/ATRX, MEN1, and mTOR pathway genes are frequently altered in pancreatic neuroendocrine tumors. Science 2011; 331(6021):1199–203.

55. Corbo V, Dalai I, Scardoni M, et al. MEN1 in pancreatic endocrine tumors: anal-ysis of gene and protein status in 169 sporadic neoplasms reveals alterations in the vast majority of cases. Endocr Relat Cancer 2010;17(3):771–83.

56. Gortz B, Roth J, Krahenmann A, et al. Mutations and allelic deletions of the MEN1 gene are associated with a subset of sporadic endocrine pancreatic and neuroendocrine tumors and not restricted to foregut neoplasms. Am J Pathol 1999;154(2):429–36.

57. de Wilde RF, Heaphy CM, Maitra A, et al. Loss of ATRX or DAXX expression and concomitant acquisition of the alternative lengthening of telomeres phenotype

are late events in a small subset of MEN-1 syndrome pancreatic neuroendocrine tumors. Mod Pathol 2012;25(7):1033–9.

58. Heaphy CM, de Wilde RF, Jiao YC, et al. Altered telomeres in tumors with ATRX and DAXX mutations. Science 2011;333(6041):425.

59. Marinoni I, Kurrer AS, Vassella E, et al. Loss of DAXX and ATRX are associated with chromosome instability and reduced survival of patients with pancreatic neuroendocrine tumors. Gastroenterology 2014;146(2):453–60.e5.

60. Chen SF, Kasajima A, Yazdani S, et al. Clinicopathologic significance of immunostaining of alpha-thalassemia/mental retardation syndrome X-linked protein and death domain-associated protein in neuroendocrine tumors. Hum Pathol 2013;44:2199–203.

61. Yuan F, Shi M, Shi H, et al. KRAS and DAXX/ATRX gene mutations are correlated with the clinicopathological features, advanced disease and poor prognosis in Chinese patients with pancreatic neuroendocrine tumors. Int J Biol Sci 2014; 10(9):957–65.

62. de Wilde RF, Edil BH, Hruban RH, et al. Well-differentiated pancreatic neuroendocrine tumors: from genetics to therapy. Nat Rev Gastroenterol Hepatol 2012; 9(4):199–208.

63. Elsasser SJ, Allis CD, Lewis PW. New epigenetic drivers of cancers. Science 2011;331(6021):1145–6.

64. Drane P, Ouararhni K, Depaux A, et al. The death-associated protein DAXX is a novel histone chaperone involved in the replication-independent deposition of H3.3. Genes Dev 2010;24(12):1253–65.

65. Goldberg AD, Banaszynski LA, Noh KM, et al. Distinct factors control histone variant H3.3 localization at specific genomic regions. Cell 2010;140(5):678–91.

66. Wong LH, McGhie JD, Sim M, et al. ATRX interacts with H3.3 in maintaining telomere structural integrity in pluripotent embryonic stem cells. Genome Res 2010; 20(3):351–60.

67. Cusanelli E, Chartrand P. Telomeric repeat-containing RNA TERRA: a noncoding RNA connecting telomere biology to genome integrity. Front Genet 2015;6:143.

68. Azzalin CM, Reichenbach P, Khoriauli L, et al. Telomeric repeat-containing RNA and RNA surveillance factors at mammalian chromosome ends. Science 2007; 318(5851):798–801.

69. Vinagre J, Pinto V, Celestino R, et al. Telomerase promoter mutations in cancer: an emerging molecular biomarker? Virchows Arch 2014;465(2):119–33.

70. Lovejoy CA, Li WD, Reisenweber S, et al. Loss of ATRX, genome instability, and an altered DNA damage response are hallmarks of the alternative lengthening of telomeres pathway. PLoS Genet 2012;8(7):e1002772.

71. Raj NP, Soumerai T, Valentino E, et al. Next-generation sequencing (NGS) in advanced well differentiated pancreatic neuroendocrine tumors (WD pNETs): a study using MSK-IMPACT. J Clin Oncol 2016;34(4):246.

72. Dalgliesh GL, Furge K, Greenman C, et al. Systematic sequencing of renal carcinoma reveals inactivation of histone modifying genes. Nature 2010;463(7279): 360–3.

73. Meeker A, Heaphy C. Gastroenteropancreatic endocrine tumors. Mol Cell Endocrinol 2014;386(1–2):101–20.

74. Karpathakis A, Dibra H, Thirlwell C. Neuroendocrine tumours: cracking the epigenetic code. Endocr Relat Cancer 2013;20(3):R65–82.

75. House MG, Herman JG, Guo MZ, et al. Aberrant hypermethylation of tumor suppressor genes in pancreatic endocrine neoplasms. Ann Surg 2003;238(3): 423–31.

76. Luco RF, Allo M, Schor IE, et al. Epigenetics in alternative Pre-mRNA splicing. Cell 2011;144(1):16–26.
77. Ohki R, Saito K, Chen Y, et al. PHLDA3 is a novel tumor suppressor of pancreatic neuroendocrine tumors. Proc Natl Acad Sci U S A 2014;111(23):E2404–13.
78. Cao YN, Gao ZB, Li L, et al. Whole exome sequencing of insulinoma reveals recurrent T372R mutations in YY1. Nat Commun 2013;4:2810.
79. Wang H, Bender A, Wang P, et al. Insights into beta cell regeneration for diabetes via integration of molecular landscapes in human insulinomas. Nat Commun 2017;8:767.
80. Blattler SM, Cunningham JT, Verdeguer F, et al. Yin Yang 1 deficiency in skeletal muscle protects against rapamycin-induced diabetic-like symptoms through activation of insulin/IGF signaling. Cell Metab 2012;15(4):505–17.
81. Cunningham JT, Rodgers JT, Arlow DH, et al. mTOR controls mitochondrial oxidative function through a YY1-PGC-1 alpha transcriptional complex. Nature 2007;450(7170):736–40.
82. Missiaglia E, Dalai I, Barbi S, et al. Pancreatic endocrine tumors: expression profiling evidences a role for AKT-mTOR pathway. J Clin Oncol 2010;28(2):245–55.
83. Samuels Y, Wang ZH, Bardelli A, et al. High frequency of mutations of the PIK3CA gene in human cancers. Science 2004;304(5670):554.
84. Rindi G, Falconi M, Klersy C, et al. TNM staging of neoplasms of the endocrine pancreas: results from a large international cohort study. J Natl Cancer Inst 2012;104(10):764–77.
85. Gleeson FC, Voss JS, Kipp BR, et al. Assessment of pancreatic neuroendocrine tumor cytologic genotype diversity to guide personalized medicine using a custom gastroenteropancreatic next-generation sequencing panel. Oncotarget 2017;8(55):93464–75.
86. Capdevila J, Casanovas O, Salazar R, et al. Translational research in neuroendocrine tumors: pitfalls and opportunities. Oncogene 2017;36(14):1899–907.
87. Roldo C, Missiaglia E, Hagan JP, et al. MicroRNA expression abnormalities in pancreatic endocrine and acinar tumors are associated with distinctive pathologic features and clinical behavior. J Clin Oncol 2006;24(29):4677–84.
88. Oberg K, Casanovas O, Castano JP, et al. Molecular pathogenesis of neuroendocrine tumors: implications for current and future therapeutic approaches. Clin Cancer Res 2013;19(11):2842–9.
89. Yachida S, Vakiani E, White CM, et al. Small cell and large cell neuroendocrine carcinomas of the pancreas are genetically similar and distinct from well-differentiated pancreatic neuroendocrine tumors. Am J Surg Pathol 2012;36(2):173–84.
90. Al-Tassan N, Chmiel NH, Maynard J, et al. Inherited variants of MYH associated with somatic G: C-->T: a mutations in colorectal tumors. Nat Genet 2002;30(2):227–32.
91. Hill JS, McPhee JT, McDade TP, et al. Pancreatic neuroendocrine tumors: the impact of surgical resection on survival. Cancer-Am Cancer Soc 2009;115(4):741–51.
92. Strosberg JR, Fine RL, Choi J, et al. First-line chemotherapy with capecitabine and temozolomide in patients with metastatic pancreatic endocrine carcinomas. Cancer 2011;117(2):268–75.
93. Cakir M, Dworakowska D, Grossman A. Somatostatin receptor biology in neuroendocrine and pituitary tumours: part 1–molecular pathways. J Cell Mol Med 2010;14(11):2570–84.

94. Schmid HA, Silva AP. Short- and long-term effects of octreotide and SOM230 on GH, IGF-I, ACTH, corticosterone and ghrelin in rats. J Endocrinol Invest 2005; 28(11 Suppl International):28–35.

95. Walter T, Brixi-Benmansour H, Lombard-Bohas C, et al. New treatment strategies in advanced neuroendocrine tumours. Dig Liver Dis 2012;44(2):95–105.

96. Martin-Richard M, Massuti B, Pineda E, et al. Antiproliferative effects of lanreotide autogel in patients with progressive, well-differentiated neuroendocrine tumours: a Spanish, multicentre, open-label, single arm phase II study. BMC Cancer 2013;13:427.

97. Palazzo M, Lombard-Bohas C, Cadiot G, et al. Ki67 proliferation index, hepatic tumor load, and pretreatment tumor growth predict the antitumoral efficacy of lanreotide in patients with malignant digestive neuroendocrine tumors. Eur J Gastroenterol Hepatol 2013;25(2).232–0.

98. Theodoropoulou M, Stalla GK. Somatostatin receptors: from signaling to clinical practice. Front Neuroendocrinol 2013;34(3):228–52.

99. Grozinsky-Glasberg S, Shimon I, Korbonits M, et al. Somatostatin analogues in the control of neuroendocrine tumours: efficacy and mechanisms. Endocr Relat Cancer 2008;15(3):701–20.

100. Sampedro-Nunez M, Luque RM, Ramos-Levi AM, et al. Presence of sst5TMD4, a truncated splice variant of the somatostatin receptor subtype 5, is associated to features of increased aggressiveness in pancreatic neuroendocrine tumors. Oncotarget 2016;7(6):6593–608.

101. Duran-Prado M, Saveanu A, Luque RM, et al. A Potential inhibitory role for the new truncated variant of somatostatin receptor 5, sst5TMD4, in pituitary adenomas poorly responsive to somatostatin analogs. J Clin Endocrinol Metab 2010;95(5):2497–502.

102. Duran-Prado M, Gahete MD, Hergueta-Redondo M, et al. The new truncated somatostatin receptor variant sst5TMD4 is associated to poor prognosis in breast cancer and increases malignancy in MCF-7 cells. Oncogene 2012;31(16): 2049–61.

103. Caplin ME, Pavel M, Cwikla JB, et al. Lanreotide in metastatic enteropancreatic neuroendocrine tumors. N Engl J Med 2014;371(3):224–33.

104. Caplin ME, Pavel M, Cwikla JB, et al. Anti-tumour effects of lanreotide for pancreatic and intestinal neuroendocrine tumours: the CLARINET open-label extension study. Endocr Relat Cancer 2016;23(3):191–9.

105. Ramundo V, Del Prete M, Marotta V, et al. Impact of long-acting octreotide in patients with early-stage MEN1-related duodeno-pancreatic neuroendocrine tumours. Clin Endocrinol (Oxf) 2014;80(6):850–5.

106. Bodei L, Cremonesi M, Grana CM, et al. Peptide receptor radionuclide therapy with (1)(7)(7)Lu-DOTATATE: the IEO phase I-II study. Eur J Nucl Med Mol Imaging 2011;38(12):2125–35.

107. Claringbold PG, Price RA, Turner JH. Phase I-II study of radiopeptide 177Lu-octreotate in combination with capecitabine and temozolomide in advanced low-grade neuroendocrine tumors. Cancer Biother Radiopharm 2012;27(9):561–9.

108. Ezziddin S, Khalaf F, Vanezi M, et al. Outcome of peptide receptor radionuclide therapy with 177Lu-octreotate in advanced grade 1/2 pancreatic neuroendocrine tumours. Eur J Nucl Med Mol Imaging 2014;41(5):925–33.

109. Imhof A, Brunner P, Marincek N, et al. Response, survival, and long-term toxicity after therapy with the radiolabeled somatostatin analogue [90Y-DOTA]-TOC in metastasized neuroendocrine cancers. J Clin Oncol 2011;29(17):2416–23.

110. Sansovini M, Severi S, Ambrosetti A, et al. Treatment with the radiolabelled so-matostatin analog Lu-DOTATATE for advanced pancreatic neuroendocrine tu-mors. Neuroendocrinology 2013;97(4):347–54.

111. Villard L, Romer A, Marincek N, et al. Cohort study of somatostatin-based radio-peptide therapy with [(90)Y-DOTA]-TOC versus [(90)Y-DOTA]-TOC plus [(177) Lu-DOTA]-TOC in neuroendocrine cancers. J Clin Oncol 2012;30(10):1100–6.

112. Qian ZR, Ter-Minassian M, Chan JA, et al. Prognostic significance of MTOR pathway component expression in neuroendocrine tumors. J Clin Oncol 2013; 31(27):3418–25.

113. Yao JC, Shah MH, Ito T, et al. Everolimus for advanced pancreatic neuroendo-crine tumors. N Engl J Med 2011;364(6):514–23.

114. Lombard-Bohas C, Yao JC, Hobday T, et al. Impact of prior chemotherapy use on the efficacy of everolimus in patients with advanced pancreatic neuroendo-crine tumors: a subgroup analysis of the phase III RADIANT-3 trial. Pancreas 2015;44(2):181–9.

115. Yao JC, Pavel M, Lombard-Bohas C, et al. Everolimus for the treatment of advanced pancreatic neuroendocrine tumors: overall survival and circulating biomarkers from the randomized, phase III RADIANT-3 study. J Clin Oncol 2016;34(32):3906–13.

116. Oh DY, Kim TW, Park YS, et al. Phase 2 study of everolimus monotherapy in pa-tients with nonfunctioning neuroendocrine tumors or pheochromocytomas/para-gangliomas. Cancer 2012;118(24):6162–70.

117. Meric-Bernstam F, Akcakanat A, Chen HQ, et al. PIK3CA/PTEN mutations and Akt activation as markers of sensitivity to allosteric mTOR inhibitors. Clin Cancer Res 2012;18(6):1777–89.

118. Hanahan D, Christofori G, Naik P, et al. Transgenic mouse models of tumour angiogenesis: the angiogenic switch, its molecular controls, and prospects for preclinical therapeutic models. Eur J Cancer 1996;32A(14):2386–93.

119. Scoazec JY. Angiogenesis in neuroendocrine tumors: therapeutic applications. Neuroendocrinology 2013;97(1):45–56.

120. Raymond E, Dahan L, Raoul JL, et al. Sunitinib malate for the treatment of pancreatic neuroendocrine tumors. N Engl J Med 2011;364(6):501–13.

121. Ahn HK, Choi JY, Kim KM, et al. Phase II study of pazopanib monotherapy in metastatic gastroenteropancreatic neuroendocrine tumours. Br J Cancer 2013;109(6):1414–9.

122. Yao JC, Phan A. Overcoming antiangiogenic resistance. Clin Cancer Res 2011; 17(16):5217–9.

123. Wiedmer T, Blank A, Pantasis S, et al. Autophagy inhibition improves sunitinib efficacy in pancreatic neuroendocrine tumors via a lysosome-dependent mech-anism. Mol Cancer Ther 2017;16(11):2502–15.

124. Wiedemann T, Pellegata NS. Animal models of multiple endocrine neoplasia. Mol Cell Endocrinol 2016;421:49–59.

125. Bertolino P, Tong WM, Galendo D, et al. Heterozygous Men1 mutant mice develop a range of endocrine tumors mimicking multiple endocrine neoplasia type 1. Mol Endocrinol 2003;17(9):1880–92.

126. Bertolino P, Tong WM, Herrera PL, et al. Pancreatic beta-cell-specific ablation of the multiple endocrine neoplasia type 1 (MEN1) gene causes full penetrance of insulinoma development in mice. Cancer Res 2003;63(16):4836–41.

127. Biondi CA, Gartside MG, Waring P, et al. Conditional inactivation of the MEN1 gene leads to pancreatic and pituitary tumorigenesis but does not affect normal development of these tissues. Mol Cell Biol 2004;24(8):3125–31.

128. Crabtree JS, Scacheri PC, Ward JM, et al. A mouse model of multiple endocrine neoplasia, type 1, develops multiple endocrine tumors. Proc Natl Acad Sci U S A 2001;98(3):1118–23.
129. Crabtree JS, Scacheri PC, Ward JM, et al. Of mice and MEN1: insulinomas in a conditional mouse knockout. Mol Cell Biol 2003;23(17):6075–85.
130. Gannon M, Shiota C, Postic C, et al. Analysis of the Cre-mediated recombination driven by rat insulin promoter in embryonic and adult mouse pancreas. Genesis 2000;26(2):139–42.
131. Harding B, Lemos MC, Reed AA, et al. Multiple endocrine neoplasia type 1 knockout mice develop parathyroid, pancreatic, pituitary and adrenal tumours with hypercalcaemia, hypophosphataemia and hypercorticosteronaemia. Endocr Relat Cancer 2009;16(4):1313–27.
132. Li F, Su Y, Cheng Y, et al. Conditional deletion of Men1 in the pancreatic beta-cell leads to glucagon-expressing tumor development. Endocrinology 2015;156(1):48–57.
133. Loffler KA, Biondi CA, Gartside M, et al. Broad tumor spectrum in a mouse model of multiple endocrine neoplasia type 1. Int J Cancer 2007;120(2):259–67.
134. Walls GV, Lemos MC, Javid M, et al. MEN1 gene replacement therapy reduces proliferation rates in a mouse model of pituitary adenomas. Cancer Res 2012;72(19):5060–8.
135. Smith TL, Yuan Z, Cardo-Vila M, et al. AAVP displaying octreotide for ligand-directed therapeutic transgene delivery in neuroendocrine tumors of the pancreas. Proc Natl Acad Sci U S A 2016;113(9):2466–71.
136. Kumar R, Li DQ, Muller S, et al. Epigenomic regulation of oncogenesis by chromatin remodeling. Oncogene 2016;35(34):4423–36.
137. Lines KE, Stevenson M, Filippakopoulos P, et al. Epigenetic pathway inhibitors represent potential drugs for treating pancreatic and bronchial neuroendocrine tumors. Oncogenesis 2017;6(5):e332.
138. Wong C, Laddha SV, Tang L, et al. The bromodomain and extra-terminal inhibitor CPI203 enhances the antiproliferative effects of rapamycin on human neuroendocrine tumors. Cell Death Dis 2014;5:e1450.
139. Jiang X, Cao Y, Li F, et al. Targeting beta-catenin signaling for therapeutic intervention in MEN1-deficient pancreatic neuroendocrine tumours. Nat Commun 2014;5:5809.
140. Xia SH, Forman LW, Faller DV. Protein kinase C delta is required for survival of cells expressing activated p21(RAS). J Biol Chem 2007;282(18):13199–210.
141. Xia SH, Chen ZH, Forman LW, et al. PKC delta survival signaling in cells containing an activated p21(Ras) protein requires PDK1. Cell Signal 2009;21(4):502–8.
142. Chen ZH, Forman LW, Miller KA, et al. Protein kinase C delta inactivation inhibits cellular proliferation and decreases survival in human neuroendocrine tumors. Endocr Relat Cancer 2011;18(6):759–71.
143. Berruti A, Fazio N, Ferrero A, et al. Bevacizumab plus octreotide and metronomic capecitabine in patients with metastatic well-to-moderately differentiated neuroendocrine tumors: the XELBEVOCT study. BMC Cancer 2014;14:184.
144. Chan JA, Stuart K, Earle CC, et al. Prospective study of bevacizumab plus temozolomide in patients with advanced neuroendocrine tumors. J Clin Oncol 2012;30(24):2963–8.
145. Ducreux M, Dahan L, Smith D, et al. Bevacizumab combined with 5-FU/streptozocin in patients with progressive metastatic well-differentiated pancreatic endocrine tumours (BETTER trial)–a phase II non-randomised trial. Eur J Cancer 2014;50(18):3098–106.

146. Mitry E, Walter T, Baudin E, et al. Bevacizumab plus capecitabine in patients with progressive advanced well-differentiated neuroendocrine tumors of the gastro-intestinal (GI-NETs) tract (BETTER trial)–a phase II non-randomised trial. Eur J Cancer 2014;50(18):3107–15.

147. Paez-Ribes M, Allen E, Hudock J, et al. Antiangiogenic therapy elicits malignant progression of tumors to increased local invasion and distant metastasis. Cancer Cell 2009;15(3):220–31.

148. Casanovas O, Hicklin DJ, Bergers G, et al. Drug resistance by evasion of anti-angiogenic targeting of VEGF signaling in late-stage pancreatic islet tumors. Cancer Cell 2005;8(4):299–309.

149. Bill R, Fagiani E, Zumsteg A, et al. Nintedanib is a highly effective therapeutic for neuroendocrine carcinoma of the pancreas (PNET) in the Rip1Tag2 transgenic mouse model. Clin Cancer Res 2015;21(21):4856–67.

150. Sennino B, Ishiguro-Oonuma T, Wei Y, et al. Suppression of tumor invasion and metastasis by concurrent inhibition of c-Met and VEGF signaling in pancreatic neuroendocrine tumors. Cancer Discov 2012;2(3):270–87.

151. Chu X, Gao X, Jansson L, et al. Multiple microvascular alterations in pancreatic islets and neuroendocrine tumors of a Men1 mouse model. Am J Pathol 2013; 182(6):2355–67.

152. Rinke A, Muller HH, Schade-Brittinger C, et al. Placebo-controlled, double-blind, prospective, randomized study on the effect of octreotide LAR in the control of tumor growth in patients with metastatic neuroendocrine midgut tumors: a report from the PROMID Study Group. J Clin Oncol 2009;27(28):4656–63.

153. Rinke A, Wittenberg M, Schade-Brittinger C, et al. Placebo-controlled, double-blind, prospective, randomized study on the effect of octreotide LAR in the control of tumor growth in patients with metastatic neuroendocrine midgut tumors (PROMID): results of long-term survival. Neuroendocrinology 2017;104(1): 26–32.

154. Walls GV, Stevenson M, Soukup BS, et al. Pasireotide therapy of multiple endocrine neoplasia type 1-associated neuroendocrine tumors in female mice deleted for an men1 allele improves survival and reduces tumor progression. Endocrinology 2016;157(5):1789–98.

155. Quinn TJ, Yuan Z, Adem A, et al. Pasireotide (SOM230) is effective for the treatment of pancreatic neuroendocrine tumors (PNETs) in a multiple endocrine neoplasia type 1 (MEN1) conditional knockout mouse model. Surgery 2012; 152(6):1068–77.

156. Cioppi F, Cianferotti L, Masi L, et al. The LARO-MEN1 study: a longitudinal clinical experience with octreotide Long-acting release in patients with multiple endocrine neoplasia type 1 syndrome. Clin Cases Miner Bone Metab 2017; 14(2):123–30.

When and How to Use Somatostatin Analogues

Wouter W. de Herder, MD, PhD

KEYWORDS

- Somatostatin • Receptor • Octreotide • Lanreotide • Pasireotide • Neuroendocrine

KEY POINTS

- Somatostatin analogues are the first-line treatment for control of hormonal excess by hormone-producing neuroendocrine tumors of the gastrointestinal tract and pancreas.
- Somatostatin analogues are the first-line treatment for tumor control of neuroendocrine tumors of the gastrointestinal tract and pancreas.
- To be effective, somatostatin analogues need somatostatin receptor expression on the gastroenteropancreatic neuroendocrine tumor cells.

The research group of the winner of the 1977 Nobel Prize in Physiology or Medicine, Roger Guillemin, discovered the peptide hormone somatostatin.[1] Somatostatin exerts an inhibitory role in the hormone secretion by the pituitary, pancreas, and gastrointestinal tract. It acts via interaction with specific somatostatin receptor (SSTR) subtypes expressed on target tissues. Five human SSTR subtypes have been recognized (named SSTR1–5), each being involved a distinct signaling pathway.[2] SSTR2 predominates in gastrointestinal and pancreatic neuroendocrine tumors (GEP-NETs).[3]

Octreotide was the first biologically stable somatostatin analogue (SSA) that became available.[4] This compound binds with high, low, and moderate affinity to SSTR2, SSTR3, and SSTR5, respectively.[5] A short-acting immediate-release formulation of octreotide (Sandostatin, Novartis, Basel, Switzerland) was initially developed. A long-acting repeatable depot formulation, Sandostatin LAR (Novartis), is currently indicated for long-term treatment of the severe diarrhea and flushing episodes associated with the carcinoid syndrome and long-term treatment of the profuse watery diarrhea associated with VIPomas, as well as for the improvement of progression-free survival (PFS) in patients with unresectable, well-differentiated or moderately differentiated, locally advanced or metastatic NETs from a midgut origin.[6]

Disclosure Statement: The author has served on advisory boards for Novartis, Ipsen, and Advanced Accelerator Applications. The author has received research support from Novartis and Ipsen.
Department of Internal Medicine, Sector of Endocrinology, ENETS Center of Excellence for Neuroendocrine Tumors, Erasmus MC, Dr. Molewaterplein 40, Rotterdam 3015 GD, The Netherlands
E-mail address: w.w.deherder@erasmusmc.nl

Endocrinol Metab Clin N Am 47 (2018) 549–555
https://doi.org/10.1016/j.ecl.2018.04.010
0889-8529/18/© 2018 Elsevier Inc. All rights reserved.

Lanreotide is another SSA that has demonstrated a similar binding profile to the SSTRs to that of octreotide.[5,6] Two different formulations, Lanreotide SR (Ipsen, Boulogne-Billancourt, France) and a long-acting depot formulation, Somatuline Autogel (Ipsen Biopharmaceuticals) are currently available. Somatuline Autogel is, like octreotide, currently indicated for the treatment of the carcinoid syndrome and for the improvement of PFS in patients with unresectable, well-differentiated or moderately differentiated, locally advanced or metastatic GEP-NETs (**Fig. 1**).[6]

INDICATION 1: HORMONAL HYPERSECRETION

SSAs are currently the first-line therapy to control hormone excess and their related syndromes in patients with GEP-NETs. Pooled data from studies using different octreotide and lanreotide formulations in gastrointestinal NET (carcinoid) patients indicate that up to 67% to 74% of patients experience symptomatic relief with SSA treatment.[7–11] Proven efficacy of SSAs for symptom control was also demonstrated in pancreatic NETS, like insulinomas, glucagonomas, VIPomas, and ectopic adrenocorticotrophic hormone, growth hormone receptor hormone, and parathyroid hormone-related peptide-secreting tumors.[12–16] In insulinomas, it is important to closely monitor the blood glucose levels after a therapeutic challenge with a short-acting SSA (octreotide), because, in the potential absence of the expression of specific SSTRs on these tumors, a paradoxic decrease in blood glucose levels can be observed.[17] The latter is

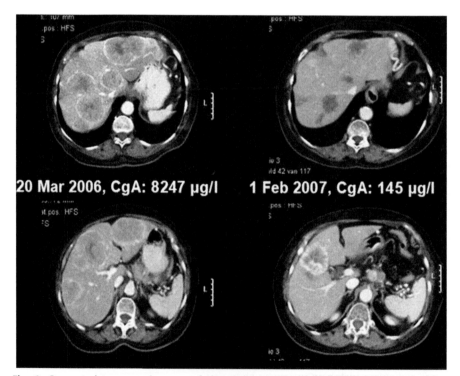

20 Mar 2006, CgA: 8247 µg/l   **1 Feb 2007, CgA: 145 µg/l**

Fig. 1. Computed tomography scan of the abdomen showing extensive liver metastases from a neuroendocrine tumor. Impressive tumor response after the administration of a long-acting somatostatin analogue paralleled by a decrease in circulating chromogranin A (CgA) levels.

caused by the suppression of the counterregulatory hormones by SSAs.[17,18] Current recommendations indicate the use of Sandostatin LAR at a dose of 20 to 30 mg per 4 weeks intramuscularly, or Somatuline Autogel at a dose of 90 to 120 mg per 4 weeks subcutaneously. However, most NET experts tend to increase these dosages, or reduce dose intervals, as required to obtain better symptom control.

INDICATION 2: ANTITUMOR EFFECT

PROMID (Study to Investigate the Antiproliferative Effect of Octreotide in Patients With Metastasized Neuroendocrine Tumors of the Midgut) was the first randomized trial to confirm the antitumor effect of Octreotide LAR in patients with well-differentiated metastatic GEP-NET of the midgut.[19] The median time to tumor progression (14.3 months) was significantly extended with Octreotide LAR 30 mg intramuscularly per 4 weeks as compared with placebo (6 months). Stable disease was achieved in 67% and 37% of patients treated with Octreotide LAR and placebo, respectively. The antitumor response was more pronounced in patients with a limited ($\leq$10%) hepatic tumor burden.[19] It is currently unclear as to whether Octreotide LAR therapy improves overall survival in patients with GEP-NET of midgut origin. CLARINET was the second large randomized trial designed to study the antitumor effect of SSAs.[20] Patients with well-differentiated or moderately differentiated nonfunctioning GEP-NETs received either placebo or Somatuline Autogel 120 mg subcutaneously per 4 weeks. The median PFS was not reached with Somatuline Autogel, whereas this was 18 months with placebo. After 2 years of treatment, estimated rates of PFS were 65.1% and 33.0% in the Somatuline Autogel and placebo groups, respectively.[20] The molecular basis of the antiproliferative effect of SSAs in GEP-NETs is largely unknown.[21]

QUESTION 1: WHEN TO INCREASE THE SOMATOSTATIN ANALOGUE DOSE, OR SHORTEN THE DOSE INTERVAL?

The beneficial effects of long-acting SSAs in patients with metastatic, well-differentiated GEP NETs are well-described. However, a substantial number of these patients, who did show an initial response to SSA therapy, will experience escape from treatment within months. This can either be a loss of symptomatic control, monitored as an increase in bowel movements, loose stools, increased flushing periods or frequency, or tumor growth, or an increasing number of metastases as documented by radiology. The potential mechanisms involved in these losses of responsiveness are yet largely unknown. These may include downregulation of SSTRs, or the outgrowth of clones lacking specific SSTR expression.[22] But, in many patients increasing the dose of the SSA, or shortening of the dose interval might again prove beneficial both for symptomatic progression, or tumor progression.[23–25] The maximum SSA doses that can be used or the minimum dose intervals are currently undefined. It generally concerns more a practical issue with regard to the administration of these drugs, which needs the care of a trained medical professional. Guidelines are currently lacking and most recommendations are, therefore, expert or experience based. It is yet unclear when to consider switching to other (second-line) therapeutic modalities, like everolimus, the only registered drug for the tumor control of GEP-NETs (although also symptomatic/hormonal improvement has been reported with the use of this drug), sunitinib (for tumor control of pancreatic NETs), or peptide receptor radiotherapy.[26–31] After switching to these therapies, it is also unclear whether the SSAs should be continued or discontinued. The general feeling is that, in the case of hormonal hypersecretion, it might be indicated to continue the SSAs, but at what dose? It is also important to realize that diarrhea in patients with metastatic gastrointestinal NETs (mostly derived from the primitive midgut) and the carcinoid syndrome is not necessarily a result of this syndrome. Other causes of diarrhea include bile salt–induced diarrhea (which can be controlled by cholestyramine), bacterial overgrowth (which might respond to antibiotics), short-bowel syndrome (after surgery), or pancreatic insufficiency (which might be caused by the SSA treatment itself); these causes should be considered and, if possible, excluded or treated. Generally, dose escalation of SSAs is well-tolerated in patients with GEP NET and might lead again to disease control. However, prospective studies are needed. Not all GEP NETs express specific SSTRs. This finding implies that these tumors will not respond to SSAs. This phenomenon is called primary failure to SSAs in contrast with the above-mentioned secondary failure. SSTR expression on GEP NETs can be demonstrated using PET with computed tomography with ^{68}Ga-DOTA–coupled SSAs, or using the less sensitive OctreoScan, using ^{111}In-pentetreotide, for single photon emission computed tomography imaging.[32,33] Negative SSTR imaging usually indicates that SSA therapy will fail. In some patients, the presence of both SSTR-positive and -negative lesions can be demonstrated. Currently, there are no recommendations whether or not to initiate SSA treatment in these particular patients.

QUESTION 2: WHEN IS THERE AN INDICATION FOR ESCAPE DOSES OF SOMATOSTATIN ANALOGUES?

Patients with the carcinoid syndrome are at risk for developing a carcinoid crisis during either minor or major surgery, or other types of interventions, such as diagnostic procedures, like endoscopy, embolization, radiofrequency ablation, or peptide receptor radiotherapy.[34] A rapid reversal of a carcinoid crisis after intravenous administration of octreotide has been reported. The therapeutic goal with octreotide prophylaxis is to prevent mediator release during the intervention.[34,35] For patients already treated with long-acting SSAs, these medications should be continued. However, because intraoperative carcinoid calamities are not predictable, there is no standard regimen for octreotide administration and various schemes have been proposed. Recent guidelines give recommendations on the use of intravenous octreotide schedules, although none of these schedules is evidence based.[34] Perioperative prophylactic treatment with intravenous octreotide at a starting dose of 50 to 100 μg/h (mean dose 100–200 μg/h) is generally recommended.[34]

QUESTION 3: CAN WE USE THE NEW GENERATION OF SOMATOSTATIN ANALOGUES IN PATIENTS WITH GASTROINTESTINAL TRACT AND PANCREAS NEUROENDOCRINE TUMORS?

Pasireotide is currently the only a next-generation SSA that is available for clinical use. It is a multi-SSTR targeting SSA with high affinity for SSTR-1, -2, -3, and -5.[36] Two formulations of pasireotide have been developed: a short-acting immediate release formulation for subcutaneous administration and a long-acting sustained-release formulation (Pasireotide LAR, Novartis). Based on its receptor affinity one might expect a good clinical response in patients with GEP NET after administration of this next-generation SSA. Furthermore, pasireotide LAR has a similar safety profile to that of first-generation SSAs, except for a higher frequency and degree of hyperglycemia.[37,38] Indeed, in a phase II study in patients with advanced gastrointestinal NETs with symptoms refractory or resistant to Octreotide LAR, treatment with short-acting immediate release pasireotide resulted in relief of symptoms (diarrhea and flushing) in 27% of these patients.[39] However, in a phase III study of Pasireotide LAR versus high-dose (40 mg) Octreotide LAR for symptom control in patients with advanced

GEP-NETs whose disease-related symptoms were uncontrolled by first-generation SSAs at maximum approved doses, Pasireotide LAR was not superior to Octreotide LAR.[40] In the phase II prospective LUNA study (Efficacy and safety of long-acting pasireotide or everolimus alone or in combination in patients with advanced carcinoids of the lung and thymus) in advanced (unresectable or metastatic), progressive, well-differentiated carcinoid tumors of the lung or thymus, Pasireotide LAR treatment resulted in an objective tumor response in 39% of patients.[37] Further investigations into the role of Pasireotide LAR in the treatment of GEP-NETs are, therefore, needed.[41] In view of the hyperglycemic potency of pasireotide, combination with everolimus (which also can cause hyperglycemia) will warrant regular blood glucose monitoring.[37,38]

REFERENCES

1. Guillemin R. Peptides in the brain. The new endocrinology of the neuron. Nobel Lecture. 1977. Available at: http://www.nobelprize.org/nobel_prizes/medicine/laureates/1977/guillemin-lecture.pdf.
2. Patel YC. Somatostatin and its receptor family. Front Neuroendocrinol 1999;20(3): 157–98.
3. de Herder WW, Hofland LJ, van der Lely AJ, et al. Somatostatin receptors in gastroentero-pancreatic neuroendocrine tumours. Endocr Relat Cancer 2003; 10(4):451–8.
4. Bauer W, Briner U, Doepfner W, et al. SMS 201–995: a very potent and selective octapeptide analogue of somatostatin with prolonged action. Life Sci 1982; 31(11):1133–40.
5. Hofland LJ, Lamberts SW. The pathophysiological consequences of somatostatin receptor internalization and resistance. Endocr Rev 2003;24(1):28–47.
6. Oberg K, Lamberts SW. Somatostatin analogues in acromegaly and gastroenteropancreatic neuroendocrine tumours: past, present and future. Endocr Relat Cancer 2016;23(12):R551–66.
7. Modlin IM, Pavel M, Kidd M, et al. Review article: somatostatin analogues in the treatment of gastroenteropancreatic neuroendocrine (carcinoid) tumours. Aliment Pharmacol Ther 2010;31(2):169–88.
8. Oberg K, Kvols L, Caplin M, et al. Consensus report on the use of somatostatin analogs for the management of neuroendocrine tumors of the gastroenteropancreatic system. Ann Oncol 2004;15(6):966–73.
9. Ito T, Lee L, Jensen RT. Carcinoid-syndrome: recent advances, current status and controversies. Curr Opin Endocrinol Diabetes Obes 2018;25(1):22–35.
10. Massironi S, Conte D, Rossi RE. Somatostatin analogues in functioning gastroenteropancreatic neuroendocrine tumours: literature review, clinical recommendations and schedules. Scand J Gastroenterol 2016;51(5):513–23.
11. Riechelmann RP, Pereira AA, Rego JF, et al. Refractory carcinoid syndrome: a review of treatment options. Ther Adv Med Oncol 2017;9(2):127–37.
12. Lamberts SW, de Herder WW, Krenning EP, et al. A role of (labeled) somatostatin analogs in the differential diagnosis and treatment of Cushing's syndrome. J Clin Endocrinol Metab 1994;78(1):17–9.
13. de Herder WW, Lamberts SW. Is there a role for somatostatin and its analogs in Cushing's syndrome? Metabolism 1996;45(8 Suppl 1):83–5.
14. de Herder WW, Lamberts SW. Octapeptide somatostatin-analogue therapy of Cushing's syndrome. Postgrad Med J 1999;75(880):65–6.

15. van Schaik E, van Vliet EI, Feelders RA, et al. Improved control of severe hypoglycemia in patients with malignant insulinomas by peptide receptor radionuclide therapy. J Clin Endocrinol Metab 2011;96(11):3381–9.

16. Kamp K, Feelders RA, van Adrichem RC, et al. Parathyroid hormone-related peptide (PTHrP) secretion by gastroenteropancreatic neuroendocrine tumors (GEP-NETs): clinical features, diagnosis, management, and follow-up. J Clin Endocrinol Metab 2014;99(9):3060–9.

17. Vezzosi D, Bennet A, Courbon F, et al. Short- and long-term somatostatin analogue treatment in patients with hypoglycaemia related to endogenous hyperinsulinism. Clin Endocrinol (Oxf) 2008;68(6):904–11.

18. de Herder WW, Krenning EP, van Eijck CH, et al. Considerations concerning a tailored, individualized therapeutic management of patients with (neuro)endocrine tumours of the gastrointestinal tract and pancreas. Endocr Relat Cancer 2004;11(1):19–34.

19. Rinke A, Muller HH, Schade-Brittinger C, et al. Placebo-controlled, double-blind, prospective, randomized study on the effect of octreotide LAR in the control of tumor growth in patients with metastatic neuroendocrine midgut tumors: a report from the PROMID Study Group. J Clin Oncol 2009;27(28):4656–63.

20. Caplin ME, Pavel M, Cwikla JB, et al. Lanreotide in metastatic enteropancreatic neuroendocrine tumors. N Engl J Med 2014;371(3):224–33.

21. Merola E, Panzuto F, Delle FG. Antiproliferative effect of somatostatin analogs in advanced gastro-entero-pancreatic neuroendocrine tumors: a systematic review and meta-analysis. Oncotarget 2017;8(28):46624–34.

22. Feelders RA, Lamberts SW, Hofland LJ, et al. Luteinizing hormone (LH)-responsive Cushing's syndrome: the demonstration of LH receptor messenger ribonucleic acid in hyperplastic adrenal cells, which respond to chorionic gonadotropin and serotonin agonists in vitro. J Clin Endocrinol Metab 2003; 88(1):230–7.

23. Strosberg JR, Benson AB, Huynh L, et al. Clinical benefits of above-standard dose of octreotide LAR in patients with neuroendocrine tumors for control of carcinoid syndrome symptoms: a multicenter retrospective chart review study. Oncologist 2014;19(9):930–6.

24. Chan DL, Ferone D, Albertelli M, et al. Escalated-dose somatostatin analogues for antiproliferative effect in GEPNETS: a systematic review. Endocrine 2017; 57(3):366–75.

25. Strosberg J, El Haddad G, Wolin E, et al. Phase 3 Trial of (177)Lu-Dotatate for midgut neuroendocrine tumors. N Engl J Med 2017;376(2):125–35.

26. Hicks RJ, Kwekkeboom DJ, Krenning E, et al. ENETS consensus guidelines for the standards of care in neuroendocrine neoplasia: peptide receptor radionuclide therapy with radiolabeled somatostatin analogues. Neuroendocrinology 2017;105(3):295–309.

27. Brabander T, Teunissen JJ, van Eijck CH, et al. Peptide receptor radionuclide therapy of neuroendocrine tumours. Best Pract Res Clin Endocrinol Metab 2016;30(1):103–14.

28. Brabander T, van der Zwan WA, Teunissen JJM, et al. Long-term efficacy, survival, and safety of [(177)Lu-DOTA(0),Tyr(3)]octreotate in patients with gastroenteropancreatic and bronchial neuroendocrine tumors. Clin Cancer Res 2017; 23(16):4617–24.

29. Raymond E, Dahan L, Raoul JL, et al. Sunitinib malate for the treatment of pancreatic neuroendocrine tumors. N Engl J Med 2011;364(6):501–13.

30. Yao JC, Shah MH, Ito T, et al. Everolimus for advanced pancreatic neuroendocrine tumors. N Engl J Med 2011;364(6):514–23.
31. Yao JC, Fazio N, Singh S, et al. Everolimus for the treatment of advanced, non-functional neuroendocrine tumours of the lung or gastrointestinal tract (RADIANT-4): a randomised, placebo-controlled, phase 3 study. Lancet 2016; 387(10022):968–77.
32. Hope TA, Bergsland EK, Bozkurt MF, et al. Appropriate use criteria for somatostatin receptor PET imaging in neuroendocrine tumors. J Nucl Med 2018;59(1): 66–74.
33. van Adrichem RC, Kamp K, van Deurzen CH, et al. Is there an additional value of using somatostatin receptor subtype 2a immunohistochemistry compared to somatostatin receptor scintigraphy uptake in predicting gastroenteropancreatic neuroendocrine tumor response? Neuroendocrinology 2016;103(5):560–6.
34. Kaltsas G, Caplin M, Davies P, et al. ENETS consensus guidelines for the standards of care in neuroendocrine tumors: pre- and perioperative therapy in patients with neuroendocrine tumors. Neuroendocrinology 2017;105(3):245–54.
35. Kvols LK, Martin JK, Marsh HM, et al. Rapid reversal of carcinoid crisis with a somatostatin analogue [letter]. N Engl J Med 1985;313(19):1229–30.
36. Schmid HA. Pasireotide (SOM230): development, mechanism of action and potential applications. Mol Cell Endocrinol 2008;286(1–2):69–74.
37. Ferolla P, Brizzi MP, Meyer T, et al. Efficacy and safety of long-acting pasireotide or everolimus alone or in combination in patients with advanced carcinoids of the lung and thymus (LUNA): an open-label, multicentre, randomised, phase 2 trial. Lancet Oncol 2017;18(12):1652–64.
38. Kulke MH, Ruszniewski P, Van Cutsem E, et al. A randomized, open-label, phase 2 study of everolimus in combination with pasireotide LAR or everolimus alone in advanced, well-differentiated, progressive pancreatic neuroendocrine tumors: COOPERATE-2 trial. Ann Oncol 2017;28(6):1309–15.
39. Kvols LK, Oberg KE, O'Dorisio TM, et al. Pasireotide (SOM230) shows efficacy and tolerability in the treatment of patients with advanced neuroendocrine tumors refractory or resistant to octreotide LAR: results from a phase II study. Endocr Relat Cancer 2012;19(5):657–66.
40. Wolin EM, Jarzab B, Eriksson B, et al. Phase III study of pasireotide long-acting release in patients with metastatic neuroendocrine tumors and carcinoid symptoms refractory to available somatostatin analogues. Drug Des Dev Ther 2015; 9:5075–86.
41. Yao JC, Chan JA, Mita AC, et al. Phase I dose-escalation study of long-acting pasireotide in patients with neuroendocrine tumors. Onco Targets Ther 2017;10: 3177–86.

New Treatments for the Carcinoid Syndrome

Paul Benjamin Loughrey, MD[a,b], Dongyun Zhang, PhD[c],
Anthony P. Heaney, MD, PhD[c,d],*

KEYWORDS

- Everolimus • Medical treatment • Surgery • Peptide receptor radionuclide therapy
- Somatostatin receptor ligands • Sunitinib • Telotristat etiprate • Theranostics

KEY POINTS

- There is consensus that an individualized patient pathway agreed to by a multidisciplinary team is the optimal planning approach to treatment.
- Use of somatostatin receptor ligands as first-line therapy has been the paradigm for some time but this may now be challenged with newer trial data on mammalian target of rapamycin inhibitor and after peptide receptor radionuclide therapy (PRRT).
- It is anticipated that as PRRT becomes more widely available it may become second-line or first-line therapy.

BACKGROUND

The first multiple distal ileal neuroendocrine tumors (NETs) were found at autopsy in 1888 by Lubarsch and the name karzinoide or carcinoma-like tumor was later coined by Oberndorfer in 1907.[1–3] Carcinoid tumors are derived from enterochromaffin or Kulchitsky cells.[4,5] A variety of biochemical syndromes are associated with carcinoid tumors with foregut tumors (lungs, thymus, duodenum, and pancreas), which cause angioedema, a hive-like pink flushing or rash due to histamine, 5-hydroxytryptophan (5-HTP), and other vasoactive substances, and with serotonin-secreting midgut tumors (small intestine, appendix, and proximal colon),[6,7] which is the cause the classic carcinoid syndrome (CS) with nondiaphoretic flushing, diarrhea, and occasional wheezing due to right-sided cardiac failure following cardiac valve stenosis or

Disclosure: The authors have nothing to disclose.
[a] Department of Ophthalmology, Royal Victoria Hospital, Belfast Trust, Grosvenor Road, Belfast, BT12 6BA, UK; [b] Department of Endocrinology and Diabetes, Royal Victoria Hospital, Belfast Trust, Grosvenor Road, Belfast, BT12 6BA, UK; [c] Department of Medicine, David Geffen School of Medicine, University of California, 700 Tiverton Avenue, Los Angeles, CA 90095, USA; [d] Department of Neurosurgery, David Geffen School of Medicine, University of California, 700 Tiverton Avenue, Los Angeles, CA 90095, USA
* Corresponding author. 650 Charles E Young Drive South, Factor Building 9-240, Los Angeles, CA 90095.
E-mail address: aheaney@mednet.ucla.edu

thickening[5] (**Fig. 1**). Hindgut tumors (transverse colon, sigmoid colon, and rectum) infrequently secrete hormones and typically are either incidentally discovered on lower gastrointestinal (GI) endoscopy or present with obstructive symptoms.

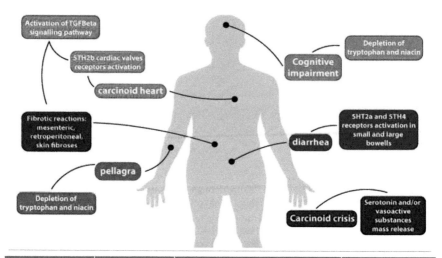

Symptoms	Frequency	Mediators	Treatment
Profound Flushing	85%–90%	Kallikrein, histamine, 5-hydroxytryptamine, prostaglandins, substance P	Somatostatin receptor ligands, Octreotide; H1 and H2 blockers, Prednisolone
Diarrhea	70%	Gastrin, histamine, 5-hydroxytryptamine, prostaglandins, vasoactive intestinal peptide	Loperamide, Diphenoxylate, Methysergide,
Abdominal Pain	35%	Small bowel obstruction due to tumor or tumor products, mesenteric ischemia, hepatomegaly	Oxycodone
Bronchospasm	15%	Histamine, 5-hydroxytryptamine,	Aminophylline
Pellagra	5%	Niacin deficiency	
Hypotension	30%	5-hydroxytryptamine, substance P	Methoxamine, Norepinephrine
Teleangiectasis	25%	N/A	

Fig. 1. Main features of midgut CS and carcinoid crisis, with treatment options. CS is usually caused by primary well-differentiated midgut NET with hepatic metastatic lesions that release vasoactive compounds. Carcinoid crisis is characterized by profound flushing, bronchospasm, tachycardia, and hypotension, and is usually precipitated by tumor cytoreductive surgery, embolization, or radio ablation. Serotonin antagonists and somatostatin receptor ligands are the major treatment options. TGF, transforming growth factor; 5HT2a, serotonin receptor 2a; 5TH2b, serotonin receptor 2b; 5TH4, serotonin receptor 4. (*Adapted from* Mota JM, Sousa LG, Riechelmann RP. Complications from carcinoid syndrome: review of the current evidence. Ecancermedicalscience 2016;10:662; with permission.)

In addition to serotonin, other tumor factors, including histamine, bradykinins, tachykinins, prostaglandins, kallikrein, substance P, dopamine, and adrenocorticotrophic hormone, act synergistically to cause the clinical features of CS.[6,8–10] CS can be exacerbated by emotion, exercise, defecation, liver palpation, alcohol consumption, and ingestion of serotonin or tyramine-containing foods, especially chocolate, avocado, nuts, banana, cheese, red wine, and caffeine.[11]

The carcinoid crisis (CC), an acute life-threatening complication of CS, is characterized by severe flushing of the face and upper trunk, hemodynamic instability, cardiac arrhythmia, bronchospasm, and disorders of thermoregulation.[6,12] Encountered most commonly with foregut and midgut carcinoid tumors[10] (see **Fig. 1**), it can occur spontaneously but is sometimes precipitated by anesthesia, tumor manipulation, or following tumor cytoreductive procedures due to tumor lysis.[11,13,14] It can be prevented by administration of intravenous (IV) octreotide (50–160 q/h) and managed with supportive measures and additional octreotide. Because other vasoactive agents may be implicated in the cause of CC,[15] administration of glucocorticoids along with serotonin receptor 1 (HTR1) and serotonin receptor 2 (HTR2) antagonists can also be helpful.[6,13]

TREATMENTS
Established Therapies

Surgery
In the setting of an isolated primary tumor, surgical resection offers the possibility of cure but even in the setting of high tumor burden, surgical cytoreduction plays an important role in alleviation of carcinoid symptoms[16] and can significantly improve survival.[17]

However, surgery in midgut carcinoid tumors may present several challenges. First, the primary tumor may be small and difficult to locate and is often encased in fibrotic tissue, causing bowel stricture, lymphatic obstruction, and mesenteric ischemia.[9] Second, in cases in which right-sided carcinoid heart disease has affected tricuspid and pulmonary valve function, elevated central venous pressure increases bleeding from the hepatic veins, complicating resection of hepatic metastases.[16]

Locoregional therapies
Because NET liver metastases receive 80% to 90% of their blood supply from the hepatic artery, whereas normal liver tissue is supplied by the portal vein,[18–20] therapies such as bland embolization, chemoembolization, selective internal radiotherapy, and/or radiofrequency ablation can be very effective to not only debulk hepatic disease but also to rapidly (within 24 hours) improve CS symptoms[8,19–27] and improve survival.[21,28,29] Liver-directed radiation is also a safe procedure[29–31] and has been shown to improve symptoms, decrease tumor markers,[24] and offer excellent response rates[23,30] in neuroendocrine liver metastases.[23,30] Female gender, well-differentiated NETs, and a low number of metastases limited to the liver portend a better response to ^{90}yttrium (^{90}Y) therapy.[32,33]

Liver-directed therapies are generally well-tolerated with low mortality rates,[23,29,30] although some patients experience a postembolization syndrome with fever and fatigue being the most common (80%–90%).[19] Other complications include bile duct injury with radiofrequency ablation. Lung shunting of beads,[21,30] liver fibrosis, and radiation gastritis can be seen in selective internal radiotherapy.[21] Sepsis can complicate all liver-directed procedures but particularly bland embolization and chemoembolization. Bowel or liver ischemia with liver abscess and hepatorenal failure can be serious complications.[19] Despite these risks, liver-directed therapies can be very effective treatments for CS control.[20]

Medical

For many years before the availability of somatostatin receptor ligands (SRLs), simple medical therapies, such as the antidiarrheal agents loperamide,[6] diphenoxylate, atropine, and opium tincture,[9] histamine 1 and 2 receptor blockers were the mainstay of symptom control.[34,35]

First-generation somatostatin receptor ligands Due to its short half-life, naturally occurring somatostatin has no clinical utility as a therapeutic agent. The first-generation subcutaneously administered SRL octreotide (150 μg 3 times a day) was demonstrated in 1986 to improve CS symptoms[12,36–39] in 88% of treated subjects.[38] Monthly administered octreotide long-acting release (LAR) and lanreotide Autogel have equivalent affinity for somatostatin receptors (SSTRs) subtypes 2, 3, and 5,[6,12] and exhibit multiple antitumor effects via inhibition of angiogenesis,[40–42] interaction with the immune system,[12,42,43] inhibition of growth factors,[44] and blockade of tumor cell proliferation.[42] Well-tolerated, even at high doses, their most common side effects are nausea, abdominal discomfort, loose stools, and gallbladder dysfunction with gallstones or biliary sludge.[45]

One drawback to treatment with SRLs is that, over time, patients can become less responsive to the drug (so-called tachyphylaxis). The mechanism of this phenomenon is not fully understood but internalization or downregulation of SSTR2,[6,46] upregulation of other SSTRs not targeted by octreotide and lanreotide,[12,47,48] variable SSTR phosphorylation, heterodimerization of the SSTRs with other receptors, and the effects of β-arrestins on SSTR signaling, have all been proposed.[49] However, despite tachyphylaxis, SRLs remain a mainstay of medical treatment for CS[6,37,50] and have significantly improved survival in NETs.[51]

Mammalian target of rapamycin inhibition The mammalian target of rapamycin (mTOR) signaling pathway integrates extracellular and intracellular signals to regulate cell proliferation, metabolism, and survival (**Fig. 2**). Everolimus (formerly RAD001, Novartis), a once-daily oral mTOR inhibitor, is now approved to treat NETs.[52] The RAD001 in Advanced Neuroendocrine Tumors (RADIANT) trials assessed everolimus in many hundreds of subjects with NETs. RADIANT-1 focused on metastatic pancreatic NETS (PNETs) which had progressed during or after cytotoxic chemotherapy.[53] Subjects were stratified according to prior octreotide therapy or ongoing octreotide therapy. In those with prior therapy, (n = 115) treatment with everolimus at a median dosage of 9.9 mg per day resulted in partial response in 9.6%, stable disease in 67.8%, and progression in 9.6%, as assessed by Response Evaluation Criteria in Solid Tumors (RECIST).[53] In combination with octreotide, everolimus induced a partial response in 4.4%, stable disease in 80%, and no disease progression was seen in any subject.[53]

RADIANT-2 was a larger study comparing everolimus plus 30 mg octreotide LAR every 28 days with placebo plus 30 mg octreotide LAR every 28 days in 429 subjects with advanced NETs with associated CS.[54] Median progression-free survival (PFS) was 16.4 months (95% CI 13.7–21.2) in the everolimus plus octreotide LAR group and 11.3 months (95% CI 8.4–14.6) in the placebo plus octreotide LAR group with a hazard ratio (HR) of 0.77 (95% CI 0.59–1.00; 1-sided log-rank test, $P = .026$).[54]

RADIANT-3 compared everolimus (n = 207) to placebo (n = 203) in progressive, advanced PNETs and showed significant improvements in median PFS (11 months vs 4.6 months, $P<.001$).[55] Most recently, RADIANT-4 evaluated everolimus in progressive and advanced nonfunctioning lung and GI NETs in 302 subjects. Treatment with everolimus 10 mg (or 5 mg on alternate days) resulted in an improved median PFS of 11 months versus 3.9 months in placebo and a 52% reduction in estimated risk of progression or death (P<.00001).[56]

Side effects of mTOR inhibition include pneumonitis, thrombocytopenia, stomatitis, rash, diarrhea, renal failure, peripheral edema, and hyperglycemia.[57] Use of everolimus after peptide radionuclide therapy (PRRT) seems to be associated with an increased risk of toxicity.[57]

Sunitinib NETs, including midgut carcinoids, are particularly vascular and express high levels of vascular endothelial growth factor (VEGF),[58] making angiogenesis pathways potential treatment targets (see **Fig. 2**). Sunitinib is an orally administered multireceptor tyrosine kinase inhibitor that targets VEGF receptor, platelet-derived growth factor receptor, stem cell factor receptor, glial cell-line-derived neurotrophic factor receptor rearranged during transfection, colony-stimulating factor receptor type 1, and FMS-like tyrosine kinase 3 receptor.[12,59]

Sunitinib therapy (37.5 mg daily) led to significantly improved PFS, overall survival, and objective response rates[59] in 171 subjects with progressive PNETs compared with placebo. Evidence is less convincing for carcinoid tumors with sunitinib therapy at a median dosage of 50 mg daily in 6 week cycles, demonstrating an objective response rate of only 2.4% (1 of 41 subjects) in carcinoid tumors, and the study was unable to definitively determine sunitinib activity.[60] Side effects include diarrhea, nausea, vomiting, fatigue, and hypertension in some patients but the drug is generally well-tolerated.[12]

Cytotoxic chemotherapy Cytotoxic chemotherapy has shown some promise in PNETs but response rates are generally low for GI NETs.[61,62] Streptozotocin, cyclophosphamide, fluorouracil, doxorubicin, cisplatin, and etoposide have been trialed in GI NETs.[63–66] Although cytotoxic chemotherapy is of limited value in CS, it may be an option for more poorly differentiated aggressive disease.[67] A trial in progress is evaluating the efficacy and toxicity of [177]lutetium (^{177}Lu) PRRT in combination with metronomic capecitabine chemotherapy in subjects with aggressive [18]fluorodeoxyglucose-positive gastroentero-PNETs.[68]

Interferon alpha Interferon alpha has been demonstrated to have effects on cell proliferation, differentiation, apoptosis, and angiogenesis.[6] It may also induce intratumoral fibrosis in metastatic disease and particularly in hepatic lesions.[6] Symptom relief was reported in 7 of 10 subjects with CS treated with interferon,[69] and combination with interferon (5 million units 3 times weekly) and lanreotide (1 mg 3 times a day) resulted in significant (P = .037) symptomatic improvement in functional NETs.[70] Interferon may synergize with SRLs[71]; however, other data have demonstrated that the combination of interferon alpha and octreotide is not superior to octreotide treatment alone.[70,72]

Interferon alpha side effects include pyrexia, fatigue, depression, anorexia, weight loss, flu-like symptoms, myelosuppression, and autoimmune disease, including systemic lupus erythematosus, thyroid dysfunction, and polymyalgia.[6,9,73]

New Therapies

Next-generation somatostatin receptor ligands
Unlike the first-generation SRLs sandostatin and lanreotide, which primarily target the SSTR2, pasireotide has higher affinity to SSTRs 1, 3, and 5 (40 times)[9,37,46,74] but 2.5 times lower affinity for SSTR2.[9,37,75] Approved for the treatment of acromegaly and Cushing disease,[76,77] it has demonstrated lower rates of tachyphylaxis for growth

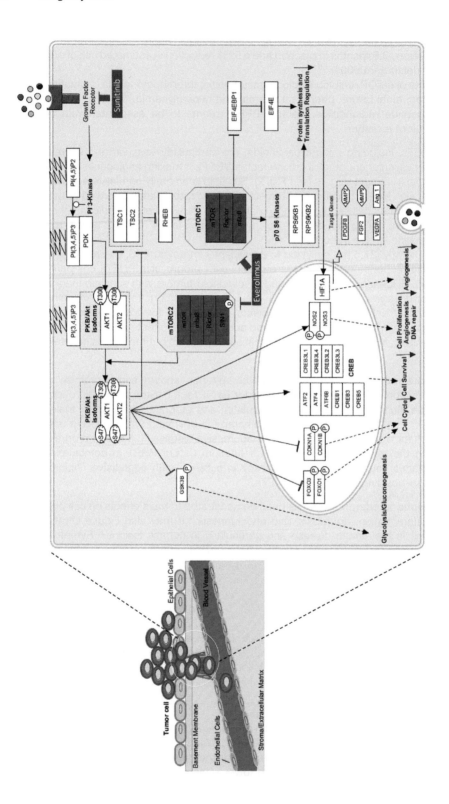

hormone and insulin-like growth factor 1 inhibition in animal studies. This benefit may extend to human subjects with carcinoid tumors.[46,78,79]

An open-label, single-arm, phase II prospective trial in 29 NET subjects, 5 of whom had CS, examined treatment with 60 mg of intramuscular pasireotide every 4 weeks.[80] The primary end point of the study was PFS assessed with computerized tomography (CT) and MRI using RECIST.[80] The median PFS was 11 months and subjects with low hepatic disease burden, normal chromogranin A (CgA), and high SSTR5 seemed to receive most benefit; 4 of the 5 subjects with CS-derived symptomatic improvement.[80] The most common side effect of the drug was hyperglycemia (65%), which required management with oral hypoglycemic agents or insulin in 13 of 22 subjects.[80] Only 1 subject had a medical history of diabetes at commencement of the study.[80]

In a phase II open-label multicenter trial in subjects with CS whose symptoms were inadequately controlled by octreotide-LAR, pasireotide was trialed with dosage escalation from 150 mg twice a day to maximum 1200 mg twice a day until a clinical improvement was observed.[74] In this study, pasireotide at a dosage of 600 to 900 mg twice a day achieved complete or partial symptom control of diarrhea and flushing in 27% of these subjects who were inadequately controlled by first-generation SRL therapy.[74] Tumor response as assessed by RECIST found 43% had stable disease, whereas 57% exhibited disease progression.[74]

However, a subsequent randomized double-blind phase III study compared pasireotide LAR 60 mg every 28 days with octreotide LAR 40 mg every 28 days in subjects with carcinoid symptoms refractory to first-generation SRLs. The study was concluded early due to low probability of the study meeting its primary endpoint.[50] No significant difference in symptom control or PFS was reported at study close.[50] Again, the major side effect of pasireotide was hyperglycemia; 9.4% for pasireotide-treated and 1.6% in octreotide-treated subjects, respectively.[50] The lack of clear superiority of pasireotide versus octreotide for symptom control in combination with its frequent induction and/or worsening of hyperglycemia has tempered its use in CS in most patients.[81]

◀————————————————————————————————

Fig. 2. The mechanisms for the antiproliferation and antiangiogenesis effects of sunitinib and everolimus. Vascular endothelial growth factor (VEGF) and platelet-derived growth factor (PDGF) are the potent growth factors involved in tumor invasion and metastasis that drive downstream secondary messengers, including phosphatidylinositol 3-kinase (PI3K)-AKT–activated mTOR complex 1 (mTORC1) and mTOR complex 2 (mTORC2). Sunitinib is an oral small molecule multitargeted receptor tyrosine kinase inhibitor that inhibits the action of VEGF to induce angiogenesis. mTOR is a serine-threonine kinase and functions as a key component of 2 multifunctional signal-transducing enzymes, downstream of the growth factor–regulated PI3K-AKT pathway, influencing the translation, cell cycle progression, survival, and angiogenesis during cancer development and progression. When mTOR is associated with raptor and mLST8 to form a complex mTORC1, it regulates cap-dependent translation by phosphorylation and activation of ribosomal S6 kinase-1 (p70S6K), and phosphorylation and inactivation of 4E-BP1, initiating the classic translation process for many proteins known to be important in cancer, such as hypoxia-inducible factor (HIF)-1. Everolimus binds mTOR and inhibits signaling downstream of mTORC1. Prolonged or high dosage of everolimus treatment can also inhibit mTORC2 formed by mTOR, rictor, sin1, and mLST8, and it blocks AKT pathway activation, inhibiting downstream cell survival and proliferation signal. (*Data from* Kutmon M, van Iersel MP, Bohler A, et al. PathVisio 3: an extendable pathway analysis toolbox. PLoS Comput Biol 2015;11(2):e1004085; and van Iersel MP, Kelder T, Pico AR, et al. Presenting and exploring biological pathways with PathVisio. BMC Bioinformatics 2008;25(9):399.)

Tryptophan hydroxylase inhibition

5-HTP is synthesized from ingested dietary tryptophan and converted to serotonin, although most dietary tryptophan is used to manufacture nicotinic acid and only a fraction for 5-HTP synthesis[6,12,49,82] (**Fig. 3**). Serotonin is then metabolized to 5-hydroxyindoleacetic acid (5-HIAA) by the action of liver and renal-derived monoamine oxidase and aldehyde dehydrogenases, and is excreted in the urine.[6,8] In the body, 95% of serotonin is found in the GI tract and 5% is found in the brain.[82] In carcinoid tumors there is an imbalance toward the production of 5-HTP. Whenever the 5-HTP bypasses the portal circulation, as in the setting of hepatic metastases, or derives directly from bronchial or ovarian carcinoid tumors, the classic features of CS may become evident.[8,12]

Telotristat ethyl (formerly LX1606 or telotristat etiprate) is an orally administered drug that inhibits tryptophan hydroxylase (TPH), the rate-limiting step in serotonin synthesis.[49,83,84] The molecule does not cross the blood–brain barrier and is, therefore, unable to act on TPH2,[49] which limits potential adverse effects on the central nervous system.[84] Previous attempts at TPH inhibition with drugs such as parachlorophenylalanine resulted in significant central nervous system adverse events.[85]

Several studies have now examined the utility of telotristat in diarrhea symptom control. A prospective randomized study compared telotristat ethyl versus placebo in subjects with CS and greater than 4 bowel motions per day, despite maximally approved octreotide LAR, over a 4 week period[86] and found that 5 of 18 (28%) subjects achieved a greater than or equal to 30% reduction in mean daily bowel motions, 9 of 16 (56%) demonstrated a greater than or equal to 50% reduction or normalization in 24-hour urinary 5-HIAA, and 10 of 18 (56%) reported symptom (diarrhea) relief during at least 1 of the first 4 weeks of treatment. No placebo-treated subjects achieved any of the aforementioned outcomes.[86]

In a small single-arm multicenter trial over a 12-week period, 14 of 15 subjects experienced a reduction in bowel motions with a reduction of greater than or equal to 50% in 43% of subjects and urinary 5-HIAA levels decreased by a mean of 74.2 mg per day from baseline.[83]

The Telotristat Etiprate for Somatostatin Analogue Not Adequately Controlled Carcinoid Syndrome (TELESTAR) multicenter randomized double-blind placebo-controlled trial had 3 arms with 45 subjects with CS not adequately controlled by SRL therapy. Each subject received placebo, telotristat ethyl 250 mg 3 times a day or telotristat ethyl 500 mg 3 times a day.[84] Telotristat resulted in reduced bowel movement of −0.81 and −0.69 for the 250 mg 3 times a day and 500 mg 3 times a day groups, respectively, versus placebo (P<.001). Mean urinary 5-HIAA levels were also significantly reduced in both dosages of telotristat ethyl in comparison with placebo (P<.001). Treatment-related adverse events were similar in all 3 groups, although nausea frequency and a dose-related increase in hepatic enzymes, particularly gamma glutamyl transferase, were observed in the telotristat 500 mg 3 times a day group.

The most commonly seen side effects and adverse events associated with telotristat are nausea, vomiting, constipation, flatulence, anorexia, elevated transaminases and gamma glutamyl transferase, headache, depression, pyrexia, and peripheral edema.[83,84,87]

Telotristat ethyl is now approved for use in CS with diarrhea refractory to treatment with standard SRL therapy[87] at a recommended dosage of 250 mg 3 times a day consumed with food.[83,84] Results are awaited from the Telotristat Etiprate for Carcinoid Syndrome Therapy (TELECAST) trial, which is evaluating the effect of telotristat ethyl versus placebo on the incidence of treatment-emergent adverse events and on urinary 5-HIAA levels[88]; and the Telotristat Etiprate–Expanded Treatment for

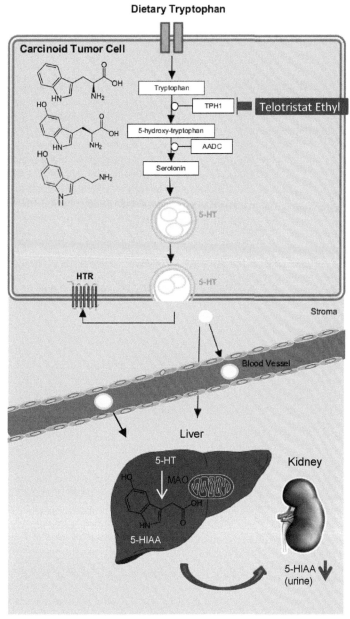

Fig. 3. Serotonin synthesis from dietary tryptophan. Serotonin is a monoamine neurotransmitter majorly synthesized in the GI tract that is derived from dietary tryptophan, which is converted to 5-HTP by tryptophan hydroxylase (TPH). 5-HTP is then catalyzed by L-aromatic amino acid decarboxylase (AADC) to serotonin (5-HT), which is then metabolized to 5-hydroxyindoleacetic acid (5-HIAA) by the action of liver and renal-derived monoamine oxidase (MAO) and aldehyde dehydrogenases and is excreted in the urine. Telotristat ethyl is an inhibitor of tryptophan hydroxylase, the rate-limiting step in serotonin biosynthesis, and can minimize serotonin-related symptoms. (*Data from* Kutmon M, van Iersel MP, Bohler A, et al. PathVisio 3: an extendable pathway analysis toolbox. PLoS Comput Biol 2015;11(2):e1004085; and van Iersel MP, Kelder T, Pico AR, et al. Presenting and exploring biological pathways with PathVisio. BMC Bioinformatics 2008;25(9):399.)

Patients with Carcinoid Syndrome Symptoms (TELEPATH) trial, which is evaluating the long-term safety and tolerability of orally administered telotristat ethyl.[89]

Bevacizumab

Bevacizumab is a monoclonal antibody to the VEGF-A ligand and is well-established in the treatment of malignancy. Trials in NETs have generally focused on combination therapies, including with everolimus, to enable dual inhibition of the mTOR and VEGF pathways. Data have been slightly more promising in PNETs. In 56 subjects with well-differentiated or moderately differentiated PNETs treated with weekly temsirolimus 25 mg IV in combination with 2 weekly 10 mg bevacizumab IV, there was confirmed response rate in 23 (41%) subjects and PFS at 6 months in 44 subjects (79%).[90] Initial evidence suggested that bevacizumab may be more effective than interferon[91] but a subsequent study of 427 subjects assessed combination therapy for octreotide LAR 20 mg with bevacizumab 15 mg/kg 3 times weekly (n = 214) or interferon 5 million units 3 times weekly (n = 213) and showed no superiority in advanced NETs.[92]

Somatostatin receptor-based theranostics: octreoscan-somatostatin receptor PET and peptide receptor radionuclide therapy

Most carcinoid tumors overexpress the G-protein-coupled SSTRs, particularly SSTR2. In light of this SSTR expression, NETs lend themselves well to theranostics whereby radiolabeled octreotide binds to the SSTRs, providing a more sensitive imaging tool than conventional structural imaging with CT and/or MRI,[93] with 80% to 100% sensitivity[12,94,95] for primary carcinoid tumors and 90% sensitivity for carcinoid hepatic metastases.[12] However, not only is SSTR-based imaging useful for diagnosis, staging, and follow-up of carcinoid tumors,[94] it can also predict efficacy of SRL treatment and the suitability for PRRT again using an SRL as a carrier for radioisotopes (see later discussion).[94,95]

For several decades, SSTR scintigraphy–octreoscan has been the standard SSTR-based option but limitations include relatively low spatial resolution, poor sensitivity to detect small tumors,[96] and that it is typically a 3-day procedure with increased cost. SSTR scintigraphy is rapidly being superseded by SSTR-based PET-CT.[95] The most widely available form of SSTR-PET uses gallium-68 (^{68}Ga)[9,95] and this study (NETSPOT) was recently approved in the United States. It provides greater sensitivity and resolution when compared with traditional single-photon emission CT (SPECT) scanning (octreoscan),[95,97] with a sensitivity of 97%, specificity of 92%, and accuracy of 96% in subjects with known or suspected NETs[97] (Fig. 4).

PRRT consists of a radionuclide, a chelator, and a cyclic octapeptide[98] that can either be administered as a systemic treatment or delivered in a directed fashion to the liver, for example.[12,31,98–101] Initially, auger electron-emitting ^{111}indium-octreotide was used[100,101] and provided some symptom relief but there was little evidence of objective tumor response, perhaps due to its short range of action,[101,102] and inadequate tissue penetration.[99,102,103] Following this, ^{90}Y, a beta-emitting radionuclide[94,99,103] with a penetration of 12 mm and half-life of 2.7 days, making it more suitable for larger tumors,[98,103] was evaluated in multiple trials[104–110] in metastatic NETs. Most ^{90}Y studies have had low enrollment numbers; however, in a large study of 1109 subjects with metastatic NETs 378 (34.1%) experienced morphologic response, 172 (14.4%) a biochemical response, and 329 (29.7%) a clinical response at 23 months.[110] Longer survival was correlated with morphologic (median survival 44.7 vs 18.3 months; $P<.001$), biochemical (median survival 35.3 vs 25.7 months; $P = .023$), and clinical response (median survival 36.8 vs 23.5 months; $P<.001$).[110] Tumor uptake on pretreatment SSTR scintigraphy predicted response to treatment

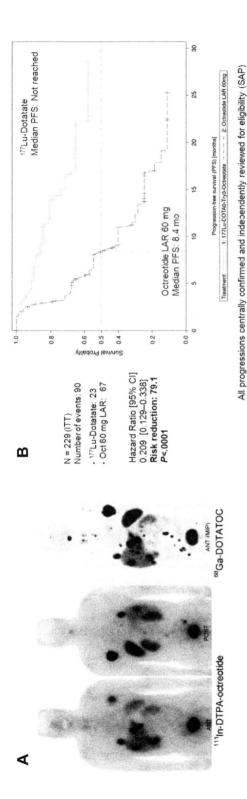

Fig. 4. Theranostics based on the SSTR. (*A*) Whole body imaging using ^{68}Ga-DOTATOC (NETSPOT) with PET imaging can minimize serotonin-related symptoms (*right panel*) and provide greater sensitivity, specificity, and accuracy compared with ^{111}In-DTPA-octreotide (SPECT, *left 2 panels*). (*B*) Somatostatin chelated radioisotopes, such as the low-energy beta and gamma emitter ^{177}Lu, can be used as therapy, as elucidated in the Neuroendocrine Tumors Therapy (NETTER) phase III randomized trial in which ^{177}Lu-DOTATOC treatment exhibited higher response rates than high-dose octreotide long-acting release (LAR) in patients with advanced midgut NETS. (*Data from* Strosberg J, El-Haddad G, Wolin E, et al. Phase 3 trial of 177Lu-dotatate for midgut neuroendocrine tumors. N Engl J Med 2017;376:125–35; and Maecke HR, André JP. 68Ga-PET Radiopharmacy: a generator-based alternative to 18F-Radiopharmacy. In: Schubiger PA, Lehmann L, Friebe M, editors. PET chemistry: the driving force in molecular imaging. Berlin: Springer Berlin; 2007:215–42.)

(HR 0.45, 95% CI 0.29–0.69, $P<.001$) and, likewise, pretreatment renal uptake predicted renal toxicity (HR 1.59, 95% CI 1.17–2.17, $P = .003$).[110] Overall, these studies indicate ^{90}Y is a safe treatment with good CS symptom improvement.[107,108]

^{177}Lu is a low-energy beta-emitter and gamma-emitter with a half-life of 6.7 days and tissue penetration of 2 mm, potentially making it more suitable for treatment of smaller tumors.[100] In the recent large Neuroendocrine Tumors Therapy (NETTER) phase III randomized trial, 229 subjects with well-differentiated midgut NETs treated with sandostatin-LAR 30 mg every 28 days were randomly assigned to receive 4 ^{177}Lu-dototate treatments at a dosage of 7.4 GBq every 8 weeks (n = 116) compared with octreotide LAR 60 mg intramuscular alone (n = 113).[111] At 20 weeks PFS in the ^{177}Lu-dototate group was 65.2% (CI 50–76.8) versus 10.8% (CI 3.5–23) in the group treated with high-dose cold octreotide alone.[111] Grade 3 or 4 neutropenia, thrombocytopenia, and leukopenia occurred at rates of 3%, 4%, and 9%, respectively, in the group treated with ^{177}Lu-dototate.[111]

Renal function is the dose-limiting factor in PRRT because radiation is reabsorbed by the proximal tubules and can induce inflammation and fibrosis.[98,112] Concomitant infusion of the positively charged amino acids lysine and arginine were administered in the radiopharmaceutical group, which reduced the reabsorption of the radiopeptide, and renal function was stable at interim analysis.[111] Age, impaired baseline renal function, hypertension, diabetes mellitus, and renal morphologic abnormalities are risk factors for renal dysfunction in PRRT and more caution may be prudent in these patients.[98,113] Overall, PRRT is a relatively safe[112,114,115] and well-tolerated treatment[98–100,105] with generally mild side effects.[100,102] ^{90}Y side effects include liver toxicity, myelodysplastic syndrome (MDS), leukemia,[116] cytopenia, male infertility, and acute renal insult with possible progression to endstage renal failure.[105–107] The shorter tissue penetration of ^{90}Y may result in less myelotoxicity.[117] Response rates to ^{90}Yttrium-labeled-tetra-azacyclododecane tetraacetic acid (DOTA)-Phe^1-Tyr^3-octreotide (TOC) (^{90}Y-DOTATOC) and ^{177}Lutetium-labeled-tetra-azacyclododecane tetraacetic acid (DOTA)-Tyr^3-octreotate (TATE) (^{177}Lu-DOTATATE) range from 15% to 35%.[103–105]

Other side effects of ^{177}Lu include liver toxicity, hematological toxicity, renal failure,[98] MDS, hair loss,[100] male infertility, and a tumor lysis presentation with hormone-related crises (rare).[99,103,118] Acute side effects of nausea, vomiting, and abdominal pain around the time of PRRT administration are due to the administration of amino acids rather than the PRRT itself.[100,103]

Higher baseline performance score, high uptake on pretreatment octreoscan, and low hepatic disease load,[103] suggest favorable responses to ^{90}Y and treatment response may also be predicted by ^{68}Ga-DOTATOC uptake.[119]

PREVENTION OF CARCINOID CRISIS DURING INTERVENTIONAL PROCEDURES

CC is an exaggerated form of CS that may precipitated during interventional procedures that involve hemodynamic fluctuations or manipulation, resection, or destruction of tumor, such as may occur during anesthesia, surgery, locoregional therapies, and PRRT. In the perioperative setting, the goal is to prevent mediator release by avoiding anxiety, hypercapnia, hypothermia, and hypotension.[120] In general, histamine-releasing drugs and succinylcholine, which can cause the release of various bioactive peptides, should be avoided because bronchospasm and hypotension can occur perioperatively.[121] Similarly, caution is needed in using sympathomimetic drugs and bronchodilators, such as β2 agonists that can activate kallikrein, leading to synthesis and release of bradykinin, resulting in vasodilatation and hypotension.

Recommendations for appropriate prophylactic use of octreotide vary in regard to timing, duration, dosage, and patient selection. Some surgeons recommend a preoperative subcutaneous dose of 100 μg of octreotide and another 100 μg intravenously just before induction of anesthesia[120]; others advise a single preoperative dose of 150 to 500 μg of octreotide only for symptomatic patients.[122] United Kingdom guidelines recommend octreotide in a constant infusion of 50 μg per hour for 12 hours before and until 14 to 48 hours after surgical intervention for all patients with a functioning carcinoid tumor.[14] The North American Neuroendocrine Tumor Society (NANETS) consensus guidelines recommend a preoperative bolus of octreotide 250 to 500 μg IV with extra doses available throughout procedure in patients with suspected CS undergoing major procedures.[123] However, these recommendations are largely derived from case reports. This has not been studied in a prospective manner and, despite use of octreotide therapy, some patients may still develop life-threatening cardiorespiratory complications that can challenge even the most experienced anesthetist.[10,124] Other agents, such as phenylephrine and vasopressin, may be needed to treat hypotension and α-blocking and β-blocking drugs to avoid severe complications due to bronchospasm or tachyarrhythmia.

FUTURE DIRECTIONS

Future refinements with individualized dosimetric analysis to inform maximal PRRT dosage, combination therapies with radiosensitizing agents, and the development of multireceptor PRRT will help define the optimal approach for the treatment of CS.[98] Development of oncolytic replication-selective adenoviruses under the control of the CgA promoter to specifically target NET cells is another promising strategy in development. Preclinical studies have been encouraging and early phase I experience has not noted worrisome toxicity signals radiosensitizing[125]; however, this concept will require extensive additional studies before it can be translated into routine clinical practice.[126,127]

SUMMARY

The other aspect of managing CS in the setting of NETs that is presently unclear is the utilization or sequence of the now several different treatment options available. There is general consensus that an individualized patient pathway agreed to by a multidisciplinary team is the optimal planning approach to treatment. In settings in which potential cure is attainable, such as surgery for an isolated primary tumor, the best treatment option is clear cut. In other instances in which widespread functional NET is present, use of SRL as first-line therapy has been the paradigm for some time but this may now be challenged with newer trial data on mTOR inhibition and PRRT. The authors anticipate that, as PRRT with individualized dosimetric analysis becomes more widely available, in the United States at least, it may become second-line or first-line therapy in unresectable disease, either alone or in various combinations.

REFERENCES

1. Lubarsch O. Ueber den primären Krebs des Ileum, nebst Bemerkungen über das gleichzeitige Vorkommen von Krebs und Tuberkolose. Virchows Arch 1888;111:280–317.
2. Zuetenhorst JM, Taal BG. Metastatic carcinoid tumors: a clinical review. Oncologist 2005;10(2):123–31.
3. Modlin IM, Shapiro MD, Kidd M. Siegfried Oberndorfer: origins and perspectives of carcinoid tumors. Hum Pathol 2004;35(12):1440–51.

4. Baxi AJ, Chintapalli K, Katkar A, et al. Multimodality imaging findings in carcinoid tumors: a head-to-toe spectrum. Radiographics 2017;37(2):516–36.
5. Ganim RB, Norton JA. Recent advances in carcinoid pathogenesis, diagnosis and management. Surg Oncol 2000;9(4):173–9.
6. Kaltsas GA, Besser GM, Grossman AB. The diagnosis and medical management of advanced neuroendocrine tumors. Endocr Rev 2004;25(3):458–511.
7. Mota JM, Sousa LG, Riechelmann RP. Complications from carcinoid syndrome: review of the current evidence. Ecancermedicalscience 2016;10:662.
8. Kulke MH, Mayer RJ. Carcinoid tumors. N Engl J Med 1999;340(11):858–68.
9. Liu EH, Solorzano CC, Katznelson L, et al. AACE/ACE disease state clinical review: diagnosis and management of midgut carcinoids. Endocr Pract 2015; 21(5):534–45.
10. Guo LJ, Tang CW. Somatostatin analogues do not prevent carcinoid crisis. Asian Pac J Cancer Prev 2014;15(16):6679–83.
11. Tomassetti P, Migliori M, Lalli S, et al. Epidemiology, clinical features and diagnosis of gastroenteropancreatic endocrine tumours. Ann Oncol 2001; 12(Suppl 2):S95–9.
12. Oberg K, Castellano D. Current knowledge on diagnosis and staging of neuroendocrine tumors. Cancer Metastasis Rev 2011;30(Suppl 1):3–7.
13. Plockinger U, Rindi G, Arnold R, et al. Guidelines for the diagnosis and treatment of neuroendocrine gastrointestinal tumours. A consensus statement on behalf of the European Neuroendocrine Tumour Society (ENETS). Neuroendocrinology 2004;80(6):394–424.
14. Ramage JK, Ahmed A, Ardill J, et al. Guidelines for the management of gastroenteropancreatic neuroendocrine (including carcinoid) tumours (NETs). Gut 2012;61(1):6–32.
15. Condron ME, Pommier SJ, Pommier RF. Continuous infusion of octreotide combined with perioperative octreotide bolus does not prevent intraoperative carcinoid crisis. Surgery 2016;159(1):358–65.
16. Sarmiento JM, Heywood G, Rubin J, et al. Surgical treatment of neuroendocrine metastases to the liver: a plea for resection to increase survival. J Am Coll Surg 2003;197(1):29–37.
17. Que FG, Nagorney DM, Batts KP, et al. Hepatic resection for metastatic neuroendocrine carcinomas. Am J Surg 1995;169(1):36–42 [discussion: 42–3].
18. Nazario J, Gupta S. Transarterial liver-directed therapies of neuroendocrine hepatic metastases. Semin Oncol 2010;37(2):118–26.
19. Vogl TJ, Naguib NN, Zangos S, et al. Liver metastases of neuroendocrine carcinomas: interventional treatment via transarterial embolization, chemoembolization and thermal ablation. Eur J Radiol 2009;72(3):517–28.
20. Yang TX, Chua TC, Morris DL. Radioembolization and chemoembolization for unresectable neuroendocrine liver metastases - a systematic review. Surg Oncol 2012;21(4):299–308.
21. Frilling A, Modlin IM, Kidd M, et al. Recommendations for management of patients with neuroendocrine liver metastases. Lancet Oncol 2014;15(1): e8–21.
22. Eriksson J, Stalberg P, Nilsson A, et al. Surgery and radiofrequency ablation for treatment of liver metastases from midgut and foregut carcinoids and endocrine pancreatic tumors. World J Surg 2008;32(5):930–8.
23. Kennedy AS, Dezarn WA, McNeillie P, et al. Radioembolization for unresectable neuroendocrine hepatic metastases using resin 90Y-microspheres: early results in 148 patients. Am J Clin Oncol 2008;31(3):271–9.

24. Paprottka PM, Hoffmann RT, Haug A, et al. Radioembolization of symptomatic, unresectable neuroendocrine hepatic metastases using yttrium-90 microspheres. Cardiovasc Intervent Radiol 2012;35(2):334–42.
25. Pericleous M, Caplin ME, Tsochatzis E, et al. Hepatic artery embolization in advanced neuroendocrine tumors: Efficacy and long-term outcomes. Asia Pac J Clin Oncol 2016;12(1):61–9.
26. Pitt SC, Knuth J, Keily JM, et al. Hepatic neuroendocrine metastases: chemo- or bland embolization? J Gastrointest Surg 2008;12(11):1951–60.
27. Strosberg JR, Choi J, Cantor AB, et al. Selective hepatic artery embolization for treatment of patients with metastatic carcinoid and pancreatic endocrine tumors. Cancer Control 2006;13(1):72–8.
28. Lacin S, Oz I, Ozkan E, et al. Intra-arterial treatment with 90yttrium microspheres In treatment-refractory and unresectable liver metastases of neuroendocrine tumors and the use of 111in-octreotide scintigraphy in the evaluation of treatment response. Cancer Biother Radiopharm 2011;26(5):631–7.
29. Memon K, Lewandowski RJ, Mulcahy MF, et al. Radioembolization for neuroendocrine liver metastases: safety, imaging, and long-term outcomes. Int J Radiat Oncol Biol Phys 2012;83(3):887–94.
30. Kalinowski M, Dressler M, Konig A, et al. Selective internal radiotherapy with Yttrium-90 microspheres for hepatic metastatic neuroendocrine tumors: a prospective single center study. Digestion 2009;79(3):137–42.
31. McStay MK, Maudgil D, Williams M, et al. Large-volume liver metastases from neuroendocrine tumors: hepatic intraarterial 90Y-DOTA-lanreotide as effective palliative therapy. Radiology 2005;237(2):718–26.
32. Shaheen M, Hassanain M, Aljiffry M, et al. Predictors of response to radioembolization (TheraSphere(R)) treatment of neuroendocrine liver metastasis. HPB (Oxford) 2012;14(1):60–6.
33. Saxena A, Chua TC, Bester L, et al. Factors predicting response and survival after yttrium-90 radioembolization of unresectable neuroendocrine tumor liver metastases: a critical appraisal of 48 cases. Ann Surg 2010; 251(5):910–6.
34. Kiesewetter B, Raderer M. Ondansetron for diarrhea associated with neuroendocrine tumors. N Engl J Med 2013;368(20):1947–8.
35. Wymenga AN, de Vries EG, Leijsma MK, et al. Effects of ondansetron on gastrointestinal symptoms in carcinoid syndrome. Eur J Cancer 1998;34(8):1293–4.
36. Bauer W, Briner U, Doepfner W, et al. SMS 201-995: a very potent and selective octapeptide analogue of somatostatin with prolonged action. Life Sci 1982; 31(11):1133–40.
37. Cives M, Strosberg J. Treatment strategies for metastatic neuroendocrine tumors of the gastrointestinal tract. Curr Treat Options Oncol 2017;18(3):14.
38. Kvols LK, Moertel CG, O'Connell MJ, et al. Treatment of the malignant carcinoid syndrome. Evaluation of a long-acting somatostatin analogue. N Engl J Med 1986;315(11):663–6.
39. Wood SM, Kraenzlin ME, Adrian TE, et al. Treatment of patients with pancreatic endocrine tumours using a new long-acting somatostatin analogue symptomatic and peptide responses. Gut 1985;26(5):438–44.
40. Butturini G, Bettini R, Missiaglia E, et al. Predictive factors of efficacy of the somatostatin analogue octreotide as first line therapy for advanced pancreatic endocrine carcinoma. Endocr Relat Cancer 2006;13(4):1213–21.
41. Garcia de la Torre N, Wass JA, Turner HE. Antiangiogenic effects of somatostatin analogues. Clin Endocrinol (Oxf) 2002;57(4):425–41.

42. Grozinsky-Glasberg S, Shimon I, Korbonits M, et al. Somatostatin analogues in the control of neuroendocrine tumours: efficacy and mechanisms. Endocr Relat Cancer 2008;15(3):701–20.

43. Susini C, Buscail L. Rationale for the use of somatostatin analogs as antitumor agents. Ann Oncol 2006;17(12):1733–42.

44. Macaulay VM. Insulin-like growth factors and cancer. Br J Cancer 1992;65(3): 311–20.

45. Trendle MC, Moertel CG, Kvols LK. Incidence and morbidity of cholelithiasis in patients receiving chronic octreotide for metastatic carcinoid and malignant islet cell tumors. Cancer 1997;79(4):830–4.

46. Schmid HA. Pasireotide (SOM230): development, mechanism of action and potential applications. Mol Cell Endocrinol 2008;286(1–2):69–74.

47. Ronga G, Salerno G, Procaccini E, et al. 111In-octreotide scintigraphy in metastatic medullary thyroid carcinoma before and after octreotide therapy: in vivo evidence of the possible down-regulation of somatostatin receptors. Q J Nucl Med 1995;39(4 Suppl 1):134–6.

48. Li M, Li W, Kim HJ, et al. Characterization of somatostatin receptor expression in human pancreatic cancer using real-time RT-PCR. J Surg Res 2004;119(2): 130–7.

49. Molina-Cerrillo J, Alonso-Gordoa T, Martinez-Saez O, et al. Inhibition of peripheral synthesis of serotonin as a new target in neuroendocrine tumors. Oncologist 2016;21(6):701–7.

50. Wolin EM, Jarzab B, Eriksson B, et al. Phase III study of pasireotide long-acting release in patients with metastatic neuroendocrine tumors and carcinoid symptoms refractory to available somatostatin analogues. Drug Des Devel Ther 2015; 9:5075–86.

51. Anthony L, Freda PU. From somatostatin to octreotide LAR: evolution of a somatostatin analogue. Curr Med Res Opin 2009;25(12):2989–99.

52. Riechelmann RP, Pereira AA, Rego JF, et al. Refractory carcinoid syndrome: a review of treatment options. Ther Adv Med Oncol 2017;9(2):127–37.

53. Yao JC, Lombard-Bohas C, Baudin E, et al. Daily oral everolimus activity in patients with metastatic pancreatic neuroendocrine tumors after failure of cytotoxic chemotherapy: a phase II trial. J Clin Oncol 2010;28(1):69–76.

54. Pavel ME, Hainsworth JD, Baudin E, et al. Everolimus plus octreotide long-acting repeatable for the treatment of advanced neuroendocrine tumours associated with carcinoid syndrome (RADIANT-2): a randomised, placebo-controlled, phase 3 study. Lancet 2011;378(9808):2005–12.

55. Yao JC, Shah MH, Ito T, et al. Everolimus for advanced pancreatic neuroendocrine tumors. N Engl J Med 2011;364(6):514–23.

56. Yao JC, Fazio N, Singh S, et al. Everolimus for the treatment of advanced, non-functional neuroendocrine tumours of the lung or gastrointestinal tract (RADIANT-4): a randomised, placebo-controlled, phase 3 study. Lancet 2016; 387(10022):968–77.

57. Panzuto F, Rinzivillo M, Fazio N, et al. Real-world study of everolimus in advanced progressive neuroendocrine tumors. Oncologist 2014;19(9):966–74.

58. Terris B, Scoazec JY, Rubbia L, et al. Expression of vascular endothelial growth factor in digestive neuroendocrine tumours. Histopathology 1998;32(2):133–8.

59. Raymond E, Dahan L, Raoul JL, et al. Sunitinib malate for the treatment of pancreatic neuroendocrine tumors. N Engl J Med 2011;364(6):501–13.

60. Kulke MH, Lenz HJ, Meropol NJ, et al. Activity of sunitinib in patients with advanced neuroendocrine tumors. J Clin Oncol 2008;26(20):3403–10.

61. Walter T, Brixi-Benmansour H, Lombard-Bohas C, et al. New treatment strategies in advanced neuroendocrine tumours. Dig Liver Dis 2012;44(2):95–105.
62. Weatherstone K, Meyer T. Streptozocin-based chemotherapy is not history in neuroendocrine tumours. Target Oncol 2012;7(3):161–8.
63. Moertel CG, Hanley JA. Combination chemotherapy trials in metastatic carcinoid tumor and the malignant carcinoid syndrome. Cancer Clin Trials 1979; 2(4):327–34.
64. Moertel CG, Kvols LK, O'Connell MJ, et al. Treatment of neuroendocrine carcinomas with combined etoposide and cisplatin. Evidence of major therapeutic activity in the anaplastic variants of these neoplasms. Cancer 1991;68(2): 227–32.
65. Dahan L, Bonnetain F, Rougier P, et al. Phase III trial of chemotherapy using 5-fluorouracil and streptozotocin compared with interferon alpha for advanced carcinoid tumors: FNCLCC-FFCD 9710. Endocr Relat Cancer 2009;16(4): 1351–61.
66. Sun W, Lipsitz S, Catalano P, et al, Eastern Cooperative Oncology Group. Phase II/III study of doxorubicin with fluorouracil compared with streptozocin with fluorouracil or dacarbazine in the treatment of advanced carcinoid tumors: Eastern Cooperative Oncology Group Study E1281. J Clin Oncol 2005;23(22):4897–904.
67. Engstrom PF, Lavin PT, Moertel CG, et al. Streptozocin plus fluorouracil versus doxorubicin therapy for metastatic carcinoid tumor. J Clin Oncol 1984;2(11): 1255–9.
68. Clinical Trials.gov. Peptide receptor radionuclide therapy with 177Lu-Dotatate associated with metronomic capecitabine in patients affected by aggressive gastro-etero-pancreatic neuroendocrine tumors (LuX). 2017; Available at: https://clinicaltrials.gov/ct2/show/NCT02736500. Accessed December 03, 2017.
69. Pavel ME, Baum U, Hahn EG, et al. Efficacy and tolerability of pegylated IFN-alpha in patients with neuroendocrine gastroenteropancreatic carcinomas. J Interferon Cytokine Res 2006;26(1):8–13.
70. Faiss S, Pape UF, Bohmig M, et al. Prospective, randomized, multicenter trial on the antiproliferative effect of lanreotide, interferon alfa, and their combination for therapy of metastatic neuroendocrine gastroenteropancreatic tumors–the International Lanreotide and Interferon Alfa Study Group. J Clin Oncol 2003;21(14): 2689–96.
71. Kolby L, Persson G, Franzen S, et al. Randomized clinical trial of the effect of interferon alpha on survival in patients with disseminated midgut carcinoid tumours. Br J Surg 2003;90(6):687–93.
72. Arnold R, Rinke A, Klose KJ, et al. Octreotide versus octreotide plus interferon-alpha in endocrine gastroenteropancreatic tumors: a randomized trial. Clin Gastroenterol Hepatol 2005;3(8):761–71.
73. Dimitriadis GK, Weickert MO, Randeva HS, et al. Medical management of secretory syndromes related to gastroenteropancreatic neuroendocrine tumours. Endocr Relat Cancer 2016;23(9):R423–36.
74. Kvols LK, Oberg KE, O'Dorisio TM, et al. Pasireotide (SOM230) shows efficacy and tolerability in the treatment of patients with advanced neuroendocrine tumors refractory or resistant to octreotide LAR: results from a phase II study. Endocr Relat Cancer 2012;19(5):657–66.
75. Schmid HA, Schoeffter P. Functional activity of the multiligand analog SOM230 at human recombinant somatostatin receptor subtypes supports its usefulness in neuroendocrine tumors. Neuroendocrinology 2004;80(Suppl 1):47–50.

76. Colao A, Petersenn S, Newell-Price J, et al. A 12-month phase 3 study of pasireotide in Cushing's disease. N Engl J Med 2012;366(10):914–24.

77. Colao A, Bronstein MD, Freda P, et al. Pasireotide versus octreotide in acromegaly: a head-to-head superiority study. J Clin Endocrinol Metab 2014;99(3):791–9.

78. Bruns C, Lewis I, Briner U, et al. SOM230: a novel somatostatin peptidomimetic with broad somatotropin release inhibiting factor (SRIF) receptor binding and a unique antisecretory profile. Eur J Endocrinol 2002;146(5):707–16.

79. Weckbecker G, Briner U, Lewis I, et al. SOM230: a new somatostatin peptidomimetic with potent inhibitory effects on the growth hormone/insulin-like growth factor-I axis in rats, primates, and dogs. Endocrinology 2002; 143(10):4123–30.

80. Cives M, Kunz PL, Morse B, et al. Phase II clinical trial of pasireotide long-acting repeatable in patients with metastatic neuroendocrine tumors. Endocr Relat Cancer 2015;22(1):1–9.

81. Breitschaft A, Hu K, Hermosillo Resendiz K, et al. Management of hyperglycemia associated with pasireotide (SOM230): healthy volunteer study. Diabetes Res Clin Pract 2014;103(3):458–65.

82. Lesurtel M, Soll C, Graf R, et al. Role of serotonin in the hepato-gastrointestinal tract: an old molecule for new perspectives. Cell Mol Life Sci 2008;65(6):940–52.

83. Pavel M, Horsch D, Caplin M, et al. Telotristat etiprate for carcinoid syndrome: a single-arm, multicenter trial. J Clin Endocrinol Metab 2015;100(4):1511–9.

84. Kulke MH, Horsch D, Caplin ME, et al. Telotristat Ethyl, a tryptophan hydroxylase inhibitor for the treatment of carcinoid syndrome. J Clin Oncol 2017;35(1):14–23.

85. Engelman K, Lovenberg W, Sjoerdsma A. Inhibition of serotonin synthesis by para-chlorophenylalanine in patients with the carcinoid syndrome. N Engl J Med 1967;277(21):1103–8.

86. Kulke MH, O'Dorisio T, Phan A, et al. Telotristat etiprate, a novel serotonin synthesis inhibitor, in patients with carcinoid syndrome and diarrhea not adequately controlled by octreotide. Endocr Relat Cancer 2014;21(5):705–14.

87. Choy M. Pharmaceutical approval update. P T 2017;42(5):304–5.

88. Clinical Trials.gov. Telotristat etiprate for carcinoid syndrome therapy (TELECAST). 2017. Available at: https://clinicaltrials.gov/ct2/show/NCT02063659?term=NCT02063659&rank=1. Accessed December 03, 2017.

89. Clinical Trials.gov. Telotristat etiprate - expanded treatment for patients with carcinoid syndrome symptoms (TELEPATH). 2017. Available at: https://clinicaltrials.gov/ct2/show/NCT02026063. Accessed 12/03, 2017.

90. Hobday TJ, Qin R, Reidy-Lagunes D, et al. Multicenter phase II trial of temsirolimus and bevacizumab in pancreatic neuroendocrine tumors. J Clin Oncol 2015;33(14):1551–6.

91. Yao JC, Phan A, Hoff PM, et al. Targeting vascular endothelial growth factor in advanced carcinoid tumor: a random assignment phase II study of depot octreotide with bevacizumab and pegylated interferon alpha-2b. J Clin Oncol 2008;26(8):1316–23.

92. Yao JC, Guthrie KA, Moran C, et al. Phase III prospective randomized comparison trial of depot octreotide plus interferon Alfa-2b versus depot octreotide plus bevacizumab in patients with advanced carcinoid tumors: SWOG S0518. J Clin Oncol 2017;35(15):1695–703.

93. Chiti A, Fanti S, Savelli G, et al. Comparison of somatostatin receptor imaging, computed tomography and ultrasound in the clinical management of neuroendocrine gastro-entero-pancreatic tumours. Eur J Nucl Med 1998;25(10): 1396–403.

94. Chatal JF, Le Bodic MF, Kraeber-Bodere F, et al. Nuclear medicine applications for neuroendocrine tumors. World J Surg 2000;24(11):1285–9.
95. Rufini V, Calcagni ML, Baum RP. Imaging of neuroendocrine tumors. Semin Nucl Med 2006;36(3):228–47.
96. Orlefors H, Sundin A, Garske U, et al. Whole-body (11)C-5-hydroxytryptophan positron emission tomography as a universal imaging technique for neuroendocrine tumors: comparison with somatostatin receptor scintigraphy and computed tomography. J Clin Endocrinol Metab 2005;90(6):3392–400.
97. Gabriel M, Decristoforo C, Kendler D, et al. 68Ga-DOTA-Tyr3-octreotide PET in neuroendocrine tumors: comparison with somatostatin receptor scintigraphy and CT. J Nucl Med 2007;48(4):508–18.
98. Bergsma H, Lom KV, Konijnenberg M, et al. Therapy-related hematological malignancies after peptide receptor radionuclide therapy with 177Lu-DOTA-Octreotate: incidence, course & predicting factors in patients with GEP-NETs. J Nucl Med 2017.
99. Kwekkeboom DJ, de Herder WW, Kam BL, et al. Treatment with the radiolabeled somatostatin analog [177 Lu-DOTA 0,Tyr3]octreotate: toxicity, efficacy, and survival. J Clin Oncol 2008;26(13):2124–30.
100. Brabander T, Teunissen JJ, Van Eijck CH, et al. Peptide receptor radionuclide therapy of neuroendocrine tumours. Best Pract Res Clin Endocrinol Metab 2016;30(1):103–14.
101. Anthony LB, Woltering EA, Espenan GD, et al. Indium-111-pentetreotide prolongs survival in gastroenteropancreatic malignancies. Semin Nucl Med 2002;32(2):123–32.
102. Kam BL, Teunissen JJ, Krenning EP, et al. Lutetium-labelled peptides for therapy of neuroendocrine tumours. Eur J Nucl Med Mol Imaging 2012;39(Suppl 1):S103–12.
103. van der Zwan WA, Bodei L, Mueller-Brand J, et al. GEPNETs update: radionuclide therapy in neuroendocrine tumors. Eur J Endocrinol 2015;172(1):R1–8.
104. Cwikla JB, Sankowski A, Seklecka N, et al. Efficacy of radionuclide treatment DOTATATE Y-90 in patients with progressive metastatic gastroenteropancreatic neuroendocrine carcinomas (GEP-NETs): a phase II study. Ann Oncol 2010;21(4):787–94.
105. Waldherr C, Pless M, Maecke HR, et al. The clinical value of [90Y-DOTA]-D-Phe1-Tyr3-octreotide (90Y-DOTATOC) in the treatment of neuroendocrine tumours: a clinical phase II study. Ann Oncol 2001;12(7):941–5.
106. Bodei L, Cremonesi M, Zoboli S, et al. Receptor-mediated radionuclide therapy with 90Y-DOTATOC in association with amino acid infusion: a phase I study. Eur J Nucl Med Mol Imaging 2003;30(2):207–16.
107. Bushnell DL Jr, O'Dorisio TM, O'Dorisio MS, et al. 90Y-edotreotide for metastatic carcinoid refractory to octreotide. J Clin Oncol 2010;28(10):1652–9.
108. Forrer F, Waldherr C, Maecke HR, et al. Targeted radionuclide therapy with 90Y-DOTATOC in patients with neuroendocrine tumors. Anticancer Res 2006;26(1B):703–7.
109. Valkema R, Pauwels S, Kvols LK, et al. Survival and response after peptide receptor radionuclide therapy with [90Y-DOTA0,Tyr3]octreotide in patients with advanced gastroenteropancreatic neuroendocrine tumors. Semin Nucl Med 2006;36(2):147–56.
110. Imhof A, Brunner P, Marincek N, et al. Response, survival, and long-term toxicity after therapy with the radiolabeled somatostatin analogue [90Y-DOTA]-TOC in metastasized neuroendocrine cancers. J Clin Oncol 2011;29(17):2416–23.
111. Strosberg J, El-Haddad G, Wolin E, et al. Phase 3 trial of 177Lu-Dotatate for midgut neuroendocrine tumors. N Engl J Med 2017;376(2):125–35.

112. Faggiano A, Lo Calzo F, Pizza G, et al. The safety of available treatments options for neuroendocrine tumors. Expert Opin Drug Saf 2017;16(10):1149–61.
113. Bodei L, Cremonesi M, Ferrari M, et al. Long-term evaluation of renal toxicity after peptide receptor radionuclide therapy with 90Y-DOTATOC and 177Lu-DOTATATE: the role of associated risk factors. Eur J Nucl Med Mol Imaging 2008; 35(10):1847–56.
114. Gulenchyn KY, Yao X, Asa SL, et al. Radionuclide therapy in neuroendocrine tumours: a systematic review. Clin Oncol (R Coll Radiol) 2012;24(4):294–308.
115. Pfeifer AK, Gregersen T, Gronbaek H, et al. Peptide receptor radionuclide therapy with Y-DOTATOC and (177)Lu-DOTATOC in advanced neuroendocrine tumors: results from a Danish cohort treated in Switzerland. Neuroendocrinology 2011;93(3):189–96.
116. Merola E, Capurso G, Campana D, et al. Acute leukaemia following low dose peptide receptor radionuclide therapy for an intestinal carcinoid. Dig Liver Dis 2010;42(6):457–8.
117. Sierra ML, Agazzi A, Bodei L, et al. Lymphocytic toxicity in patients after peptide-receptor radionuclide therapy (PRRT) with 177Lu-DOTATATE and 90Y-DOTATOC. Cancer Biother Radiopharm 2009;24(6):659–65.
118. Bodei L, Cremonesi M, Grana CM, et al. Peptide receptor radionuclide therapy with (1)(7)(7)Lu-DOTATATE: the IEO phase I-II study. Eur J Nucl Med Mol Imaging 2011;38(12):2125–35.
119. Oksuz MO, Winter L, Pfannenberg C, et al. Peptide receptor radionuclide therapy of neuroendocrine tumors with (90)Y-DOTATOC: is treatment response predictable by pre-therapeutic uptake of (68)Ga-DOTATOC? Diagn Interv Imaging 2014;95(3):289–300.
120. Dierdorf SF. Carcinoid tumor and carcinoid syndrome. Curr Opin Anaesthesiol 2003;16:343–7.
121. Kroigaard M, Garvey LH, Gillberg L, et al. Scandinavian clinical practice guidelines on the diagnosis, management and follow-up of anaphylaxis during anaesthesia. Acta Anaesthesiol Scand 2007;51:655–70.
122. Massimino K, Harrskog O, Pommier S. Pommier R Octreotide LAR and bolus octreotide are insufficient for preventing intraoperative complications in carcinoid patients. J Surg Oncol 2013;107:842–6.
123. Strosberg JR, Halfdanarson TR, Bellizzi AM, et al. Consensus guidelines for the management and treatment of neuroendocrine tumors. Pancreas 2017;46: 707–14.
124. Kinney MA, Warner ME, Nagorney DM, et al. Perianaesthetic risks and outcomes of abdominal surgery for metastatic carcinoid tumours. Br J Anaesth 2001;87:447–52.
125. Leja J, Dzojic H, Gustafson E, et al. A novel chromogranin-A promoter-driven oncolytic adenovirus for midgut carcinoid therapy. Clin Cancer Res 2007;13(8): 2455–62.
126. Leja J, Nilsson B, Yu D, et al. Double-detargeted oncolytic adenovirus shows replication arrest in liver cells and retains neuroendocrine cell killing ability. PLoS One 2010;5(1):e8916.
127. Leja J, Yu D, Nilsson B, et al. Oncolytic adenovirus modified with somatostatin motifs for selective infection of neuroendocrine tumor cells. Gene Ther 2011; 18(11):1052–62.

Gastrinomas
Medical or Surgical Treatment

Jeffrey A. Norton, MD[a], Deshka S. Foster, MD[a], Tetsuhide Ito, MD, PhD[b],
Robert T. Jensen, MD[c],*

KEYWORDS

- Zollinger-Ellison syndrome • Gastrinoma • Neuroendocrine tumor • Acid secretion
- Proton pump inhibitors • Multiple endocrine neoplasia type 1

KEY POINTS

- Zollinger-Ellison syndrome (ZES) is caused by a gastrin-secreting neuroendocrine tumor that results in marked acid hypersecretion.
- All patients with ZES have 2 management problems that must both be dealt with: control of the acid hypersecretion, which causes refractory peptic disease, and control of the gastrinoma, which is malignant in 60% to 90% of cases.
- Twenty percent to 25% of patients with ZES have it as part of the multiple endocrine neoplasia type 1 syndrome that needs to be recognized, as its management differs from sporadic cases (75%–80%).
- Over the years, surgical and medical approaches have played varying roles in the treatment of each aspect of ZES.
- Presently, the roles of medical and surgical approaches are generally complementary; however, in several areas the selective use of one over the other is controversial.

The relationship between surgical treatments and medical treatments in the various management aspects of the Zollinger-Ellison syndrome (ZES) has taken many forms. In some aspects of ZES at different times, only one of these approaches has been used, whereas at other times both are available and used to different extents by different groups; thus, they have had a somewhat adversarial relationship, whereas in other cases they are complementary. The latter is the situation at present in most instances; however, there remain management aspects whereby the exact role of surgery or medical treatment remains unclear and contentious. In this article, these

Disclosure: The authors have nothing to disclose.
[a] Department of Surgery, Stanford University School of Medicine, 291 campus Drive, Stanford, CA 94305-5101, USA; [b] Neuroendocrine Tumor Centra, Fukuoka Sanno Hospital, International University of Health and Welfare, 3-6-45 Momochihama, Sawara-Ku, Fukuoka 814-0001, Japan; [c] Digestive Diseases Branch, NIDDK, National Institutes of Health, Building 10, Room 9C-103, Bethesda, MD 20892-1804, USA
* Corresponding author.
E-mail address: robertj@bdg10.niddk.nih.gov

aspects are discussed showing changes over time but generally concentrating on the role of each in the current management of ZES.

GENERAL/DEFINITIONS

ZES was first described in 1955 in 2 patients by 2 surgeons at the Ohio State University, RM Zollinger and EH Ellison; 6 additional cases were described by other surgeons in the discussion of this article.[1] A later review of the literature before this time concluded at least 4 cases of probable gastrinomas had been described previously,[2] but it was Zollinger/Ellison who made the critical hypothesis that the gastric acid hypersecretion was due to secretion of the pancreatic neuroendocrine tumor (panNET).[1,2] At present, it is known that ZES is due to the ectopic secretion of gastrin by a neuroendocrine tumor (NET) (gastrinoma) resulting in gastric acid hypersecretion,[3–5] which characteristically causes advanced gastroesophageal reflux disease (GERD) and/or peptic ulcer disease, often refractory in nature.[1,6] The terms *gastrinoma* and *ZES* are frequently used synonymously; however, historically gastrinoma referred to the NET secreting gastrin and ZES to the clinical manifestations of the disease. Numerous tumors, including non-NET neoplasms, synthesize gastrin; in most it is not fully processed to biologically active gastrin-17 to 34; consequently, these do not cause ZES because they do not secrete sufficient amounts of fully processed gastrin and, thus, are generally not called gastrinomas by most clinicians and in most classifications of panNETs.[7,8]

Gastrinomas, like all other functional panNETs (F-panNETs) secreting biologically active peptides causing a functional syndrome (insulinomas, VIPomas, glucagonomas, and so forth), differ from other more common neoplasms (colon, pancreatic adenocarcinomas, and so forth) in presenting to the clinician 2 different treatment problems.[8–11] In each syndrome, the hormone excess state needs to be controlled (ie, gastric acid hypersecretion in gastrinomas) and the tumor itself dealt with, because in all cases except insulinomas, F-panNETs are malignant in greater than 50% of cases (ie, 60%–90% for gastrinomas) (**Fig. 1**A).[8–11] Whereas complete surgical resection would treat both of these problems with one approach, as is the usual case with patients with insulinomas,[10,12,13] unfortunately surgical cure in ZES, even today, is seen in less than 50% of all patients with ZES in most series.[4,14–16] Thus, both treatment of gastric acid hypersecretion and the tumor per se have remained separate treatment problems in most patients with ZES; surgical and medical approaches have played variably important roles in the treatment of each over the years.[4,17,18]

ROLES OF MEDICAL AND SURGICAL TREATMENT IN CONTROL OF GASTRIC ACID HYPERSECRETION IN PATIENTS WITH ZOLLINGER-ELLISON SYNDROME: PAST VERSUS PRESENT
General Points: Acid Hypersecretion

Since the first description of patients with ZES and detailed reports from the original ZES registry and various early series,[1,9,19,20] the morbidity of the devastating effects of uncontrolled acid hypersecretion in patients with ZES has become clear. This result occurs because patients with ZES have on average a basal acid output (BAO) that is elevated 4- to 6-fold and in some patients increased up to greater than 10-fold, combined with an increased maximal ability to secrete acid (MAO) (**Fig. 1**B) due to the stimulatory and trophic effects of chronic hypergastrinemia on the parietal cells, gastric enterochromaffin-like cells, and other gastric mucosal cells.[3,9,21–23] In almost all cases the initial clinical symptoms of patients with ZES are due to the effects of acid hypersecretion, with pain due to peptic ulcer disease (73%–98%), heartburn

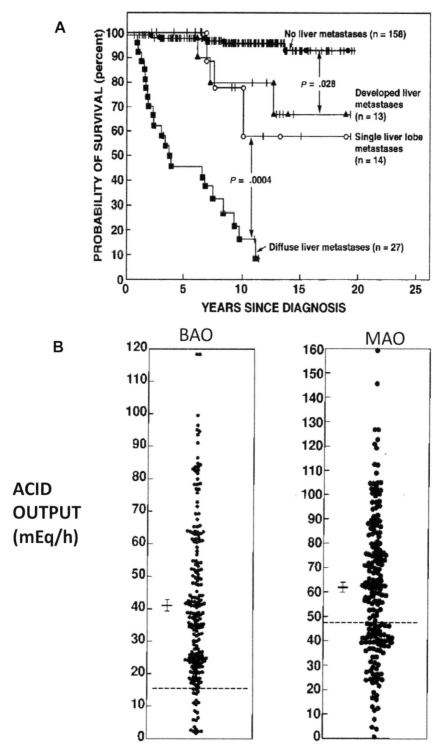

Fig. 1. Extent of disease effect on survival and acid hypersecretion in patients with ZES. (*A*) Shown are results from 212 patients with ZES prospectively followed. (*B*) Results are from

(52–56%-recent series), diarrhea (60%–75% recent series), weight loss (7%–53%), and symptoms due to the complications of acid hypersecretion (bleeding, strictures, perforation, penetration).[6] These early studies as well as later studies have taught clinicians that patients with ZES require control of gastric acid hypersecretion at all times, both acutely when first seen and long-term.[9,16,24–27]

Past: Control of Acid Hypersecretion: Medical Versus Surgical

Initially, medical therapy had no role in the control of acid hypersecretion in patients with ZES, with anticholinergic drugs, radiation, and other drugs being ineffective.[9,28] Surgery, ultimately only total gastrectomy (ie, removal of the primary target for gastrin), proved to be the only effective treatment in most patients because it was not possible to surgically cure the patients in most cases by removing the gastrinoma resulting in a long-term cure.[4,9,25,29,30] Thus, a surgical approach was the only effective treatment of gastric acid hypersecretion until the development of histamine H_2-receptor antagonists in the 1970s.[9,31,32]

The histamine H_2 receptor antagonists (metiamide, cimetidine, ranitidine, nizalidine, famotidine, and so forth) were all effective in different series at reducing acid hypersecretion; but results in different series reported a 0% to 60% failure rate,[18,26,31–33] which was primarily due to a failure to use established criteria for acid control and to titrate the dose in different patients.[18,24] The National Institutes of Health's studies demonstrated that if a sufficient drug was used to control the acid hypersecretion to less than 10 mEq/h before the next drug dose (<5 mEq/h if patients have previous gastric acid-reducing surgery), then the acid secretion could be controlled in 100% of the patients and peptic lesions healed and the development of new ones prevented.[18,26,27,31,33] Unfortunately, in many patients this took high, frequent doses of the histamine H_2 receptor antagonists, and it was true for all members of this class with the dosing only varying by their potency.[18,26,27,31,33] Similarly, during times of surgery and when patients could not take oral medications, parenteral administration of histamine H_2 receptor antagonists required relatively high doses given by continuous intravenous administration.[18] Furthermore, patients treated long-term with histamine H_2 receptor antagonists required yearly reassessment of acid control and on average required one dosing change (usually an increase) once per year.[18,33,34] Because of the requirement for dose titration in all patients coupled with the decreasing availability of gastric acid analysis in the United States and in other countries until the development and availability of proton pump inhibitors (PPIs) in the 1980s,[35] both histamine H_2 receptor antagonists and the continued use of total gastrectomy and other surgical products, such as parietal cell vagotomy coupled with the use of histamine H_2 receptor antagonists, were used by different groups to control acid hypersecretion in patients with ZES from the 1970s to 1990s.[18,24,26,33,36]

Present: Control of Acid Hypersecretion: Medical Versus Surgical

At present the pendulum has swung almost 180° from the initial use of only surgical treatments to control acid hypersecretion in patients with ZES to the almost

---

205 patients with ZES without previous gastric acid reducing surgery. Each point represents data from one patient. The dotted line is the upper limit of normal. The mean ± standard error of the mean is shown for each. BAO, basal acid output; MAO, maximal ability to secrete acid. (*Data from* Refs.[3,15,58])

exclusive use of medical therapy. Currently, except for rare patients (<1%) who cannot or will not reliably take oral medications, PPIs have become the drugs of choice.[8,18,22,35,37] This change has occurred because PPIs have a long duration of action allowing once- or twice-a-day dosing in most patients, little tachyphylaxis is seen with less than 1 dosing change per year, and in most patients acid hypersecretion is adequately controlled without requiring dose titration with measurement of gastric acid secretory rates on the drug.[17,18,22,31] All PPIs (omeprazole, esomeprazole, lansoprazole, pantoprazole, rabeprazole) have been shown to be efficacious in ZES for controlling acid hypersecretion. PPIs have been proven safe and effective for greater than 10 years of treatment; except for low vitamin B_{12} levels in some patients, no side effects have limited their use.[17,18,21,31,38,39] From epidemiologic studies on patients without ZES taking long-term PPIs (GERD, idiopathic peptic ulcer disease, and so forth), several side effects of PPIs have been proposed, including bone fractures, dementia, hypomagnesemia, decrease nutrient absorption (vitamin B_{12}, iron, calcium, and so forth), interstitial renal disease, various bacterial overgrowths in the gut (clostridia and so forth), and interference with metabolism or absorption of several drugs.[40,41] There are no specific reports of these occurring with increased frequency in patients with ZES or limiting further PPI treatment.

In cases whereby patients cannot take oral medications (ie, during surgery, surgical recovery, and so forth), parenteral PPIs have also become the agents of choice because of their potency and long duration of action.[18,42] They can be given by intermittent intravenous injections, which are more convenient than prolonged continuous infusion of histamine H_2 receptor antagonists.[18,42]

Histamine H_2 receptor antagonists remain effective and can be used in rare patients who cannot take PPIs; however, they are rarely used today because of the need for high doses, frequent dosing, assessment of acid control to determine proper dosing, and for continuous infusion with parenteral administration.[8,18]

Although surgery is not the primary method for acute or long-term control of acid hypersecretion in patients without ZES, it plays a long-term role in its effect on gastric hypersecretion after curative resection of the gastrinoma. As mentioned earlier, cure is generally not possible in greater than 60% of all patients (**Fig. 2**) (discussed in detail in a later section); nevertheless, a significant proportion of patients can be rendered disease free after gastrinoma resection.[8,14,15,43–47] There are relatively few studies of the effect of the curative resection on acid secretory rates, but in several reports a proportion of disease-free patients are able to stop or significantly decrease all antisecretory drugs.[8,14,15,43–46,48] Four detailed prospective studies[42,48–50] of the effect of curative resection of the gastrinoma on disease-free status have been reported and provided some important findings. First, after a curative gastrinoma resection, the mean BAO decreased by 75% and the MAO by 50% and remained at similar levels for up to 4 years. Second, even though the BAO and MAO markedly decreased after curative resection, 67% of patients continued to show mild hypersecretion for up to 4 years even though the patients remained disease free (normal fasting serum gastrin levels, negative imaging, negative secretin tests) (**Fig. 3**A). Third, after curative resection the ranitidine daily dose could be reduce by 66% and 40% of patients could be removed from all antisecretory drugs. These results demonstrate that curative resection of the gastrinoma has a profound effect on the acid secretory rates, although some patients continue to show mild-moderate hypersecretion and require, by an unknown mechanism, low doses of antisecretory drugs at present, even though they are cured.

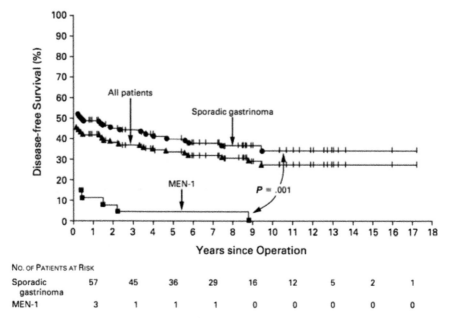

No. of Patients at Risk

Sporadic gastrinoma	57	45	36	29	16	12	5	2	1
MEN-1	3	1	1	1	0	0	0	0	0

Fig. 2. Disease-free survival after surgery (enucleation, resection) in patients with ZES with or without MEN1. Data are from 123 patients with sporadic ZES and 28 patients with MEN1/ZES. Patients were treated by a fixed protocol involving enucleation of tumor, local tumor resection, and distal pancreatectomy where indicated but without Whipple resections. (*Adapted from* Norton JA, Fraker DL, Alexander HR, et al. Surgery to cure the Zollinger-Ellison syndrome. N Engl J Med 1999;341:641; with permission.)

ROLES OF MEDICAL AND SURGICAL TREATMENT IN TREATMENT OF SPORADIC GASTRINOMA: PAST VERSUS PRESENT
General Points: Treatment Directed at Gastrinoma

Most patients with ZES have a sporadic, noninherited form (75%–80%), whereas the remainder (20%–25%) have it as part of the multiple endocrine neoplasia type 1 syndrome (MEN1/ZES), an autosomal dominant disorder.[51,52] This distinction is important for many aspects of the treatment, both directed at the acid hypersecretion and the gastrinoma itself.[51–53] In this section, treatment directed at the gastrinoma in sporadic cases is discussed; in a later section, the special aspects in the use of surgical or medical approaches for the treatment of MEN1/ZES are considered, and several are contentious.[16,53–56]

Initially, it was thought that almost all sporadic gastrinomas occurred in the pancreas, similar to insulinomas; however, it is now established that most (60%–95%) occur in the duodenum; in a recent series they were 3- to 9-fold more frequent than pancreatic gastrinomas.[15,45] Duodenal and pancreatic gastrinomas differ in their biological behavior in that both are associated with frequent lymph node metastases (30%–70%)[16,57,58]; however, the pancreatic tumors have a much higher rate of liver metastases,[57,58] which is one of the primary determinants of long-term survival (see **Fig. 1A**), with the result that patients with pancreatic gastrinomas have a worse prognosis.[57–59] Sporadic gastrinomas as a group are malignant in 60% to 90% of cases; approximately 13% to 53% (mean 34%) of patients have liver metastases at presentation, with most being diffuse liver involvement.[57–60]

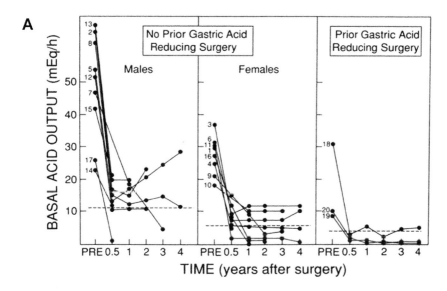

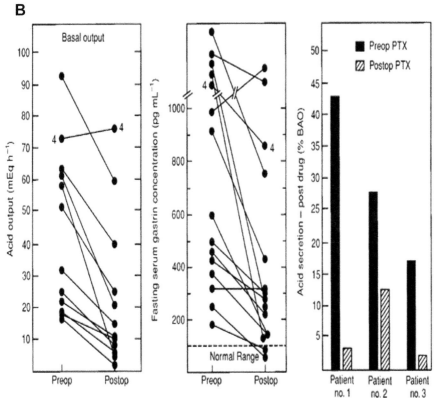

Fig. 3. Effect of curative gastrinoma resection on BAO (*A*) and effect of parathyroidectomy (PTX) (*B*) on basal acid hypersecretion, fasting serum gastrin levels, and responsiveness to antisecretory drugs in patients with MEN1/ZES with hyperparathyroidism. (*A*) Shown are results from 20 patients surgically rendered disease free. Mean preoperative (preop) BAO was

Past: Treatment Directed at Sporadic Gastrinoma: Nonsurgical Versus Surgical Approach

With the increased ability to medically control acid hypersecretion in patients with sporadic ZES since the 1980s, attention has shifted increasingly to the possible role of surgery for curative resection. Initially, several authorities recommended a nonoperative approach in patients with sporadic ZES with either small or no tumors imaged.[61,62] This approach was based on the fact that patients at that time were rarely cured, no gastrinoma was found at surgery in 30% to 60% of patients,[9,61,62] and because these patients generally did very well with long-term acid suppression alone.[61,62] This situation occurred primarily because it was not yet clear that most of the sporadic gastrinomas were in the duodenum and that only with a careful search could they be found (mobilization of duodenum, duodenotomy, transillumination of duodenum)[45,63–66] because they were often less than 1 cm in diameter[45,57,67] (**Fig. 4**A). Furthermore, it was not appreciated in patients with MEN1/ZES that the gastrinomas were also in the duodenum, the imaged pancreatic tumors were usually nonfunctional-panNETs(NF-panNETs), and that these patients could rarely be cured because of the multiplicity of the duodenal gastrinomas (see **Fig. 2**) without aggressive resections, such as a Whipple resection, which was not routinely recommended.[8,14,15,53,56,68]

Present: Treatment Directed at Sporadic Gastrinoma: Nonsurgical Versus Surgical Approach

In direct contrast to the treatment of gastric acid hypersecretion in sporadic ZES, which has changed from surgical to largely medical, the approach to the tumor has changed in most centers and has become increasingly surgical, with decreasing numbers of patients with potentially resectable sporadic disease followed medically with control of acid hypersecretion only. All existing guidelines, including from the European Neuroendocrine Tumor Society (ENET), the North American Neuroendocrine Tumor Society (NANET), the European Society for Medical Oncology, and the National Comprehensive Cancer Network,[8,12,13,69,70] recommend that in sporadic ZES surgical resection should be carried out if a complete tumor removal can be performed and there are no accompanying medical conditions limiting life expectancy or increasing surgical risks to unacceptable levels.

---

39 mEq/h, and the mean serum fasting gastrin 1020 pg/mL (nL <100). By 3 to 6 months postoperatively (postop) BAO had decreased 75% and remained unchanged. Dotted lines show upper limit of normal in these studies. (*B*) Shown are results from 10 consecutive patients with MEN1/ZES with hyperparathyroidism with BAO, fasting serum gastrin levels (FSG), and sensitivity to antisecretory drugs (histamine H_2 receptor antagonists determined before and a different times after parathyroidectomy. All patients except patient 4 became normocalcemic after parathyroidectomy. After parathyroidectomy, 9 of 10 (90%) had a decrease in BAO; 7 out of 10 showed a decrease in FSG, including to normal levels in 2 patients. Acid responsiveness was expressed as the percent of the BAO at a given time after taking the same dose of histamine H_2 receptor antagonist. In each of the 3 patients studied, the given dose of histamine H_2 receptor antagonist caused greater acid suppression after parathyroidectomy. (*Adapted from* [A] Pisegna JR, Norton JA, Slimak G, et al. Effects of curative resection on gastric secretory function and antisecretory drug requirement in the Zollinger-Ellison syndrome. Gastroenterology 1992;102:772, with permission; and [B] Norton JA, Cornelius MJ, Doppman JL, et al. Effect of parathyroidectomy in patients with hyperparathyroidism, Zollinger-Ellison syndrome and multiple endocrine neoplasia Type I: A prospective study. Surgery 1987;102:958–66, with permission.)

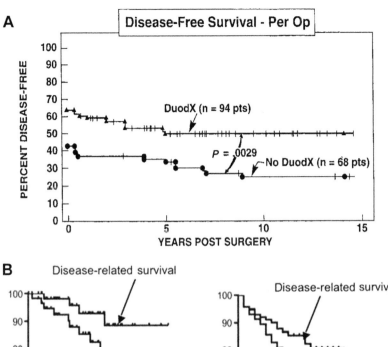

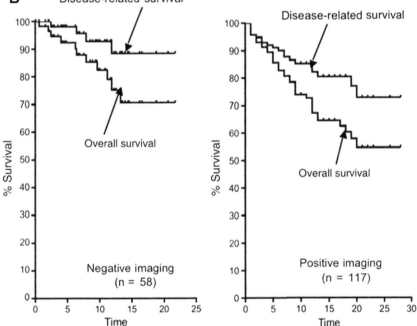

Fig. 4. Results of performing a duodenotomy (A) on disease-free status and results of surgical exploration for possible cure in patients with ZES with or without positive preoperative imaging studies (B). (A) Effect of duodenotomy (DUODX) on disease-free status in 142 patients with ZES without MEN1. With DUODX, gastrinomas were found in 98% and duodenal gastrinomas in 62%; the cure rate postoperatively was 65% compared with patients without DUODX (P <.01) in whom gastrinomas were found in 76%;18% had duodenal gastrinomas found, and 44% were cured after resection. Results expressed as the percentage of each operated rendered disease free (per op). Modified and drawn from data in.[45] (B) Surgical results from 117 patients with sporadic ZES with positive imaging are compared with results in 58 patients with sporadic ZES with negative preoperative imaging. Postoperatively 63% of the patients with negative imaging were disease free postoperatively, whereas it was

This change in approach to the sporadic gastrinoma to an increasing surgical option, whenever possible, has occurred for several reasons. First, acid hypersecretion can now be well controlled throughout the surgical period, whereas in the past, the lack of effective medical therapies for this resulted in mortalities as high as 30%.[9,25,30] Second, tumor imaging modalities (discussed later) have markedly improved in sensitivity making it possible to better localize the primary and stage the disease, preventing unnecessary surgery.[8,54,71] Third, more recent surgical studies have demonstrated increasing disease-free rates approaching 40% to 63% of patients operated on without Whipple resections[44–47,58] (see **Fig. 2**) and higher in patients with Whipple resections.[15,72] Fourth, importantly, 2 studies[73,74] have provided evidence that surgical resection in sporadic ZES leads to a decreased rate of the development of liver metastases, which is the most important determinate of long-term survival[57–59] (see **Fig. 1**A); also one study[74] demonstrated increased disease-related survival with surgery. Fifth, the surgical approach to find duodenal gastrinomas has been studied and demonstrated that specific techniques are needed to find this tumor (duodenotomy, mobilization of duodenum, intraoperative transillumination of duodenum in some cases)[45,63–66](see **Fig. 4**A). Sixth, a recent study demonstrates that even in patients with sporadic ZES with negative preoperative imaging studies, an experienced surgeon will find gastrinoma in 98% of the patients with 50% rendered disease free, which is not different from the results in patients with positive imaging preoperatively[44] (**Fig. 4**B). Seventh, the importance of routine lymphadenectomy in sporadic ZES has been emphasized in the number of studies and is now routinely recommended. The presence of lymph node primary gastrinomas is controversial, even though several studies have reported long-term (up to 20 years) disease-free survival after resection of only a lymph node.[75–78] Studies have reported increased disease-free survival when lymph nodes are routinely resected in patients with sporadic ZES.[47] Furthermore, in 2 studies,[14,77] the recurrence or relapse rate after achieving disease-free status after resection of a primary lymph node gastrinoma was lower than that after resection of a duodenal or pancreatic primary. Therefore, routine removal of lymph nodes cannot only increase the disease-free survival rate but the number of positive lymph nodes or the lymph node ratio also has important prognostic significance in gastrinomas and other panNETs.[12,79–83]

Present: Surgical Treatment Directed at Sporadic Gastrinoma: Controversies

Despite the general recommendation that patients with sporadic ZES should undergo surgical resection if possible, there are several specific areas in the surgical management that are controversial. In addition to the question of primary lymph node gastrinomas, which is discussed in the previous paragraph, other areas of controversy include the role of Whipple resection (cephalic pancreaticoduodenectomy); the role of laparoscopic surgery in patients with sporadic gastrinomas; the role of surgical resections in patients with advanced disease or disease possibly involving mesenteric

---

seen in 54% with positive imaging and at a 20-year follow-up, the negative imaging patients had a better survival (71% vs 58%) and better disease-related survival (88% vs 73% [$P = .15$]). pts, patients. (*From* [A] Norton JA, Alexander HR, Fraker DL, et al. Does the use of routine duodenotomy (DUODX) affect rate of cure, development of liver metastases or survival in patients with Zollinger-Ellison syndrome (ZES)? Ann Surg 2004;239:623, with permission; and [B] Norton JA, Fraker DL, Alexander HR, et al. Value of surgery in patients with negative imaging and sporadic zollinger-ellison syndrome. Ann Surg 2012;256:514, with permission.)

blood vessels; and the extent/timing of imaging in patients without tumors on cross-sectional imaging before or after surgical procedures.

Currently, in the different guidelines the preferred approach, if possible, is enucleation, local resection for pancreatic head lesions, or distal pancreatectomy when necessary for distal pancreatic lesions.[8,12,13,69,70] Whipple resections are generally reserved for large pancreatic head or duodenal lesions that are unable to be adequately removed with enucleation.[8,12,13,15,69,70] One of the main problems with rendering patients disease free is that lymph node metastases are found in 30% to 70% of cases and are, therefore, often missed without more extensive surgery, such as a Whipple resection. Studies support an increased disease-free rate with Whipple resection[15,72]; but because of possible long-term complications, coupled with the excellent prognosis of patients who are not cured but with small residual disease, more aggressive general use of Whipple resections is currently not generally recommended.[8,12,13,69,70]

Laparoscopic surgery is increasingly being used in patients with panNETs, especially those with localized insulinomas, NF-panNETs, and MEN1 with panNETs.[84–89] In contrast to these other panNETs, only a small number of patients with gastrinomas have been treated with laparoscopic surgery.[16,84,87,90–92] This circumstance is in large part because of the need for an extensive exploration with a Kocher maneuver, duodenotomy (see **Fig. 4**A), routine lymphadenectomy, and exploration of the gastrinoma triangle and liver as well as the biliary system that are required in patients with ZES.[16,55]

Similar to other advanced NETs, the role of surgical resection in patients with ZES with advanced metastatic disease or even with extensive invasive localized disease is not well defined. Unfortunately, most patients presenting with hepatic metastases with gastrinomas have metastases in both hepatic lobes, with only 5% to 15% having localized hepatic metastases.[57,58,60] If imaging studies support the resectability of the metastases, then surgical resection is generally recommended, if patients are operative candidates without other medical conditions precluding surgery.[8,12,43] Similarly, if most or all imaginable disease is thought surgically resectable, surgery is generally recommended.[8,12,43] Patients with gastrinomas, as well as other malignant panNETs/NETs not uncommonly present with local invasion and/or vessel encasement or possible involvement, which has led them to frequently not being considered surgical candidates.[93] A few recent studies have challenged this thinking.[93–95] One recent study[93] demonstrated 17% of all gastrinomas fall into this category demonstrating possible major vascular involvement (**Fig. 5**); in 42 patients a panNET could be resected, with only 9 patients requiring vascular reconstruction; 30% showed long-term disease-free status, and after resection the patients had a 10-year survival of 60%. This result[93] led the investigators to conclude that surgical resection of panNETs with vascular abutment/invasion is indicated and generally successful without requiring vascular reconstruction and, thus, should not be a contraindication to surgery.

Originally, cross-sectional imaging studies (computed tomography [CT], MRI, ultrasound) were primarily used to attempt to localize the primary tumor and establish the extent of the tumor involvement in patients with ZES. Even with dramatic improvements in sensitivity, most small gastrinomas (<1.0–1.5 cm) were missed[10,60,96,97]; other approaches were increasingly used, such as functional studies assessing gastrin gradients either after selective portal venous sampling or hepatic venous sampling after selective intra-arterial secretin injection,[60,98,99] which had sensitivities of 71% to 86%. The development of somatostatin receptor imaging (SRI), using the fact that gastrinomas, similar to most NETs, overexpress somatostatin receptors (primarily somatostatin receptor subtype 2 [sst2]), has largely replaced functional imaging studies, such as gastrin sampling.[8,16] Initially, indium-111−pentetreotide was used with single-

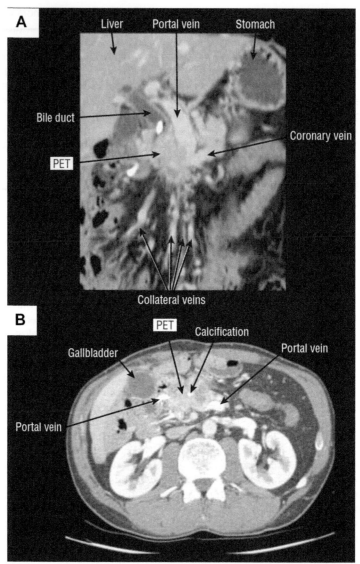

Fig. 5. Imaging results in a patient with a panNET obstructing the proximal portal vein. (*A*) A coronal planar view and (*B*) a transverse view of the computed tomography scan. The label PET shows the location of a panNET obstructing the proximal portal vein and with the development of extensive collateral veins. This patient had the tumor and a portion of the portal vein resected with venous reconstruction. This patient is representative of a subgroup of gastrinomas and other PanNET that are thought by many to be unresectable because of the vascular involvement; however, a recent study[93] shows most are resectable. (*Adapted from* Norton JA, Harris EJ, Chen Y, et al. Pancreatic endocrine tumors with major vascular abutment, involvement, or encasement and indication for resection. Arch Surg 2011;146:725; with permission.)

photon emission CT/CT imaging and shown to be more sensitive that any cross-sectional imaging study to allow whole-body scans at one time and to be the most sensitive modality for localizing distant metastases in patients with advanced ZES.[12,16,100–102] Recently, this is being replaced by gallium-68 (^{68}Ga)-DOTATATE-somatostatin peptide PET/CT, which has even greater sensitivity and is now approved for use in both the United States and Europe.[71,96,103,104] Endoscopic ultrasound (EUS) is the most sensitive modality for detecting intrapancreatic lesions, but its utility is limited in patients with sporadic ZES because most gastrinomas are duodenal and these are missed on EUS.[8,15] In general, almost all patients with sporadic ZES undergo a conventional imaging study; it is recommended that they also should have SRI, preferably with ^{68}Ga-DOTATATE-somatostain peptide PET/CT, especially if a surgical procedure is considered.[12,16,71,96] At present, the best timing of imaging tests postsurgically is not established or whether they will be more sensitive than functional studies (ie, assessing serum gastrin, secretin testing) in detecting recurrences postoperatively in patients with ZES.

ROLES OF MEDICAL AND SURGICAL TREATMENT IN TREATMENT OF MULTIPLE ENDOCRINE NEOPLASIA TYPE 1/ZOLLINGER-ELLISON SYNDROME: PAST VERSUS PRESENT

General Points: Treatment of Multiple Endocrine Neoplasia Type 1/Zollinger-Ellison Syndrome

The 20% to 25% of patients with ZES due to MEN1 (MEN1/ZES) have several specific problems due to the presence of MEN1 that affect the medical and surgical treatments.[51–53,55] Patients with MEN1 characteristically develop hyperplasia/tumors of multiple endocrine organs, with 98% to 100% developing multiple parathyroid adenomas with hyperparathyroidism, 80% to 100% developing panNETs, and 50% to 60% developing pituitary adenomas.[51–53,55] For the panNETs, 80% to 100% develop microscopic NF-panNETs (0%–13% -symptomatic) and 54% develop MEN1/ZES (range 20%–61%), whereas insulinomas occur in 18% (range 7%–31%), with the other F-panNET syndromes occurring in less than 3%.[51–53,55] These patients also developed tumors in other organs to a lesser extent, including adrenal adenomas/carcinomas (27%–36%), carcinoid tumors (bronchial/lung [0%–8%], gastric [7%–35%], thymic [0%–8%%]), nonendocrine tumors of the skin (angiofibromas/collagenomas [60%–90%]), central nervous system tumors (meningiomas, schwannomas, ependymomas) (0%–8%), and smooth muscle tumors (1%–7%-leiomyomas/leiomyosarcomas).[51,55,105] Characteristically, these patients present with hyperparathyroidism; however, in some recent series up to 33% present with F-panNETS.[52,106,107]

The specific features of MEN1 create several unique problems in the medical and/or surgical management of ZES in these patients. First, the hyperparathyroidism can affect the activity of the hormone excess state of the F-panNET, such as gastrin/acid secretion and the control of the acid hypersecretion in MEN1/ZES[18,108–110] (see **Fig. 3**B). Second, microscopic NF-panNETs are present in all patients with MEN1 and larger sizes in up to 80% and, thus, not only may require treatment but their presence complicates the localization of the gastrinoma.[51,53,54,111] In 85% to 100% of patients with MEN1/ZES in different series, the gastrinomas occur in the duodenum; however, in a minority of patients (0%–15%) they are reported in the pancreas.[51,53,112–114] Third, in patients with MEN1/ZES the duodenal gastrinomas are almost always multiple, frequently small (<0.5 cm), and associated with lymph node metastases in 40% to 60%.[53,113,115] The result of this is patients with MEN1/ZES cannot be cured of all their NF-panNETs or gastrinomas (see **Fig. 2**) without aggressive resections, such as Whipple resection.[51,53,54] In contrast, other

F-panNETs in patients with MEN1 (insulinomas, glucagonomas, and so forth) are generally curable.[51,53,116] Fourth, the natural history of patients with MEN1 is changing; however, it is at present largely unknown, although the mean age at death is still shortened at 55 to 60 years old in several studies.[53,105,117] Patients with MEN1 are now rarely dying of acid hypersecretion due to MEN1/ZES, which was a major cause of death in early series.[52,53,105,117] However, other tumors, such as thymic carcinoids, are now increasingly described in patients with MEN1, especially adult males, and are aggressive and an increasing cause of death.[53,105,117] The lack of the long-term natural history is particularly important for NF-panNETs and gastrinomas, because in many cases these patients are treated without surgery, as discussed later.

Present: Specific Aspects of Control of Acid Hypersecretion in Multiple Endocrine Neoplasia Type 1/Zollinger-Ellison Syndrome: Medical Versus Surgical

In general, the management of acid secretion in patients with MEN1/ZES follows the patterns discussed earlier in the paragraphs regarding acid hypersecretion in sporadic ZES, with initially only a surgical approach with total gastrectomy being effective, to later when an increasing medical approach has been used, first with histamine H_2 receptor antagonists and still later PPIs were increasingly used. At present, as for sporadic ZES, the drugs of choice both for control of the acid hypersecretion in patients with MEN1/ZES are PPIs.[8,11,13,18]

However, surgery can still play an important role in facilitating control of acid hypersecretion in patients with MEN1/ZES. In contrast to the situation in patients with sporadic ZES whereby acid hypersecretion could be markedly altered by curing a significant number of patients, cure is rare in MEN1/ZES without aggressive resections, which are not routinely recommended in any current guidelines (ENET's, NANET's).[12,51,69] Surgery can play a role in facilitating the control of acid hypersecretion in patients with MEN1/ZES by correcting the hyperparathyroidism by an appropriate parathyroidectomy (ie, 3.5 gland or 4.0 gland removal with a parathyroid implant)[51,52,108,110] (**Fig. 2**B). From acid secretory studies in patients with MEN1/ZES with hyperparathyroidism, increased relative resistance to the effects of antisecretory drugs have been reported and higher drug doses than in patients with sporadic ZES are frequently required.[118] Calcium is a potent stimulator of gastrin release from gastrinomas[119]; several studies report that patients with MEN1/ZES with hypercalcemia due to hyperparathyroidism, when the hyperparathyroidism is corrected, have a decreased magnitude of hypergastrinemia (sometimes gastrin levels return to normal), a decrease in secretin-stimulated gastrin release, and an increase in sensitivity to antisecretion drugs (see **Fig. 2**B).[108,112,120]

Present: Treatment-Directed at Multiple Endocrine Neoplasia Type 1/Pancreatic Endocrine Tumor/Gastrinoma: Nonsurgical Versus Surgical Approach

At present, this is an area of considerable disagreement between a surgical and nonsurgical approach. Whereas all agree that patients with F-panNETs with MEN1, excluding gastrinomas, should undergo routinely surgical exploration because of their high (>90%–100%) cure rate, this is not the case with patients with gastrinomas or with NF-panNETs.[12,13,51,53,116] As stated earlier, gastrinomas/NF-panNETs are almost always multiple and often small (<0.5 cm); thus, they are rarely curable unless aggressive resections are performed, such as Whipple resections or even total pancreatectomy with NF-panNETs.[15,51,53,121,122] This fact, coupled with increasing evidence that patients with panNETs or MEN1/ZES with small tumors (<1.5–2.0 cm) have an excellent long-term prognosis without surgery[8,51,53,54,121,123,124] (**Fig. 6**), has led to the current controversy on their treatment. An additional point that contributes to this

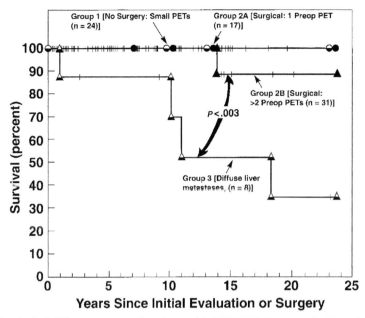

Fig. 6. Survival of different groups of patients with MEN1/ZES. Data are for 81 patients with MEN1/ZES of which 17 were in group 1 (all panNETs imaged preoperatively [preop] <2.5-cm diameter, no surgery) and group 3 (n = 8) with diffuse liver metastases and no surgical resection. Group 2 consisted of 17 patients in group 2A with a single panNET (2.5–6.0 cm in diameter) and group 2B (n = 31) with 2 or more lesions greater than 2.5 cm, who underwent laparotomy. Groups 1, 2A, and 2B had similar 15-year survival rates of 89% to 100%, which were better than patients with diffuse liver metastases in group 3 (52%). This study concluded that patients with small panNETs less than 2.5 cm with MEN1/ZES can be followed without surgery (15-year survival = 100%) and that patients with larger lesions should have them resected if possible. (*Adapted from* Norton JA, Alexander HR, Fraker DL, et al. Comparison of surgical results in patients with advanced and limited disease with multiple endocrine neoplasia type 1 and Zollinger-Ellison syndrome. Ann Surg 2001;234:503; with permission.)

controversy is that these patients frequently present at younger ages than seen with sporadic forms of these tumors and are often asymptomatic in the case of NF-panNETs. Not only are these resections associated with morbidity/mortality but long-term complications can also occur. Also, recent studies report patients with MEN1 have an increased incidence of diabetes/glucose intolerance, which is not uncommon after pancreatic resections, reported in 24% to 86% of patients with MEN1 after resection and 17% to 25% after pancreaticoduodenectomy.[53]

Current recommendations from several societies, including the ENET, the NANET, and the Endocrine Society,[8,12,13,125] recommend that small panNETs (<1.5–2.0 cm) in patients with NF-panNETs or MEN1/ZES be treated conservatively. All agree that if patients with these small panNETs are treated conservatively, it is important that they be closely monitored. How to best monitor these small panNETs in patients with MEN1 is also an area of contention.[54] Cross-sectional imaging studies will miss greater than 50% of lesions less than 1.5 cm; however, SRI has greater sensitivity, but it is not established to be reliable for assessing serial changes in tumor size; the issue of repeated radiation exposure can be a factor in these patients.[53,54] Numerous studies show that for intrapancreatic NETs, such as NF-panNETs, EUS is the most sensitive modality for their detection and allows accurate assessment of changes in NET size on repeated examinations.[54,89,126–128] Serial studies show that most pan-NETs in patients with MEN1 less than 2 cm are relatively stable and uncommonly increase rapidly in size.[54,127,129–131] In MEN1/ZES with imaged NETs less than 2 cm, the role of EUS is much more limited because these NETs are not intrapancreatic and often missed by EUS; thus, they are usually followed by repeated cross-sectional imaging studies.[54] Although recent studies demonstrate that ^{68}Ga-DOTATATE-PET/CT is much more sensitive for detecting lesions in patients with MEN1 than cross-sectional imaging, at present its exact role initially and in follow-up is unclear and controversial in patients with MEN1.[54,132–135]

One of the most pressing problems is to identify predictors in patients with NF-pan-NETs or gastrinomas, which will identify those patients whose tumors will pursue an aggressive course in patients with MEN1.[53,105,136] Although numerous factors (both clinical and tumoral features) have been reported to have prognostic value in patients with MEN1 for the development of a panNETs or their aggressive behavior, similar to patients with sporadic panNETs, in general they are not particularly helpful in a given patient.[51,59,105,136–139] In sporadic panNETs, the World Health Organization's grading has been shown to have important prognostic value.[12,140,141] Preliminary studies in patients with MEN1 suggest that the histologic grade of the tumors has predictive value; however, most (>80%) are G1 and some of these can also pursue an aggressive course.[142] Recently, the predictive value of using fludeoxyglucose F-18 (^{18}F-FDG) PET/CT has been proposed for patients with MEN1 with panNETs.[143] Numerous studies demonstrate that in most well-differentiated NETs (G1, G2), the ^{18}F-FDG PET/CT is negative; but in a proportion it is positive, and this correlates with aggressive behavior.[71] In the aforementioned recent study[143] in 49 patients with MEN1 undergoing ^{18}F-FDG PET, 6 out of 8 patients (75%) with FDG-avid panNETs harbored aggressive or metastatic NETs, compared with only 1 of 41 (2.4%) without FDG avidity for a sensitivity of 86% and a specificity of 95% for identifying aggressive panNETs. Although a few genotype-phenotype correlations with prognostic value have been reported in patients with MEN1 with panNETs, including mutations in JunD, CHES1, truncation mutations in the N- or C-terminal of the MEN1 gene, missense mutations in the MEN1 gene, and the CDNK1B V109 G polymorphism, they have not been well studied prospectively and are not widely used at present.[131,139,144–148]

A laparoscopic approach is being increasingly used in MEN1 patients with insulinomas, other localized nongastrinoma panNETs and NF-panNETs, but is not generally used in patients with MEN1/ZES, except the occasional patient with a gastrinoma limited to the pancreatic tail.[86,89,149] In a meta-analysis[150] of pancreatic distal resection for all indications, the laparoscopic approach resulted in a lower complication rate, less blood loss, and shorter hospital stays; however, the rate of development of postoperative fistulas was similar. Whereas the results in patients with MEN1 are more limited, the available results support the conclusions that minimally invasive approaches in patients with MEN1 with the panNETs listed earlier are safe and feasible.[86,89]

ROLES OF MEDICAL AND SURGICAL TREATMENT IN TREATMENT OF PATIENTS WITH MULTIPLE ENDOCRINE NEOPLASIA TYPE 1/ZOLLINGER-ELLISON SYNDROME WITH ADVANCED DISEASE

As discussed earlier in the section regarding the treatment of MEN1/ZES, unfortunately most patients with advanced metastatic disease with MEN1/ZES present with diffuse hepatic metastases; in only a minority (<15%) is surgical resection (ie, generally, removal of least 90% of the disease) possible and recommended.[13,57,75,124,151] The patients with advanced metastatic disease that is nonresectable and progressive have a decreased survival (see **Figs. 1** and **6**) and, thus, require treatment that involves several possible antitumor nonsurgical approaches. These approaches include medical therapy (everolimus or tyrosine kinase inhibitors, such as sunitinib), peptide radioreceptor therapy with luteium-177–labeled somatostatin analogues (which will likely be approved by the Food and Drug Administration this coming year based on a recent successful phase 3 trial in gastrointestinal midgut NETs[152]), chemotherapy, or liver-directed therapies (embolization, chemoembolization, radioembolization). These treatments are similar to those in other advanced NETs and are not specific for MEN1/ZES and have been recently reviewed in other publications,[153–157] so are not dealt with further in this article.

REFERENCES

1. Zollinger RM, Ellison EH. Primary peptic ulcerations of the jejunum associated with islet cell tumors of the pancreas. Ann Surg 1955;142:709–28.
2. Stabile BE. Gastrinoma before Zollinger and Ellison. Am J Surg 1997;174:232–6.
3. Roy PK, Venzon DJ, Feigenbaum KM, et al. Gastric secretion in Zollinger-Ellison syndrome: correlation with clinical expression, tumor extent and role in diagnosis - a prospective NIH study of 235 patients and review of the literature in 984 cases. Medicine(Baltimore) 2001;80:189–222.
4. Ellison EC, Johnson JA. The Zollinger-Ellison syndrome: a comprehensive review of historical, scientific, and clinical considerations. Curr Probl Surg 2009; 46:13–106.
5. Berna MJ, Hoffmann KM, Serrano J, et al. Serum gastrin in Zollinger-Ellison syndrome: I. Prospective study of fasting serum gastrin in 309 patients from the National Institutes of Health and comparison with 2229 cases from the literature. Medicine (Baltimore) 2006;85:295–330.
6. Roy PK, Venzon DJ, Shojamanesh H, et al. Zollinger-Ellison syndrome: clinical presentation in 261 patients. Medicine (Baltimore) 2000;79:379–411.
7. Rehfeld JF, van Solinge WW. The tumor biology of gastrin and cholecystokinin. Adv Cancer Res 1994;63:295–347.
8. Jensen RT, Niederle B, Mitry E, et al. Gastrinoma (duodenal and pancreatic). Neuroendocrinology 2006;84:173–82.
9. Jensen RT, Gardner JD. Gastrinoma. In: Go VLW, DiMagno EP, Gardner JD, et al, editors. The pancreas: biology, pathobiology and disease. New York: Raven Press Publishing Co; 1993. p. 931–78.
10. Metz DC, Jensen RT. Gastrointestinal neuroendocrine tumors:; pancreatic endocrine tumors. Gastroenterology 2008;135:1469–92.
11. Ito T, Igarashi H, Jensen RT. Pancreatic neuroendocrine tumors: clinical features, diagnosis and medical treatment: advances. Best Pract Res Clin Gastroenterol 2012;26:737–53.
12. Falconi M, Eriksson B, Kaltsas G, et al. ENETS consensus guidelines update for the management of patients with functional pancreatic neuroendocrine tumors and non-functional pancreatic neuroendocrine tumors. Neuroendocrinology 2016;103:153–71.
13. Jensen RT, Cadiot G, Brandi ML, et al. ENETS consensus guidelines for the management of patients with digestive neuroendocrine neoplasms: functional pancreatic endocrine tumor syndromes. Neuroendocrinology 2012;95:98–119.

14. Norton JA, Fraker DL, Alexander HR, et al. Surgery to cure the Zollinger-Ellison syndrome. N Engl J Med 1999;341:635–44.
15. Norton JA, Jensen RT. Resolved and unresolved controversies in the surgical management of patients with Zollinger-Ellison syndrome. Ann Surg 2004;240: 757–73.
16. Ito T, Igarashi H, Jensen RT. Zollinger-Ellison syndrome: recent advances and controversies. Curr Opin Gastroenterol 2013;29:650–61.
17. Metz DC, Strader DB, Orbuch M, et al. Use of omeprazole in Zollinger-Ellison: a prospective nine-year study of efficacy and safety. Aliment Pharmacol Ther 1993;7:597–610.
18. Ito T, Igarashi H, Uehara H, et al. Pharmacotherapy of Zollinger-Ellison syndrome. Expert Opin Pharmacother 2013;14:307–21.
19. Ellison EC, O'Dorisio TM, Woltering EA, et al. Suppression of gastrin and gastric acid secretion in the Zollinger-Ellison syndrome by long-acting somatostatin (SMS 201-995). Scand J Gastroenterol 1986;21(Suppl 119):206–11.
20. Guida PM, Todd JE, Moore SW, et al. Zollinger-Ellison syndrome with interesting variations. Am J Surg 1966;112:807–17.
21. Maton PN, Lack EE, Collen MJ, et al. The effect of Zollinger-Ellison syndrome and omeprazole therapy on gastric oxyntic endocrine cells. Gastroenterology 1990;99:943–50.
22. Jensen RT. Consequences of long-term proton pump blockade: highlighting insights from studies of patients with gastrinomas. Basic Clin Pharmacol Toxicol 2006;98:4–19.
23. Peghini PL, Annibale B, Azzoni C, et al. Effect of chronic hypergastrinemia on human enterochromaffin-like cells: insights from patients with sporadic gastrinomas. Gastroenterology 2002;123:68–85.
24. Jensen RT. Basis for failure of cimetidine in patients with Zollinger-Ellison syndrome. Dig Dis Sci 1984;29:363–6.
25. Ellison EH, Wilson SD. The Zollinger-Ellison syndrome: re-appraisal and evaluation of 260 registered cases. Ann Surg 1964;160:512–30.
26. Metz DC, Pisegna JR, Fishbeyn VA, et al. Control of gastric acid hypersecretion in the management of patients with Zollinger-Ellison syndrome. World J Surg 1993;17:468–80.
27. Raufman JP, Collins SM, Pandol SJ, et al. Reliability of symptoms in assessing control of gastric acid secretion in patients with Zollinger-Ellison syndrome. Gastroenterology 1983;84:108–13.
28. Jensen RT, Gardner JD, Raufman JP, et al. Zollinger-Ellison syndrome: current concepts and management. Ann Intern Med 1983;98:59–75.
29. Maton PN, Mackem SM, Norton JA, et al. Ovarian carcinoma as a cause of Zollinger-Ellison syndrome. Natural history, secretory products and response to provocative tests. Gastroenterology 1989;97:468–71.
30. Fox PS, Hofmann JW, Wilson SD, et al. Surgical management of the Zollinger-Ellison syndrome. Surg Clin North Am 1974;54:395–407.
31. Jensen RT. Use of omeprazole and other proton pump inhibitors in the Zollinger-Ellison syndrome. In: Olbe L, editor. Milestones in drug therapy. Basel (Switzerland): Birkhauser Verlag AG Publish. Co; 1999. p. 205–21.
32. McCarthy DM, Olinger EJ, May RJ, et al. H_2-histamine receptor blocking agents in the Zollinger-Ellison syndrome. Experience in seven cases and implications for long-term therapy. Ann Intern Med 1977;87:668–75.
33. Collen MJ, Howard JM, McArthur KE, et al. Comparison of ranitidine and cimetidine in the treatment of gastric hypersecretion. Ann Intern Med 1984;100:52–8.

34. Wolfe MM, Jensen RT. Zollinger-Ellison syndrome: current concepts in diagnosis and management. N Engl J Med 1987;317:1200–9.
35. Lamers CBHW, Lind T, Moberg S, et al. Omeprazole in Zollinger-Ellison syndrome: effects of a single dose and of long term treatment in patients resistant to histamine H_2-receptor antagonists. N Engl J Med 1984;310:758–61.
36. Brennan MF, Sloan AP, Friesen SR, et al. Is total gastrectomy still acceptable in the treatment of the Zollinger-Ellison syndrome. Langenbecks Arch Chir 1986; 367:215–21.
37. Nieto JM, Pisegna JR. The role of proton pump inhibitors in the treatment of Zollinger-Ellison syndrome. Expert Opin Pharmacother 2006;7:169–75.
38. Hirschowitz BI, Simmons J, Mohnen J. Clinical outcome using lansoprazole in acid hypersecretors with and without Zollinger-Ellison syndrome: a 13-year prospective study. Clin Gastroenterol Hepatol 2005;3:39–48.
39. Termanini B, Gibril F, Sutliff VE III, et al. Effect of long-term gastric acid suppressive therapy on serum vitamin B_{12} levels in patients with Zollinger-Ellison syndrome. Am J Med 1998;104:422–30.
40. Ito T, Jensen RT. Association of long-term proton pump inhibitor therapy with bone fractures and effects on absorption of calcium, vitamin b(12), iron, and magnesium. Curr Gastroenterol Rep 2010;12:448–57.
41. Eusebi LH, Rabitti S, Artesiani ML, et al. Proton pump inhibitors: risks of long-term use. J Gastroenterol Hepatol 2017;32:1295–302.
42. Metz DC, Benya RV, Fishbeyn VA, et al. Prospective study of the need for long-term antisecretory therapy in patients with Zollinger-Ellison syndrome following successful curative gastrinoma resection. Aliment Pharmacol Ther 1993;7(#3): 247–57.
43. Krampitz GW, Norton JA. Current management of the Zollinger-Ellison syndrome. Adv Surg 2013;47:59–79.
44. Norton JA, Fraker DL, Alexander HR, et al. Value of surgery in patients with negative imaging and sporadic Zollinger-Ellison syndrome. Ann Surg 2012; 256:509–17.
45. Norton JA, Alexander HR, Fraker DL, et al. Does the use of routine duodenotomy (DUODX) affect rate of cure, development of liver metastases or survival in patients with Zollinger-Ellison syndrome (ZES)? Ann Surg 2004;239:617–26.
46. Atema JJ, Amri R, Busch OR, et al. Surgical treatment of gastrinomas: a single-centre experience. HPB (Oxford) 2012;14:833–8.
47. Bartsch DK, Waldmann J, Fendrich V, et al. Impact of lymphadenectomy on survival after surgery for sporadic gastrinoma. Br J Surg 2012;99:1234–40.
48. Pisegna JR, Norton JA, Slimak GG, et al. Effects of curative resection on gastric secretory function and antisecretory drug requirement in the Zollinger-Ellison syndrome. Gastroenterology 1992;102:767–78.
49. Fraker DL, Norton JA, Saeed ZA, et al. A prospective study of perioperative and postoperative control of acid hypersecretion in patients with Zollinger-Ellison syndrome. Surgery 1988;104:1054–63.
50. Ojeaburu JV, Ito T, Crafa P, et al. Mechanism of acid hypersecretion post curative gastrinoma resection. Dig Dis Sci 2011;56:139–54.
51. Jensen RT, Berna MJ, Bingham MD, et al. Inherited pancreatic endocrine tumor syndromes: advances in molecular pathogenesis, diagnosis, management and controversies. Cancer 2008;113(7 suppl):1807–43.
52. Gibril F, Schumann M, Pace A, et al. Multiple endocrine neoplasia type 1 and Zollinger-Ellison syndrome. A prospective study of 107 cases and comparison with 1009 patients from the literature. Medicine (Baltimore) 2004;83:43–83.

53. Jensen RT, Norton JA. Treatment of pancreatic neuroendocrine tumors in multiple endocrine neoplasia type 1: some clarity but continued controversy. Pancreas 2017;46:589–94.

54. Ito T, Jensen RT. Imaging in multiple endocrine neoplasia type 1: recent studies show enhanced sensitivities but increased controversies. Int J Endocr Oncol 2016;3:53–66.

55. Norton JA, Krampitz G, Jensen RT. Multiple endocrine neoplasia: genetics and clinical management. Surg Oncol Clin N Am 2015;24:795–832.

56. Lopez CL, Waldmann J, Fendrich V, et al. Long-term results of surgery for pancreatic neuroendocrine neoplasms in patients with MEN1. Langenbecks Arch Surg 2011;396:1187–97.

57. Weber HC, Venzon DJ, Lin JT, et al. Determinants of metastatic rate and survival in patients with Zollinger-Ellison syndrome: a prospective long-term study. Gastroenterology 1995;108:1637–49.

58. Yu F, Venzon DJ, Serrano J, et al. Prospective study of the clinical course, prognostic factors and survival in patients with longstanding Zollinger-Ellison syndrome. J Clin Oncol 1999;17:615–30.

59. Jensen RT. Natural history of digestive endocrine tumors. In: Mignon M, Colombel JF, editors. Recent advances in pathophysiology and management of inflammatory bowel diseases and digestive endocrine tumors. Paris: John Libbey Eurotext Publishing Co; 1999. p. 192–219.

60. Jensen RT. Zollinger-Ellison syndrome. In: Doherty GM, Skogseid B, editors. Surgical endocrinology: clinical syndromes. Philadelphia: Lippincott Williams & Wilkins; 2001. p. 291–344.

61. McCarthy DM. The place of surgery in the Zollinger-Ellison syndrome. N Engl J Med 1980;302:1344–7.

62. Hirschowitz BI. Clinical course of nonsurgically treated Zollinger-Ellison syndrome. In: Mignon M, Jensen RT, editors. Endocrine tumors of the pancreas: recent advances in research and management. Frontiers of gastrointestinal research. Basel (Switzerland): S. Karger; 1995. p. 360–71.

63. Norton JA, Doppman JL, Jensen RT. Curative resection in Zollinger-Ellison syndrome: results of a 10-year prospective study. Ann Surg 1992;215:8–18.

64. Frucht H, Norton JA, London JF, et al. Detection of duodenal gastrinomas by operative endoscopic transillumination: a prospective study. Gastroenterology 1990;99:1622–7.

65. Sugg SL, Norton JA, Fraker DL, et al. A prospective study of intraoperative methods to diagnose and resect duodenal gastrinomas. Ann Surg 1993;218:138–44.

66. Thompson NW, Pasieka J, Fukuuchi A. Duodenal gastrinomas, duodenotomy, and duodenal exploration in the surgical management of Zollinger-Ellison syndrome. World J Surg 1993;17:455–62.

67. Thom AK, Norton JA, Axiotis CA, et al. Location, incidence and malignant potential of duodenal gastrinomas. Surgery 1991;110:1086–93.

68. Thompson NW, Bondeson AG, Bondeson L, et al. The surgical treatment of gastrinoma in MEN I syndrome patients. Surgery 1989;106:1081–5.

69. Kunz PL, Reidy-Lagunes D, Anthony LB, et al. Consensus guidelines for the management and treatment of neuroendocrine tumors. Pancreas 2013;42:557–77.

70. Oberg K, Knigge U, Kwekkeboom D, et al. Neuroendocrine gastro-enteropancreatic tumors: ESMO clinical practice guidelines for diagnosis, treatment and follow-up. Ann Oncol 2012;23(Suppl 7):vii124–30.

71. Ito T, Jensen RT. Molecular imaging in neuroendocrine tumors: recent advances, controversies, unresolved issues, and roles in management. Curr Opin Endocrinol Diabetes Obes 2017;24:15–24.

72. Giovinazzo F, Butturini G, Monsellato D, et al. Lymph nodes metastasis and recurrences justify an aggressive treatment of gastrinoma. Updates Surg 2013;65:19–24.

73. Fraker DL, Norton JA, Alexander HR, et al. Surgery in Zollinger-Ellison syndrome alters the natural history of gastrinoma. Ann Surg 1994;220:320–30.

74. Norton JA, Fraker DL, Alexander HR, et al. Surgery increases survival in patients with gastrinoma. Ann Surg 2006;244:410–9.

75. Norton JA, Alexander HA, Fraker DL, et al. Possible primary lymph node gastrinomas: occurrence, natural history and predictive factors: a prospective study. Ann Surg 2003;237:650–9.

76. Arnold WS, Fraker DL, Alexander HR, et al. Apparent lymph node primary gastrinoma. Surgery 1994;116:1123–30.

77. Chen Y, Deshpande V, Ferrone C, et al. Primary lymph node gastrinoma: a single institution experience. Surgery 2017;162:1088–94.

78. Harper S, Carroll RW, Frilling A, et al. Primary lymph node gastrinoma: 2 cases and a review of the literature. J Gastrointest Surg 2015;19:651–5.

79. Krampitz GW, Norton JA, Poultsides GA, et al. Lymph nodes and survival in duodenal and pancreatic neuroendocrine tumors. Arch Surg 2012;147:820–7.

80. Conrad C, Kutlu OC, Dasari A, et al. Prognostic value of lymph node status and extent of lymphadenectomy in pancreatic neuroendocrine tumors confined to and extending beyond the pancreas. J Gastrointest Surg 2016;20:1966–74.

81. Zhang X, Lu L, Shang Y, et al. The number of positive lymph node is a better predictor of survival than the lymph node metastasis status for pancreatic neuroendocrine neoplasms: a retrospective cohort study. Int J Surg 2017;48:142–8.

82. Curran T, Pockaj BA, Gray RJ, et al. Importance of lymph node involvement in pancreatic neuroendocrine tumors: impact on survival and implications for surgical resection. J Gastrointest Surg 2015;19:152–60.

83. Liu P, Zhang X, Shang Y, et al. Lymph node ratio, but not the total number of examined lymph nodes or lymph node metastasis, is a predictor of overall survival for pancreatic neuroendocrine neoplasms after surgical resection. Oncotarget 2017;8:89245–55.

84. Heniford BT, Arca MJ, Iannitii DA, et al. Laparoscopic cryoablation of hepatic metastases. Semin Surg Oncol 1998;15:194–201.

85. Shoji H, Kuroki M, Nakano E, et al. An enucleated duodenal gastrinoma with multiple type 1 endocrine neoplasia located by selective arterial calcium injection. Nihon Shokakibyo Gakkai Zasshi 2011;108:80–7.

86. Lopez CL, Albers MB, Bollmann C, et al. Minimally invasive versus open pancreatic surgery in patients with multiple endocrine neoplasia type 1. World J Surg 2016;40(7):1729–36.

87. Fernandez-Cruz L, Blanco L, Cosa R, et al. Is laparoscopic resection adequate in patients with neuroendocrine pancreatic tumors? World J Surg 2008;32:904–17.

88. Fernandez Ranvier GG, Shouhed D, Inabnet WB III. Minimally invasive techniques for resection of pancreatic neuroendocrine tumors. Surg Oncol Clin N Am 2016;25:195–215.

89. Nell S, Brunaud L, Ayav A, et al. Robot-assisted spleen preserving pancreatic surgery in MEN1 patients. J Surg Oncol 2016;114:456–61.

90. Haugvik SP, Marangos IP, Rosok BI, et al. Long-term outcome of laparoscopic surgery for pancreatic neuroendocrine tumors. World J Surg 2013;37:582–90.

91. Atalar K, Warren OJ, Jacyna M, et al. Laparoscopic resection for primary lymph node gastrinoma. Pancreas 2013;42:723–5.

92. Murase N, Uchida H, Tainaka T, et al. Laparoscopic-assisted pancreaticoduodenectomy in a child with gastrinoma. Pediatr Int 2015;57:1196–8.

93. Norton JA, Harris EJ, Chen Y, et al. Pancreatic endocrine tumors with major vascular abutment, involvement, or encasement and indication for resection. Arch Surg 2011;146:724–32.

94. Haugvik SP, Labori KJ, Waage A, et al. Pancreatic surgery with vascular reconstruction in patients with locally advanced pancreatic neuroendocrine tumors. J Gastrointest Surg 2013;17:1224–32.

95. Prakash L, Lee JE, Yao J, et al. Role and operative technique of portal venous tumor thrombectomy in patients with pancreatic neuroendocrine tumors. J Gastrointest Surg 2015;19:2011–8.

96. Sundin A, Arnold R, Baudin E, et al. ENETS consensus guidelines for the standards of care in neuroendocrine tumors: radiological, nuclear medicine & hybrid imaging. Neuroendocrinology 2017;105:212–44.

97. Krudy AG, Doppman JL, Jensen RT, et al. Localization of islet cell tumors by dynamic CT: comparison with plain CT, arteriography, sonography and venous sampling. Am J Roentgenol 1984;143:585–9.

98. Cherner JA, Doppman JL, Norton JA, et al. Selective venous sampling for gastrin to localize gastrinomas. A prospective study. Ann Intern Med 1986; 105:841–7.

99. Doppman JL, Miller DL, Chang R, et al. Gastrinomas: localization by means of selective intraarterial injection of secretin. Radiology 1990;174:25–9.

100. Gibril F, Reynolds JC, Doppman JL, et al. Somatostatin receptor scintigraphy: its sensitivity compared with that of other imaging methods in detecting primary and metastatic gastrinomas: a prospective study. Ann Intern Med 1996;125: 26–34.

101. Gibril F, Doppman JL, Reynolds JC, et al. Bone metastases in patients with gastrinomas: a prospective study of bone scanning, somatostatin receptor scanning, and MRI in their detection, their frequency, location and effect of their detection on management. J Clin Oncol 1998;16:1040–53.

102. Gibril F, Jensen RT. Diagnostic uses of radio labelled somatostatin-receptor analogues in gastroenteropancreatic endocrine tumors. Dig Liver Dis 2004;36: S106–20.

103. Oberg K, Sundin A. Imaging of neuroendocrine tumors. Front Horm Res 2016; 45:142–51.

104. Naswa N, Sharma P, Soundararajan R, et al. Diagnostic performance of somatostatin receptor PET/CT using (68)Ga-DOTANOC in gastrinoma patients with negative or equivocal CT findings. Abdom Imaging 2013;38:552–60.

105. Ito T, Igarashi H, Uehara H, et al. Causes of death and prognostic factors in multiple endocrine neoplasia type 1: a prospective study: comparison of 106 MEN1/Zollinger-Ellison syndrome patients with 1613 literature MEN1 patients with or without pancreatic endocrine tumors. Medicine (Baltimore) 2013;92:135–81.

106. Benya RV, Metz DC, Venzon DJ, et al. Zollinger-Ellison syndrome can be the initial endocrine manifestation in patients with multiple endocrine neoplasia-type 1. Am J Med 1994;97:436–44.

107. Goudet P, Dalac A, Le BA, et al. MEN1 disease occurring before 21 years old. A 160-patient cohort study from the GTE (Groupe d'etude des Tumeurs Endocrines). J Clin Endocrinol Metab 2015;100:1568–77.

108. Norton JA, Venzon DJ, Berna MJ, et al. Prospective study of surgery for primary hyperparathyroidism (HPT) in multiple endocrine neoplasia type 1 (MEN1), and Zollinger-Ellison syndrome (ZES): long-term outcome of a more virulent form of HPT. Ann Surg 2008;247:501–10.

109. Metz DC, Pisegna JR, Fishbeyn VA, et al. Currently used doses of omeprazole in Zollinger-Ellison syndrome are too high. Gastroenterology 1992;103:1498–508.

110. Norton JA, Cornelius MJ, Doppman JL, et al. Effect of parathyroidectomy in patients with hyperparathyroidism, Zollinger-Ellison syndrome and multiple endocrine neoplasia type I: a prospective study. Surgery 1987;102:958–66.

111. Polenta V, Slater EP, Kann PH, et al. Preoperative imaging overestimates the tumor size in pancreatic neuroendocrine neoplasms associated with multiple endocrine neoplasia type 1. World J Surg 2018;42(5):1440–7.

112. Jensen RT. Management of the Zollinger-Ellison syndrome in patients with multiple endocrine neoplasia type 1. J Intern Med 1998;243:477–88.

113. MacFarlane MP, Fraker DL, Alexander HR, et al. A prospective study of surgical resection of duodenal and pancreatic gastrinomas in multiple endocrine neoplasia-type 1. Surgery 1995;118:973–80.

114. Pipeleers-Marichal M, Somers G, Willems G, et al. Gastrinomas in the duodenums of patients with multiple endocrine neoplasia type 1 and the Zollinger-Ellison syndrome. N Engl J Med 1990;322:723–7.

115. Anlauf M, Garbrecht N, Henopp T, et al. Sporadic versus hereditary gastrinomas of the duodenum and pancreas: distinct clinico-pathological and epidemiological features. World J 2006;12:5440–6.

116. Vezzosi D, Cardot-Bauters C, Bouscaren N, et al. Long-term results of the surgical management of insulinoma patients with MEN1: a Groupe d'etude des Tumeurs Endocrines (GTE) retrospective study. Eur J Endocrinol 2015; 172:309–19.

117. Gibril F, Chen Y-J, Schrump DS, et al. Prospective study of thymic carcinoids in patients with multiple endocrine neoplasia type 1. J Clin Endocrinol Metab 2003; 88:1066–81.

118. Metz DC, Forsmark C, Lew EA, et al. Replacement of oral proton pump inhibitors with intravenous pantoprazole to effectively control gastric acid hypersecretion in patients with Zollinger-Ellison syndrome. Am J Gastroenterol 2001;96: 3274–80.

119. Berna MJ, Hoffmann KM, Long SH, et al. Serum gastrin in Zollinger-Ellison syndrome: II. Prospective study of gastrin provocative testing in 293 patients from the National Institutes of Health and comparison with 537 cases from the literature. Evaluation of diagnostic criteria, proposal of new criteria, and correlations with clinical and tumoral features. Medicine (Baltimore) 2006;85:331–64.

120. McCarthy DM, Peikin SR, Lopatin RN, et al. Hyperparathyroidism a reversible cause of cimetidine-resistant gastric hypersecretion. Br Med J 1979;1:1765–6.

121. Bartsch DK, Albers MB. Controversies in surgery for multiple endocrine neoplasia type-1- associated Zollinger-Ellison syndrome. Int J Endocr Oncol 2015;2:263–71.

122. Lopez CL, Falconi M, Waldmann J, et al. Partial pancreaticoduodenectomy can provide cure for duodenal gastrinoma associated with multiple endocrine neoplasia type 1. Ann Surg 2013;257:308–14.

123. Triponez F, Goudet P, Dosseh D, et al. Is surgery beneficial for MEN1 patients with small (< or = 2 cm), nonfunctioning pancreaticoduodenal endocrine tumor? An analysis of 65 patients from the GTE. World J Surg 2006;30:654–62.

124. Norton JA, Alexander HR, Fraker DL, et al. Comparison of surgical results in patients with advanced and limited disease with multiple endocrine neoplasia type 1 and Zollinger-Ellison syndrome. Ann Surg 2001;234:495–506.

125. Thakker RV, Newey PJ, Walls GV, et al. Clinical practice guidelines for multiple endocrine neoplasia type 1 (MEN1). J Clin Endocrinol Metab 2012;97: 2990–3011.

126. Donegan D, Singh Ospina N, Rodriguez-Gutierrez R, et al. Long-term outcomes in patients with multiple endocrine neoplasia type 1 and pancreaticoduodenal neuroendocrine tumours. Clin Endocrinol (Oxf) 2017;86(2):199–206.

127. D'souza SL, Elmunzer BJ, Scheiman JM. Long-term follow-up of asymptomatic pancreatic neuroendocrine tumors in multiple endocrine neoplasia type I syndrome. J Clin Gastroenterol 2014;48:458–61.

128. van Asselt SJ, Brouwers AH, van Dullemen HM, et al. EUS is superior for detection of pancreatic lesions compared with standard imaging in patients with multiple endocrine neoplasia type 1. Gastrointest Endosc 2015;81:159–67.

129. Kann PH, Balakina E, Ivan D, et al. Natural course of small, asymptomatic neuroendocrine pancreatic tumours in multiple endocrine neoplasia type 1: an endoscopic ultrasound imaging study. Endocr Relat Cancer 2006;13:1195–202.

130. Kappelle WF, Valk GD, Leenders M, et al. Growth rate of small pancreatic neuroendocrine tumors in multiple endocrine neoplasia type 1: results from an endoscopic ultrasound based cohort study. Endoscopy 2017;49:27–34.

131. Pieterman CRC, de Laat JM, Twisk JWR, et al. Long-term natural course of small nonfunctional pancreatic neuroendocrine tumors in MEN1-results from the Dutch MEN1 study group. J Clin Endocrinol Metab 2017;102:3795–805.

132. Albers MB, Librizzi D, Lopez CL, et al. Limited value of Ga-68-DOTATOC-PET-CT in routine screening of patients with multiple endocrine neoplasia type 1. World J Surg 2017;41:1521–7.

133. Lastoria S, Marciello F, Faggiano A, et al. Role of Ga-DOTATATE PET/CT in patients with multiple endocrine neoplasia type 1 (MEN1). Endocrine 2016;52:488–94.

134. Sadowski SM, Millo C, Cottle-Delisle C, et al. Results of (68)Gallium-DOTATATE PET/CT scanning in patients with multiple endocrine neoplasia type 1. J Am Coll Surg 2015;221:509–17.

135. Morgat C, Velayoudom-Cephise FL, Schwartz P, et al. Evaluation of Ga-DOTA-TOC PET/CT for the detection of duodenopancreatic neuroendocrine tumors in patients with MEN1. Eur J Nucl Med Mol Imaging 2016;43(7):1258–66.

136. Gibril F, Venzon DJ, Ojeaburu JV, et al. Prospective study of the natural history of gastrinoma in patients with MEN1: definition of an aggressive and a nonaggressive form. J Clin Endocrinol Metab 2001;86:5282–93.

137. Maton PN, Gardner JD, Jensen RT. Cushing's syndrome in patients with Zollinger-Ellison syndrome. N Engl J Med 1986;315:1–5.

138. Mignon M, Cadiot G. Natural history of gastrinoma: lessons from the past. Ital J Gastroenterol Hepatol 1999;31:S98–103.

139. Bartsch DK, Langer P, Wild A, et al. Pancreaticoduodenal endocrine tumors in multiple endocrine neoplasia type 1: surgery or surveillance? Surgery 2000; 128:958–66.

140. van Vliet EI, Teunissen JJ, Kam BL, et al. Treatment of gastroenteropancreatic neuroendocrine tumors with peptide receptor radionuclide therapy. Neuroendocrinology 2013;97:74–85.

141. Conemans EB, Nell S, Pieterman CRC, et al. Prognostic factors for survival of MEN1 patients with duodenopancreatic tumors metastatic to the liver: results from the DMSG. Endocr Pract 2017;23:641–8.

142. Conemans EB, Brosens LAA, Raicu-Ionita GM, et al. Prognostic value of WHO grade in pancreatic neuro-endocrine tumors in multiple endocrine neoplasia type 1: results from the DutchMEN1 study group. Pancreatology 2017;17:766–72.

143. Kornaczewski Jackson ER, Pointon OP, Bohmer R, et al. Utility of FDG-PET imaging for risk stratification of pancreatic neuroendocrine tumors in MEN1. J Clin Endocrinol Metab 2017;102:1926–33.

144. Kouvaraki MA, Shapiro SE, Cote GJ, et al. Management of pancreatic endocrine tumors in multiple endocrine neoplasia type 1. World J Surg 2006;30:643–53.

145. Bartsch DK, Slater EP, Albers M, et al. Brief report: higher risk of aggressive pancreatic neuroendocrine tumors in MEN1 patients with MFN1 mutations affecting the CHES1 interacting MENIN domain. J Clin Endocrinol Metab 2014;99:E2387–91.

146. Thevenon J, Bourredjem A, Faivre L, et al. Higher risk of death among MEN1 patients with mutations in the JunD interacting domain: a Groupe d'etude des Tumeurs Endocrines (GTE) cohort study. Hum Mol Genet 2013;22:1940–8.

147. Circelli L, Ramundo V, Marotta V, et al. Prognostic role of the CDNK1B V109G polymorphism in multiple endocrine neoplasia type 1. J Cell Mol Med 2015; 19:1735–41.

148. Christakis I, Qiu W, Hyde SM, et al. Genotype-phenotype pancreatic neuroendocrine tumor relationship in multiple endocrine neoplasia type 1 patients: a 23-year experience at a single institution. Surgery 2018;163(1):212–7.

149. Kulke MH, Anthony LB, Bushnell DL, et al. NANETS treatment guidelines: well-differentiated neuroendocrine tumors of the stomach and pancreas. Pancreas 2010;39:735–52.

150. Nigri GR, Rosman AS, Petrucciani N, et al. Meta-analysis of trials comparing minimally invasive and open distal pancreatectomies. Surg Endosc 2011;25: 1642–51.

151. Norton JA, Warren RS, Kelly MG, et al. Aggressive surgery for metastatic liver neuroendocrine tumors. Surgery 2003;134:1057–65.

152. Strosberg J, El-Haddad G, Wolin E, et al. Phase 3 trial of 177Lu-dotatate for midgut neuroendocrine tumors. N Engl J Med 2017;376:125–35.

153. Ito T, Igarashi H, Jensen RT. Therapy of metastatic pancreatic neuroendocrine tumors (pNETs): recent insights and advances. J Gastroenterol 2012;47:941–60.

154. von Schrenck T, Howard JM, Doppman JL, et al. Prospective study of chemotherapy in patients with metastatic gastrinoma. Gastroenterology 1988;94: 1326–34.

155. Pavel M, O'Toole D, Costa F, et al. ENETS consensus guidelines update for the management of distant metastatic disease of intestinal, pancreatic, bronchial neuroendocrine neoplasms (NEN) and NEN of unknown primary site. Neuroendocrinology 2016;103:172–85.

156. Do Minh D, Chapiro J, Gorodetski B, et al. Intra-arterial therapy of neuroendocrine tumour liver metastases: comparing conventional TACE, drug-eluting beads TACE and yttrium-90 radioembolisation as treatment options using a propensity score analysis model. Eur Radiol 2017;27:4995–5005.

157. Cives M, Strosberg J. Treatment strategies for metastatic neuroendocrine tumors of the gastrointestinal tract. Curr Treat Options Oncol 2017;18:14.

Current Chemotherapy Use in Neuroendocrine Tumors

David L. Chan, MBBS, FRACP[a,b], Simron Singh, MD, MPH, FRCPC[a,c],*

KEYWORDS

- Chemotherapy • Neuroendocrine tumors • Metastatic

KEY POINTS

- Advanced grade 3 (G3) poorly differentiated neuroendocrine carcinomas (NECs) are usually treated with platinum/etoposide chemotherapy in the first-line setting.
- There is no consensus regarding "well differentiated G3 gastroenteropancreatic neuroendocrine tumors"; a platinum doublet or capecitabine (CAPTEM) are reasonable options in this setting.
- Chemotherapy is not routinely used as first-line therapy for G1 to G2 neuroendocrine tumors (NETs). The combination of CAPTEM and temozolomide shows promise in this setting as later-line therapy.
- There is little evidence for adjuvant chemotherapy for resected G1 to G2 NETs; adjuvant platinum/etoposide is often given for resected G3 NETs.

INTRODUCTION

The incidence of neuroendocrine tumors (NETs) has increased over the past 30 years,[1] and they are the second most prevalent gastrointestinal tumor behind colorectal cancer. NETs are heterogeneous neoplasms that most commonly arise from the gastrointestinal tract, pancreas, and lung. Their biological behavior can vary widely, and for this reason characterization of NETs relies as much on their histologic grading as the primary site of disease. Grade 1 (G1) NETs may display extremely indolent behavior, whereas grade 3 (G3) NETs may grow over a matter of weeks and require urgent treatment. Gastrointestinal tumors are graded using the World Health Organization (WHO) 2010 system, using a combination of the mitotic count and Ki-67 index. The WHO

Disclosure Statement: D.L. Chan has received travel support from Novartis and honoraria from Ipsen. S. Singh has received honoraria and travel funding from Ipsen, Pfizer and Novartis.
a Department of Medical Oncology, Sunnybrook Health Sciences Centre, 2075 Bayview Avenue, Toronto, ON M4N3M5, Canada; b Department of Medical Oncology, Royal North Shore Hospital, Level 1 ASB, Reserve Road, St Leonards, New South Wales 2065, Australia; c Department of Medicine, University of Toronto, Odette Cancer Centre, Sunnybrook Health Sciences Centre, King's College Cir, Toronto, ON M5S 1A8, Canada
* Corresponding author. Odette Cancer Centre, Sunnybrook Health Sciences Centre, 2075 Bayview Avenue, Toronto, Ontario M4N3M5, Canada.
E-mail address: Simron.singh@sunnybrook.ca

Endocrinol Metab Clin N Am 47 (2018) 603–614
https://doi.org/10.1016/j.ecl.2018.04.006
0889-8529/18/© 2018 Elsevier Inc. All rights reserved.

endo.theclinics.com

2017 system published earlier this year provides minor modifications to the grading cutoffs, as well as separating G3 pancreatic NETs into well-differentiated and poorly differentiated tumors.[2] This is due to new evidence showing that patients with G3 poorly differentiated pancreatic neuroendocrine carcinomas (PDNECs) have worse outcomes, even though the Ki-67 index of these tumors overlaps considerably with G3 well-differentiated NETs (WDNETs).[3,4]

NETs are generally treated by a multidisciplinary team, as treatments are complex and varied.[5] These may include surgery (both curative and debulking), external beam radiotherapy and peptide receptor radionuclide treatment (PRRT), liver-directed therapies (embolization, radiofrequency ablation), systemic treatments, and clinical trials. Sequencing of these modalities is a major clinical and logistical challenge due to the number of services involved. Although surgery is the standard of care for resectable NETs, up to 50% of patients present with metastatic or unresectable disease,[6] and systemic therapy is the mainstay of therapy for these patients.

Chemotherapy was one of the few systemic treatments available for NETs for much of the twentieth century. The development of other systemic treatments (such as somatostatin analogs and the targeted agents everolimus and sunitinib) have decreased the prominence of chemotherapy in the treatment of low-grade (G1–G2) NETs; however, it is still the first-line treatment of choice in high-grade NETs. Cytotoxic chemotherapy disrupts the mitotic processes of dividing cells and thus is more likely to affect rapidly proliferating malignancies. Different classes of agents exist, alkylating agents (cisplatin, temozolomide), topoisomerase inhibitors (etoposide), and thymidylate synthase inhibitors (capecitabine), for instance, with the possibility of synergistic efficacy between different classes. There remains considerable debate over the utility and sequencing of chemotherapy in the role of systemic therapy in NETs overall.

AN OVERVIEW OF RANDOMIZED CHEMOTHERAPY TRIALS IN NEUROENDOCRINE TUMORS

A systematic review investigating randomized trials of chemotherapy for NETs showed that the vast majority of trials were conducted in the 1980s and 1990s (**Table 1**).[7] These generally involved the comparison of streptozocin (usually in combination with 5-fluorouracil [5-FU]) with another chemotherapeutic regimen, as streptozocin had shown signs of clinical activity in prior single-arm trials and became adopted as a standard treatment at that time. There were no placebo-controlled randomized trials identified. Most of the trials failed to show a significant difference between the 2 treatment arms in terms of overall survival (OS) and progression-free survival (PFS), although ascertainment of response varied tremendously during this time period. The only trials that demonstrated significant differences in outcomes were Moertel and colleagues[8] and Sun and colleagues.[9] Both trials showed an OS advantage for streptozocin and doxorubicin compared with streptozocin and 5-FU, although there was no significant difference in PFS in the trial by and colleagues.[9]

It is important to note that the previously described trials need to be interpreted with caution, given the evolution in both classification and monitoring of NETs over the past 2 decades. These trials often included a very heterogeneous population of NETs, which would not be considered appropriate in today's environment. As the 3-grade system for classifying gastroenteropancreatic NETs (GEPNETs) was only published in 2007, trials before this were often limited to analysis by the degree of differentiation alone rather than using the mitotic rate and Ki-67 index, as is standard practice today. Even the most recent trial, Meyer and colleagues,[10] enrolled patients with all 3 grades of NET, perhaps reflecting the difficulty in conduct of well-designed NET trials. There

Table 1
Randomized trials of chemotherapy in neuroendocrine tumors

Study	Intervention	Comparator	PFS-Intervention	PFS-Comparator	P	OS Intervention	OS Comparator	P
Engstrom et al,[58] 1984	Doxorubicin	STZ + 5-FU	—	—	—	12.0 mo	16.1 mo	P = .25
Moertel et al,[59] 1979	STZ + Cyclophosphamide	STZ + 5-FU	7 mo	6.5 mo	NS	11.5 mo	6.8 mo	Not reported
Moertel et al,[60] 1980	STZ+5FU	STZ	—	—	NS	26 mo	16.4 mo	NS
Moertel et al,[8] 1992[a]	STZ + Dox	STZ + 5-FU	19 mo (TTP)	5 mo (TTP)	P<.01	26.4 mo	16.8 mo	P<.01
Moertel et al,[8] 1992	Chlorozotocin	STZ + 5-FU	3 mo (TTP)	5 mo (TTP)	NS	18 mo	16.8 mo	NS
Sun et al,[9] 2005	STZ + Dox	STZ + 5-FU	4.5 mo	5.3 mo	P = .17	24.3 mo	15.7 mo	P = .027
Dahan et al,[61] 2009	IFNα-2A	STZ + 5-FU	14.1 mo (6.7-21.2)	5.5 mo (2.9-25)	P = .25	44.3 mo	30.4 mo	P = .83
Meyer et al,[10] 2014	STZ + Capecitabine	STZ + Capecitabine + Cisplatin	9.7 mo	10.2 mo	Not reported; HR 0.74 (95% CI 0.46-1.20)	27.5 mo	26.7 mo	Not reported; HR 1.16 (95% CI 0.65-2.07)

Abbreviations: 5-FU, 5-fluorouracil; CI, confidence interval; Dox, doxorubicin; HR, hazard ratio; IFN, interferon; NS, not significant; OS, overall survival; PFS, progression-free survival; STZ, streptozocin; TTP, time to progression.

[a] Moertel 1992 was a three-armed trial; adapted here to show comparisons against STZ/5-FU.

Data from Wong MH, Chan DL, Lee A, et al. Systematic review and meta-analysis on the role of chemotherapy in advanced and metastatic neuroendocrine tumor (NET). PLoS One 2016;11(6):e0158140; with permission.

was no standardized evaluation of response for many of these trials; evaluation of cross-sectional imaging had not yet been standardized by the Response Evaluation Criteria In Solid Tumors (RECIST) criteria,[11] and some trials even used physical palpation or clinical benefit to determine response.

CHEMOTHERAPY FOR ADVANCED GRADE 1 TO 2 GASTROENTEROPANCREATIC NEUROENDOCRINE TUMORS

The benefit from cytotoxic chemotherapy for G1-2 GEPNET remains murky and uncertain, and its role in management of GEPNETs is a matter of ongoing debate. Classically, treatments including agents such as streptozocin, 5-FU, doxorubicin, and more recently capecitabine, have all been used. However, randomized trials in the past 20 years have demonstrated the efficacy of the first somatostatin analogs[12,13] and then the targeted agents everolimus[14] and sunitinib.[15] Somatostatin analogs (SSAs) remain the mainstay of treatment of G1 to G2 NETs. These agents have been used preferentially to cytotoxic chemotherapy, because of the randomized data for their efficacy, as well as their superior side-effect profile and patient preference. No randomized trial has shown the benefit of chemotherapy over best supportive care, and most randomized trials of chemotherapy in G1-2 GEPNETS failed to show a significant difference in PFS or OS between different regimens (see **Table 1**).

More recently, the orally administered combination of capecitabine, a prodrug of 5-FU, and temozolomide, an alkylating agent (CAPTEM), has shown some promise in this setting. Temozolomide is pharmacologically related to dacarbazine, another alkylating agent with known activity in pancreatic NETs, and capecitabine was postulated to be active due to its continuous release in a slowly proliferating tumor, with synergistic activity demonstrated in the BON1 neuroendocrine cell line.[16]

A single-center retrospective study of 30 patients receiving first-line CAPTEM for metastatic well-differentiated pancreatic NETs (pNETs) demonstrated a response rate of 70% and median PFS of 18 months.[17] Another retrospective study showed a response rate of 61% in 18 heavily pretreated patients with different gastrointestinal primaries (39% pancreatic). More recent retrospective series report similar results, although there are still relatively few data regarding nonpancreatic gastrointestinal NETs.[18,19]

There are mixed data and subsequent controversy regarding the role of O^6-methylguanine DNA methyltransferase (MGMT) status as a predictive biomarker for temozolomide efficacy. MGMT is an enzyme that effects DNA repair at O^6-guanine DNA sites targeted by alkylating agents such as temozolomide, and its absence (via methylation of the promoter gene) is associated with temozolomide efficacy in gliomas.[20] Two early studies suggested that patients with MGMT-deficient tumors may respond better to temozolomide-based treatment.[21,22] However, a subsequent study of 143 patients with advanced pNET showed no correlation between MGMT methylation and response.[23]

The National Comprehensive Cancer Network guidelines[24] recommend consideration of chemotherapy (such as 5-FU, capecitabine, dacarbazine, oxaliplatin, streptozocin, and temozolomide) in patients with progressive disease and no other treatment options. The European Neuroendocrine Tumor Society (ENETS) guidelines recommend consideration of chemotherapy in bulky or progressive pancreatic NETs, and certain nonpancreatic NETs (Ki-67 >15%, aggressive clinical behavior or somatostatin receptor [SSTR] negative).[25] Both the North American Neuroendocrine Tumor Society (NANETS) and the Canadian consensus guidelines recommend CAPTEM or streptozocin-based therapy (especially in the setting or rapid growth) for pNETs.[26,27] All these guidelines are unfortunately more based on consensus rather than available level 1 evidence. We agree that chemotherapy (apart from CAPTEM for pNETs) should be considered only after failure of other systemic options, such as SSAs and targeted agents.

CHEMOTHERAPY FOR ADVANCED GRADE 3 GASTROENTEROPANCREATIC NEUROENDOCRINE TUMORS

Chemotherapy plays a more prominent role in G3 GEPNETS compared with their G1-2 counterparts, as the higher proliferative index of these tumors means more cells are susceptible to the effects of chemotherapy. There are no randomized data to date regarding chemotherapy in G3 GEPNETs, with regimens being extrapolated from the setting of small cell lung cancer (SCLC). For example, some patients with locally advanced disease may be treated for chemoradiation with cisplatin/etoposide, despite the paucity of evidence in GEPNETs. Platinum-based doublets remain the standard of care, but there have been increasing data regarding the efficacy of other regimens.

There is increasing evidence pointing to the difference between well-differentiated G3 neuroendocrine tumors (so-called WDNETs) and poorly differentiated neuroendocrine carcinomas (NECs). WDNETS may be morphologically and clinically distinct from NECs, with superior clinical outcomes and potentially differing responses to cytotoxic chemotherapy. Most studies to date in this field have investigated pancreatic NETs, leading to its reclassification in the WHO 2017 schema.[2]

Platinum-Based Doublet Therapy

A platinum-based (cisplatin or carboplatin) doublet is the usual standard of care for PDNEC. This is usually given for 4 to 6 cycles. As mentioned previously, there is no randomized trial that investigates this regimen, but several retrospective studies confirm the efficacy and safety of this approach.[28,29] The efficacy of chemotherapy in well-differentiated G3 NETs remains undefined.

The largest series of patients with G3 NETs receiving chemotherapy included 252 patients, 89% of whom received platinum-based chemotherapy with either cisplatin or carboplatin.[30] The response rate to first-line chemotherapy was 31%; however, a significant difference in response rate was noted between patients with a Ki-67 index greater than 55% and those less than 55% (response rate 42% vs 15%, $P<.001$). Cisplatin carries a higher risk of neurotoxicity and nephrotoxicity, whereas carboplatin is associated with more hematological toxicity.[31] Some clinicians may prefer cisplatin over carboplatin in first-line treatment, extrapolating from clinical data in SCLC showing slightly superior response rates with cisplatin.

Several predictive biomarkers have been suggested for platinum/etoposide chemotherapy. Two studies have suggested higher Ki-67 (with cutoffs of 60% and 55%, respectively) might predict for increased response rates.[30,32] Interestingly, the degree of differentiation did not influence the response rate.[32] KRAS mutation and the loss of expression of retinoblastoma may also predict for the efficacy of platinum-based chemotherapy in this setting.[33]

Another regimen that has been investigated is cisplatin/irinotecan. A retrospective study of patients with advanced NECs included patients treated with both cisplatin/irinotecan and cisplatin/etoposide.[34] The response rate and OS (13.0 mo vs 7.3 mo) was significantly better in the cisplatin/irinotecan arm. However, these 2 arms were imbalanced with respect the primary site, which was a poor prognostic factor on analysis, and the OS difference was not statistically significant on multivariate analysis. Other studies attest to the tolerability of this regimen,[35,36] but in our view the current data do not show that this regimen is superior to platinum/etoposide.

There is recognition in major societies (ENETS, NANETS) that first-line chemotherapy is appropriate for G3 NEC and should consist of platinum-based chemotherapy (cisplatin/etoposide, carboplatin/etoposide, or cisplatin/irinotecan). Second-line regimens suggested included temozolomide-based, irinotecan-based, or oxaliplatin-based combinations.[37] Rechallenging with the original first-line regimen may be an alternative if the period between ceasing first-line treatment and progression was more than 6 months.[26] The ENETS guidelines stated that "the efficacy of chemotherapy in NET G3 is presently uncertain."

Other Therapies

There is no consensus regarding optimal second-line therapy for G3 disease, largely because available therapies are all associated with disappointing response rates. Second-line regimens have been largely extrapolated from the context of SCLC, for example, single-agent topotecan or CAV (cyclophosphamide, doxorubicin, and vincristine).[38] More recently, regimens such as CAPTEM, FOLFIRI, and FOLFOX have been used at some centres, but there are few data regarding their efficacy in G3 NETs at present. A series of 25 patients with PDNEC were treated with temozolomide-containing regimens (5 with temozolomide alone, 12 with CAPTEM, and 7 with a combination of CAPTEM and bevacizumab) with a response rate of 33% and median PFS of 6 months. The largest reported series to date had only 7 patients.[39] There are several other triplet regimens (for example, the combination of cisplatin, capecitabine, and dacarbazine, and FOLFIRINOX [folinic acid, 5-fluorouracil, irinotecan and oxaliplatin]),[40,41] but there are insufficient data to support the increased efficacy (and tolerability) of such regimens over doublet therapy at present. A randomized trial comparing cisplatin/etoposide to CAPTEM in the first-line setting for G3 gastroenteropancreatic neuroendocrine carcinoma is currently under way (NCT02595424) (**Table 2**).

CHEMOTHERAPY FOR RESECTABLE GASTROENTEROPANCREATIC NEUROENDOCRINE TUMORS

There is no evidence to support the use of neoadjuvant or adjuvant chemotherapy for resectable G1 to G2 NETs. Given the low response rates reported in the literature, neoadjuvant chemotherapy is unlikely to decrease the size of the tumor to allow for easier surgery, and no trials have shown a benefit in disease-free survival or OS from adjuvant treatment.

The role of surgery in treatment of potentially resectable G3 GEPNETs is controversial. This is because of their aggressive biological nature and propensity to metastasize; even patients with localized G3 GEPNETs are associated with a median survival of only 24 months.[44] For those patients post resection of G3 NET, adjuvant treatment with a platinum/etoposide regimen for 4 to 6 cycles has been recommended by consensus-based guidelines,[24,47] extrapolating from treatment strategies for SCLC.

CHEMOTHERAPY FOR BRONCHIAL NEUROENDOCRINE TUMORS

Bronchial NETs can be classified as typical carcinoid (TC), atypical carcinoid (AC), and neuroendocrine carcinoma–large cell (LCNEC) and small cell (otherwise known as SCLC). There are no randomized data to guide use of chemotherapy in this setting.

There is no role for adjuvant therapy after resection of TC or AC, although adjuvant platinum/etoposide therapy improves outcomes in LCNEC.[48] As for SCLC, its potential to disseminate widely means that surgery is rarely carried out. The benefit for

Table 2
Selected trials in grade 3 gastroenteropancreatic neuroendocrine tumors

Trial Name	Histology (No. Patients Treated)	Regimen	Response Rate, %	Overall Survival, mo
1. First-line studies				
Moertel et al,[29] 1991	"Anaplastic neuroendocrine carcinoma" (18)	Cisplatin/etoposide	67	19.0
Mitry et al,[28] 1999	PDNEC (41)	Cisplatin/etoposide	42	15.0
Sorbye et al,[30] 2013	GEPNEN (252)	Mostly cisplatin/ etoposide or carboplatin/ etoposide	31	11.0
Yamaguchi et al,[34] 2014	PDNEC, MiNEN, or clinical NEC (258)	Cisplatin/etoposide Cisplatin/irinotecan	28 50	7.3 13.0
Nakano et al,[35] 2012	PDNEC (28 first-line, 16 second-line or beyond)	Cisplatin/irinotecan	50	16.0
Du et al,[42] 2013	GEPNEC (11)	FOLFIRI	64	13.0
Bajetta et al,[43] 2007	PDNEC (13)	XELOX	23	5.0
Walter et al,[44] 2017	GEPNEC (152)	Platinum/etoposide (cisplatin in 113, carboplatin in 39)	50	11.6
2. Second (and subsequent)-line studies				
Hentic et al,[45] 2012	G3 NEC (19)	FOLFIRI	31	18.0
Hadoux et al,[46] 2015	G3 PDNEC (20; 12 GEPNEC, 4 thoracic)	FOLFOX	29	9.9
Welin et al,[39] 2011	PDNEC (25)	Temozolomide, CAPTEM, some with bevacizumab	33	22.0

For trials before 2010, poorly differentiated tumors (and relevant subgroups from trials investigating wide populations) were used as a surrogate for G3 disease.

Abbreviations: CAPTEM, capecitabine; FOLFIRI, 5-fluorouracil/leucovorin/irinotecan; FOLFOX, 5-fluorouracil/leucovorin/oxaliplatin; G3, grade 3; GEPNEC, gastroenteropancreatic neuroendocrine carcinoma; GEPNEN, gastroenteropancreatic neuroendocrine neoplasm; MiNEN, mixed neuroendocrine-nonneuroendocrine neoplasms; NEC, neuroendocrine carcinoma; PDNEC, poorly differentiated pancreatic neuroendocrine carcinoma; XELOX, capecitabine/oxaliplatin.

adjuvant chemotherapy in LCNEC was confirmed in a recent large database analysis including 1672 patients with resected LCNEC, with improvement in 5-year survival for LCNEC stages IB to IIIA.[49]

Advanced TC and AC are relatively resistant to chemotherapy. Similar to G1-2 GEP-NETs, agents that have been used include streptozocin, 5-FU, capecitabine, temozolomide, and doxorubicin. Temozolomide was associated with response rates of 14% in a series of 31 patients,[50] but zero responses were seen in 7 patients treated with streptozocin/5-FU.[51]

Advanced LCNEC and SCLC are usually treated with cytotoxic chemotherapy. Regarding first-line treatment, platinum-based chemotherapy is associated with response rates of 50% to 70%, superior to non–platinum-based chemotherapies,[52] with benefit regardless of large cell/small cell histology.[53]

Chemotherapy for bronchial NETs was recommended as a possible option by the ENETS guidelines in the case of a high Ki-67 index, rapid progression of disease, or failure of other therapies.[25]

CHEMOTHERAPY FOR OTHER NEUROENDOCRINE TUMORS

Neuroendocrine tumors may occur less commonly in other anatomic sites, such as the thymus and cervix. Considering their low incidence, there are understandably few data regarding the efficacy of chemotherapy in these NET subtypes. Small retrospective series support the use of temozolomide in thymic carcinoid,[50,54] as well as regimens such as cisplatin/etoposide in small cell NET of the cervix (where adjuvant chemotherapy is often combined with radiation).[55] As in GEPNETs, the degree of differentiation (or grade) should be considered when considering chemotherapy.

CURRENT AND FUTURE DIRECTIONS IN NEUROENDOCRINE TUMOR CHEMOTHERAPY

As the role of chemotherapy in well-differentiated NETs has diminished, current clinical studies generally focus on G3 NETs. In addition to the cisplatin/etoposide versus CAPTEM trial mentioned previously, another phase II study under the auspices of the Eastern Cooperative Oncology Group comparing temozolomide with CAPTEM has completed accrual, although results have not been presented to date (NCT01824875). Another phase II study is randomizing patients to carboplatin/etoposide or carboplatin/nab-paclitaxel (NCT02215447). Regarding bronchial NETs, a phase III trial is under way comparing adjuvant cisplatin/etoposide and cisplatin/irinotecan for completely resected pulmonary high-grade NEC.[56]

Other studies may look at the combination of chemotherapy with other modalities. The potential for chemotherapy to potentiate the effects of radiation has led to some centers combining chemotherapy (usually capecitabine or CAPTEM) with PRRT. Although this approach remains investigational (NCT02358356), it is vital to maximize the effect of PRRT, in view of the encouraging results of the NETTER-1 trial.[57] Finally, the identification and verification of predictive biomarkers for the efficacy of common regimens, such as cisplatin/etoposide and CAPTEM, should help clinicians sequence these therapies.

SUMMARY

Chemotherapy has had a reduced role in treatment of G1-2 GEPNETs and well-differentiated bronchial carcinoids, but remains important in the treatment of G3 GEPNETs and bronchial NECs. Platinum/etoposide and capecitabine/temozolomide are the most commonly used regimens in current practice. Further biomarker research will help predict clinical benefit from these agents and optimize the benefit gained from these therapies.

REFERENCES

1. Hallet J, Law CHL, Cukier M, et al. Exploring the rising incidence of neuroendocrine tumors: a population-based analysis of epidemiology, metastatic presentation, and outcomes. Cancer 2015;121(4):589–97.
2. Lloyd RV, Osamura RY, Klöppel G, et al, editors. WHO classification of tumours of endocrine organs. 4. Auflage. Lyon (France): International Agency for Research on Cancer; 2017.
3. Tang LH, Untch BR, Reidy DL, et al. Well-differentiated neuroendocrine tumors with a morphologically apparent high-grade component: a pathway distinct

from poorly differentiated neuroendocrine carcinomas. Clin Cancer Res 2016; 22(4):1011–7.

4. Basturk O, Yang Z, Tang LH, et al. The high-grade (WHO G3) pancreatic neuro-endocrine tumor category is morphologically and biologically heterogenous and includes both well differentiated and poorly differentiated neoplasms. Am J Surg Pathol 2015;39(5):683–90.

5. Singh S, Law C. Multidisciplinary reference centers: the care of neuroendocrine tumors. J Oncol Pract 2010;6:e11–6.

6. Dasari A, Shen C, Halperin D, et al. Trends in the incidence, prevalence, and survival outcomes in patients with neuroendocrine tumors in the United States. JAMA Oncol 2017. https://doi.org/10.1001/jamaoncol.2017.0589.

7. Wong MH, Chan DL, Lee A, et al. Systematic review and meta-analysis on the role of chemotherapy in advanced and metastatic neuroendocrine tumor (NET). Stemmer SM, ed. PLoS One 2016;11(6):e0158140.

8. Moertel CG, Lefkopoulo M, Lipsitz S, et al. Streptozocin-doxorubicin, streptozocin-fluorouracil or chlorozotocin in the treatment of advanced islet-cell carcinoma. N Engl J Med 1992;326(8):519–23.

9. Sun W, Lipsitz S, Catalano P, et al. Phase II/III study of doxorubicin with fluorouracil compared with streptozocin with fluorouracil or dacarbazine in the treatment of advanced carcinoid tumors: Eastern Cooperative Oncology Group Study E1281. J Clin Oncol 2005;23:4897–904.

10. Meyer T, Qian W, Caplin ME, et al. Capecitabine and streptozocin ± cisplatin in advanced gastroenteropancreatic neuroendocrine tumours. Eur J Cancer 2014; 50(5):902–11.

11. Eisenhauer EA, Therasse P, Bogaerts J, et al. New response evaluation criteria in solid tumours: revised RECIST guideline (version 1.1). Eur J Cancer 2009;45(2): 228–47.

12. Rinke A, Muller HH, Schade-Brittinger C, et al. Placebo-controlled, double-blind, prospective, randomized study on the effect of octreotide LAR in the control of tumor growth in patients with metastatic neuroendocrine midgut tumors: a report from the PROMID Study Group. J Clin Oncol 2009;27:4656–63.

13. Caplin ME, Pavel M, Cwikla JB, et al. Lanreotide in metastatic enteropancreatic neuroendocrine tumors. N Engl J Med 2014;371:224–33.

14. Yao JC, Fazio N, Singh S, et al. Everolimus for the treatment of advanced, non-functional neuroendocrine tumours of the lung or gastrointestinal tract (RADIANT-4): a randomised, placebo-controlled, phase 3 study. Lancet 2016; 387(10022):968–77.

15. Raymond E, Dahan L, Raoul JL, et al. Sunitinib malate for the treatment of pancreatic neuroendocrine tumors. N Engl J Med 2011;364:501–13.

16. Fine RL, Gulati AP, Krantz BA, et al. Capecitabine and temozolomide (CAPTEM) for metastatic, well-differentiated neuroendocrine cancers: the Pancreas Center at Columbia University experience. Cancer Chemother Pharmacol 2013;71(3): 663–70.

17. Strosberg JR, Fine RL, Choi J, et al. First-line chemotherapy with capecitabine and temozolomide in patients with metastatic pancreatic endocrine carcinomas. Cancer 2011;117(2):268–75.

18. Crespo G, Jiménez-Fonseca P, Custodio A, et al. Capecitabine and temozolomide in grade 1/2 neuroendocrine tumors: a Spanish multicenter experience. Future Oncol 2017;13(7):615–24.

19. Ramirez RA, Beyer DT, Chauhan A, et al. The role of capecitabine/temozolomide in metastatic neuroendocrine tumors. Oncologist 2016;21(6):671–5.

20. Hegi ME, Diserens A-C, Gorlia T, et al. MGMT gene silencing and benefit from temozolomide in glioblastoma. N Engl J Med 2005;352(10):997–1003.
21. Walter T, van Brakel B, Vercherat C, et al. O6-Methylguanine-DNA methyltransferase status in neuroendocrine tumours: prognostic relevance and association with response to alkylating agents. Br J Cancer 2015;112(3):523–31.
22. Kulke MH, Hornick JL, Frauenhoffer C, et al. O6-methylguanine DNA methyltransferase deficiency and response to temozolomide-based therapy in patients with neuroendocrine tumors. Clin Cancer Res 2009;15(1):338–45.
23. Cives M, Ghayouri M, Morse B, et al. Analysis of potential response predictors to capecitabine/temozolomide in metastatic pancreatic neuroendocrine tumors. Endocr Relat Cancer 2016;23(9):759–67.
24. Kulke MH, Shah MH, Benson AB, et al. NCCN Clinical Practice Guidelines in Oncology, Neuroendocrine Tumours, Version 3.2017 - June 13, 2017. 2017. Available at: https://www.nccn.org/professionals/physician_gls/pdf/neuroendocrine.pdf. Accessed September 6, 2017.
25. Pavel M, O'Toole D, Costa F, et al. ENETS consensus guidelines update for the management of distant metastatic disease of intestinal, pancreatic, bronchial neuroendocrine neoplasms (NEN) and NEN of unknown primary site. Neuroendocrinology 2016;103(2):172–85.
26. Kunz PL, Reidy-Lagunes D, Anthony LB, et al. Consensus guidelines for the management and treatment of neuroendocrine tumors. Pancreas 2013;42(4):557–77.
27. Singh S, Dey C, Kennecke H, et al. Consensus recommendations for the diagnosis and management of pancreatic neuroendocrine tumors: guidelines from a Canadian National Expert Group. Ann Surg Oncol 2015;22(8):2685–99.
28. Mitry E, Baudin E, Ducreux M, et al. Treatment of poorly differentiated neuroendocrine tumours with etoposide and cisplatin. Br J Cancer 1999;81:1351–5.
29. Moertel CG, Kvols LK, O'Connell MJ, et al. Treatment of neuroendocrine carcinomas with combined etoposide and cisplatin. Evidence of major therapeutic activity in the anaplastic variants of these neoplasms. Cancer 1991;68(2):227–32.
30. Sorbye H, Welin S, Langer SW, et al. Predictive and prognostic factors for treatment and survival in 305 patients with advanced gastrointestinal neuroendocrine carcinoma (WHO G3): the NORDIC NEC study. Ann Oncol 2013;24(1):152–60.
31. Rossi A, Di Maio M, Chiodini P, et al. Carboplatin- or cisplatin-based chemotherapy in first-line treatment of small-cell lung cancer: the COCIS meta-analysis of individual patient data. J Clin Oncol 2012;30(14):1692–8.
32. Kim HK, Ha SY, Lee J, et al. The impact of pathologic differentiation (well/poorly) and the degree of Ki-67 index in patients with metastatic WHO grade 3 GEP-NECs. Oncotarget 2017. https://doi.org/10.18632/oncotarget.18168.
33. Hijioka S, Hosoda W, Matsuo K, et al. Rb Loss and KRAS mutation are predictors of the response to platinum-based chemotherapy in pancreatic neuroendocrine neoplasm with grade 3: a Japanese Multicenter Pancreatic NEN-G3 Study. Clin Cancer Res 2017;23(16):4625–32.
34. Yamaguchi T, Machida N, Morizane C, et al. Multicenter retrospective analysis of systemic chemotherapy for advanced neuroendocrine carcinoma of the digestive system. Cancer Sci 2014;105(9):1176–81.
35. Nakano K, Takahashi S, Yuasa T, et al. Feasibility and efficacy of combined cisplatin and irinotecan chemotherapy for poorly differentiated neuroendocrine carcinomas. Jpn J Clin Oncol 2012;42(8):697–703.
36. Niho S, Kenmotsu H, Sekine I, et al. Combination chemotherapy with irinotecan and cisplatin for large-cell neuroendocrine carcinoma of the lung: a multicenter phase II study. J Thorac Oncol 2013;8(7):980–4.

37. Garcia-Carbonero R, Rinke A, Valle JW, et al. ENETS consensus guidelines for the standards of care in neuroendocrine neoplasms: systemic therapy—chemotherapy. Neuroendocrinology 2017;105(3):281–94.

38. von Pawel J, Schiller JH, Shepherd FA, et al. Topotecan versus cyclophosphamide, doxorubicin, and vincristine for the treatment of recurrent small-cell lung cancer. J Clin Oncol 1999;17(2):658–67.

39. Welin S, Sorbye H, Sebjornsen S, et al. Clinical effect of temozolomide-based chemotherapy in poorly differentiated endocrine carcinoma after progression on first-line chemotherapy. Cancer 2011;117(20):4617–22.

40. Bajetta E, Catena L, Biondani P, et al. Activity of a three-drug combination including cisplatin (CLOVER regimen) for poorly differentiated neuroendocrine carcinoma. Anticancer Res 2014;34(10):5657–60.

41. Zhu J, Strosberg JR, Dropkin E, et al. Treatment of high-grade metastatic pancreatic neuroendocrine carcinoma with FOLFIRINOX. J Gastrointest Cancer 2015; 46(2):166–9.

42. Du Z, Wang Y, Zhou Y, et al. First-line irinotecan combined with 5-fluorouracil and leucovorin for high-grade metastatic gastrointestinal neuroendocrine carcinoma. Tumori 2013;99(1):57–60.

43. Bajetta E, Catena L, Procopio G, et al. Are capecitabine and oxaliplatin (XELOX) suitable treatments for progressing low-grade and high-grade neuroendocrine tumours? Cancer Chemother Pharmacol 2007;59(5):637–42.

44. Walter T, Tougeron D, Baudin E, et al. Poorly differentiated gastro-enteropancreatic neuroendocrine carcinomas: are they really heterogeneous? Insights from the FFCD-GTE national cohort. Eur J Cancer 2017;79:158–65.

45. Hentic O, Hammel P, Couvelard A, et al. FOLFIRI regimen: an effective second-line chemotherapy after failure of etoposide-platinum combination in patients with neuroendocrine carcinomas grade 3. Endocr Relat Cancer 2012;19(6):751–7.

46. Hadoux J, Malka D, Planchard D, et al. Post-first-line FOLFOX chemotherapy for grade 3 neuroendocrine carcinoma. Endocr Relat Cancer 2015;22(3):289–98.

47. Strosberg JR, Coppola D, Klimstra DS, et al. The NANETS consensus guidelines for the diagnosis and management of poorly differentiated (high-grade) extrapulmonary neuroendocrine carcinomas. Pancreas 2010;39:799–800.

48. Iyoda A, Hiroshima K, Moriya Y, et al. Prospective study of adjuvant chemotherapy for pulmonary large cell neuroendocrine carcinoma. Ann Thorac Surg 2006;82(5):1802–7.

49. Kujtan LA, Muthukumar V, Toor M, et al. The role of adjuvant therapy in the management of resected large cell neuroendocrine carcinoma (LCNEC) of the lung: a National Cancer Database (NCDB) analysis. J Clin Oncol 2017;35(15_suppl): 8529.

50. Crona J, Fanola I, Lindholm DP, et al. Effect of temozolomide in patients with metastatic bronchial carcinoids. Neuroendocrinology 2013;98(2):151–5.

51. Granberg D, Eriksson B, Wilander E, et al. Experience in treatment of metastatic pulmonary carcinoid tumors. Ann Oncol 2001;12(10):1383–91.

52. Sun J-M, Ahn M-J, Ahn JS, et al. Chemotherapy for pulmonary large cell neuroendocrine carcinoma: similar to that for small cell lung cancer or non-small cell lung cancer? Lung Cancer 2012;77(2):365–70.

53. Igawa S, Watanabe R, Ito I, et al. Comparison of chemotherapy for unresectable pulmonary high-grade non-small cell neuroendocrine carcinoma and small-cell lung cancer. Lung Cancer 2010;68(3):438–45.

54. Ekeblad S, Sundin A, Janson ET, et al. Temozolomide as monotherapy is effective in treatment of advanced malignant neuroendocrine tumors. Clin Cancer Res 2007;13(10):2986–91.

55. Cohen JG, Kapp DS, Shin JY, et al. Small cell carcinoma of the cervix: treatment and survival outcomes of 188 patients. Am J Obstet Gynecol 2010;203(4): 347.e1-6.

56. Eba J, Kenmotsu H, Tsuboi M, et al. A phase III trial comparing irinotecan and cisplatin with etoposide and cisplatin in adjuvant chemotherapy for completely resected pulmonary high-grade neuroendocrine carcinoma (JCOG1205/1206). Jpn J Clin Oncol 2014;44(4):379–82.

57. Strosberg J, El-Haddad G, Wolin E, et al. Phase 3 trial of [177] Lu-Dotatate for midgut neuroendocrine tumors. N Engl J Med 2017;376(2):125–35.

58. Engstrom PF, Lavin PT, Moertel CG, et al. Streptozocin plus fluorouracil versus doxorubicin therapy for metastatic carcinoid tumor. J Clin Oncol 1984;2(11): 1255–9.

59. Moertel CG, Hanley JA. Combination chemotherapy trials in metastatic carcinoid tumor and the malignant carcinoid syndrome. Cancer Clin Trials 1979;2(4): 327–34.

60. Moertel CG, Hanley JA, Johnson LA. Streptozocin alone compared with strepto-zocin plus fluorouracil in the treatment of advanced islet-cell carcinoma. N Engl J Med 1980;303(21):1189–94.

61. Dahan L, Bonnetain F, Rougier P, et al. Phase III trial of chemotherapy using 5-fluorouracil and streptozotocin compared with interferon alpha for advanced carcinoid tumors: FNCLCC-FFCD 9710. Endocr Relat Cancer 2009;16(4): 1351–61.

Peptide Receptor Radiotherapy Comes of Age

Taymeyah Al-Toubah, MPH, Jonathan Strosberg, MD*

KEYWORDS

- PRRT • Neuroendocrine tumor • Peptide receptor radionuclide therapy • NETTER-1
- Carcinoid

KEY POINTS

- Radiolabeled somatostatin analogs are an effective treatment for patients with metastatic, progressive, somatostatin receptor–positive neuroendocrine tumors.
- The NETTER-1 study was the first randomized controlled clinical trial to evaluate the efficacy of peptide receptor radionuclide therapy in metastatic midgut neuroendocrine tumors.
- Short-term risks of radiolabeled somatostatin analogs include cytopenias, which tend to be mild and transient.
- There is a roughly 2% risk of treatment-related myelodysplastic syndrome or acute leukemia.

INTRODUCTION

Neuroendocrine tumors (NETs) are biologically and clinically heterogeneous neoplasms that arise from cells of the endocrine and nervous systems and have the ability to produce and secrete various hormones.[1,2] They are often characterized by the overexpression of somatostatin receptors (SSTR) on the cell surface.[3] The majority of NETs arise from the gastroenteropancreatic and bronchopulmonary tracts, with their incidence and prevalence increasing over the past few decades, attributable to increased awareness and improved diagnostic testing.[4] NETs can result in a wide range of symptoms secondary to the hypersecretion of various hormones including serotonin.[4,5] Therapeutic options have expanded in recent years to include somatostatin analogs (SSAs), mammalian target of rapamycin inhibitors, angiogenesis inhibitors, and new cytotoxic drugs. Peptide receptor radionuclide therapies (PRRT), consisting of radiolabeled SSAs, have exhibited promising treatment results over the past 2 decades, allowing for targeted delivery of radionuclides to tumor cells

Disclosure Statement: None (T. Al-Toubah); Novartis, Ipsen, Lexicon (J. Strosberg).
Department of GI Oncology, H. Lee Moffitt Cancer Center and Research Institute, 12902 Magnolia Drive, Tampa, FL 33612, USA
* Corresponding author.
E-mail address: Jonathan.Strosberg@Moffitt.org

Endocrinol Metab Clin N Am 47 (2018) 615–625
https://doi.org/10.1016/j.ecl.2018.04.005
0889-8529/18/© 2018 Elsevier Inc. All rights reserved.

endo.theclinics.com

with high SSTR expression.[6] PRRT has been studied in numerous early phase, single-arm clinical trials. However, the NETTER-1 trial (A Multicentre, Stratified, Open, Randomized, Comparator-controlled, Parallel-group Phase III Study Comparing Treatment With 177Lu-DOTA0-Tyr3-Octreotate to Octreotide LAR in Patients With Inoperable, Progressive, Somatostatin Receptor Positive Midgut Carcinoid Tumours) was the first randomized, phase III, clinical trial providing high-level evidence of the efficacy of PRRT in advanced NETs.[7] In this article, we discuss the evolution, clinical efficacy, and future of PRRT in NETs.

EVOLUTION OF PEPTIDE RECEPTOR RADIONUCLIDE THERAPIES

The principle of PRRT in NETs involves attachment of an SSA to a radionuclide, thereby allowing delivery of radiation to SSTR-expressing tumors. In general, low- and intermediate-grade tumors express higher levels of SSTRs than high-grade tumors.[8] Radiolabeled SSAs consist of a radionuclide isotope, an SSA, and a chelator that binds and stabilizes the complex. The most common chelators are DOTA (tetraa-zacyclododecane-tetra-acetic acid) and DTPA (diethylenetriamine penta-acetic acid). The SSAs octreotide or octreotate, which has a slightly stronger affinity to SSTR sub-type 2, are the most common carriers.[9]

Throughout the years, various radionuclides have been used in PRRT, including [111]indium (^{111}In), [90]yttrium (^{90}Y), and [177]lutetium (^{177}Lu). [111]In emits Auger and conversion electrons with very short tissue penetration of 0.02 to 10 and 200 to 500 μm, respectively. The earliest experiences with PRRT using ^{111}In-DTPA-pentetreotide resulted in symptom palliation in some cases, but disappointing tumor response results.[10,11] The 2 more commonly used isotopes, ^{90}Y and ^{177}Lu, are beta (electron) emitters, with penetration ranges of 12 and 2 mm, respectively, and a substantially superior therapeutic potential. [177]Lu is often regarded as the preferred isotope owing to its lower risk of nephrotoxicity.[12] Because ^{177}Lu also emits gamma rays, it can be used for dosimetry and monitoring tumor response during treatment.[13]

PRRT is administered to patients with evidence of SSTR expression on imaging studies, because increased response rates have been documented in patients with higher levels of radiotracer uptake on SSTR scintigraphy.[14] Patients are screened before treatment with baseline SSTR scintigraphy (OctreoScan), or more recently, ^{68}Ga DOTATOC or DOTATATE-PET scans to assess for receptor expression.[14,15] In 1 study, pretreatment ^{68}Ga-DOTATOC-PET/computed tomography predicted tumor response to PRRT with a sensitivity and specificity of 95% and 60%, respectively, using a threshold maximum standardized uptake value of greater than 16.[15]

Locations of tumor and overall tumor burden have an impact on response rates. For example, patients with pancreatic NETs have higher rates of partial radiographic response compared with patients with midgut NETs.[16] Patients with very large tumors and high hepatic tumor burden are, on average, less likely to respond.[17]

^{90}Y-DOTATOC AND [177]LU-DOTATATE

Numerous phase I and II trials as well data from institutional registries have been reported evaluating the tolerability and efficacy of [90]Y- and ^{177}Lu-radiolabeled SSAs. It is difficult to compare the studies owing to large variations in eligibility criteria, response assessments, and dosimetries. **Tables 1** and **2** provide a summary of outcomes of ^{177}Lu-based and ^{90}Y-based treatment. The range of overall response rates (ORRs) across studies using ^{90}Y-DOTATOC has varied between 4% and 38% and the median progression-free survival (PFS) ranged from 16 to 29 months.[27] Similar studies

Table 1
Outcomes of ^{177}Lu-based treatment

	Disease Control Rate (%)	Response Rate (%)	PFS or TTP (mo)	OS (mo)	No. of Patients	Patient Population	Design/Response Criteria	Phase
Bodei et al,[18] 2011	82	33	36 (95% CI, 24–50) (TTP)	NR; 68% at 36 mo	51	GEP and lung NETs	Prospective – RECIST	I–II
Delpassand et al,[19] 2014	72	31	16.1	NR	32	GEP NETs	Prospective – RECIST	II
Ezziddin et al,[20] 2014	84	72	34 (95% CI, 26–42)	53 (95% CI, 46–60)	68	pNETs	Retrospective – SWOG	NA
Danthala et al,[21] 2014	80	58	8.3 (95% CI, 6.2–10.3) ≤2 doses 45.6 (95% CI, 40.9–50.2) >2 doses	NA	40	GEP and lung NETs	Retrospective – WHO	NA
Sabet et al,[22] 2015	92	44	33 (95% CI, 25–41)	61 (95% CI NA)	61	Small bowel NETs	Retrospective – SWOG	NA
Brabander et al,[23] 2017	82	39	29 (95% CI, 26–33)	63 (95% CI, 55–72)	443	GEP and lung NETs	Prospective[a] – RECIST	NA

Abbreviations: CI, confidence interval; GEP, gastroenteropancreatic; NA, not applicable; NET, neuroendocrine tumor; NR, not reported; OS, overall survival; PFS, progression-free survival; pNET, pancreatic neuroendocrine tumor; TTP, time to progression.
[a] Dutch nationals with GEP and lung NETs selected retrospectively from prospective registry.

Table 2
Outcomes of ^{90}Y-based treatment

	Disease Control Rate (%)	Response Rate (%)	PFS or TTP (mo)	OS (mo)	No. of Patients	Patient Population	Design/Response Criteria	Phase
Waldherr et al,[24] 2002	92	23	NA	NA	39	GEP and lung NETs	Prospective – WHO	I
Bodei et al,[25] 2003	52	20	10 (TTP)	NA	21	GEP, MTC, PDTC, lymphoma, ODG, and lung NETs	Prospective – WHO	I
Paganelli et al,[26] 2003	76	28	14 (95% CI, 2–14)	NA	87	GEP, MTC, and lung NETs	Prospective – SWOG	I
Valkema et al,[27] 2006	71	21	29.3 (95% CI, 19.3–39.3)	36.7 (95% CI, 19.4–54.1)	58	GEP NETs	Prospective – SWOG	I
Bushnell et al,[28] 2010	74	4	16.3	26.9	90	GEP and lung NETs	Prospective – SWOG	II
Cwikla et al,[29] 2010	87	23	17 (95% CI, 16.4–21.2)	22 (95% CI, 20.4–26.7)	60	GEP NETs	Prospective – RECIST	II
Imhof et al,[30] 2011	39	34	12.7 (95% CI, 2.1–24.7)	94.6	1109	GEP, thymus, lung, and other rare NETs	Prospective – RECIST	II
Sowa-Staszczak et al,[31] 2011	78	31	37.4	NR; 20.3 at 12 mo (25th percentile)	46	GEP NETs + MTC	Prospective – RECIST	II
Savelliet al,[32] 2012	69	44	22.3 at 30 mo	NA	38	GEP NETs	Prospective – RECIST	II
Vinjamuri et al,[33] 2013	72	25	NA	46 (95% CI, 34–56)	57	GEP and lung NETs	Retrospective – RECIST	NA

Abbreviations: CI, confidence interval; GEP, gastroenteropancreatic; NA, not applicable; NET, neuroendocrine tumor; NR, not reported; ODG, oligodendroglioma; OS, overall survival; PDTC, poorly differentiated thyroid carcinoma; PFS, progression-free survival; TTP, time to progression.

have been completed using ^{177}Lu-DOTATATE with ORRs ranging from 18% to 44% and disease control rates ranging from 72% to 100%.[22,34]

The NETTER-1 trial was the first randomized phase III study of PRRT. Patients with midgut NETs progressing on standard dose octreotide were randomized to receive ^{177}Lu-DOTATATE followed by octreotide 30 mg every 4 weeks, or high-dose octreotide LAR (60 mg every 4 weeks).[7] A fixed dose of ^{177}Lu-DOTATATE was used: 7.4 GBq (200 mCi) every 8 weeks for 4 treatments. The primary endpoint was PFS by blinded central radiology review. At time of primary endpoint analysis, ^{177}Lu-DOTATATE therapy resulted in a 79% reduction in risk of progression or death compared with high-dose octreotide ($P<.0001$; hazard ratio, 0.21; 95% confidence interval, 0.13–0.33). The median PFS was not reached in the PRRT arm compared with 8.4 months in the control arm of the study. The ORR with ^{177}Lu-DOTATATE was 18% versus 3% with high-dose octreotide ($P<.0004$).[7] Moreover, there was early evidence suggesting improved overall survival (hazard ratio, 0.4 [$P = .004$] with $P<.000085$ as the threshold for significance on interim survival analysis). In addition to the substantial improvement in PFS, the NETTER-1 trial demonstrated that ^{177}Lu-DOTATATE provides a significant quality of life benefit for patients with midgut NETs compared with high-dose octreotide in key domains including global health status, physical functioning, role functioning, diarrhea, fatigue, and pain.[35] Based on results of the NETTER-1 study as well as single-arm registry data, ^{177}Lu-DOTATATE has been approved by the Food and Drug Administration (FDA) as well as the European Medicines Agency (EMA) for treatment of advanced, progressive gastroenteropancreatic NETs.[22]

ADMINISTRATION OF [177]LU-DOTATATE AND SELECTION OF PATIENTS

PRRT is typically administered every 8 weeks over the course of approximately 6 months for a total of 4 administrations. The standard dose, based on the NETTER-1 study, is 7.4 GBq (200 mCi) per treatment. Coadministration of positively charged amino acids (typically lysine and arginine) substantially reduces the renal toxicity induced by PRRT and is considered mandatory.

Eligible patients should have relatively normal baseline renal function (creatinine clearance >50 mL/min) and bone marrow function. The threshold criteria for SSTR expression on functional imaging is receptor uptake greater than normal liver parenchyma (Krenning grade 2 on SSTR scintigraphy). All lesions meeting size criteria for visibility on SSTR imaging should be positive. The threshold uptake for ^{68}Ga-DOTATATE is less clear.

NEW RADIONUCLIDES UNDER STUDY

In recent years, there has been significant interest in alpha particle emitting radionuclides such as [213]Bi or [225]Ac for PRRT. These radionuclides emit high-energy particles, 8.32 MeV for [213]Bi and 27.5 MeV for [225]Ac, combined with short particle ranges of only 50 to 80 μm, allowing for extremely targeted therapy and the ability to spare normal tissue from radiotoxicity. The linear energy transfer is much higher for alpha particles than beta particles (^{90}Y and ^{177}Lu), which may be of therapeutic benefit in PRRT application, particularly in micrometastatic disease.[36] Because the cytotoxic effect of alpha radiation is independent of the cell cycle and oxygen concentration, this treatment may be especially beneficial to tumors in hypoxic regions.[37] A pilot study of 3 patients in which [213]Bi-DOTATOC was administered to NET patients refractory to ^{90}Y-DOTATOC or ^{177}Lu-DOTATOC showed marked reduction in tumor vascularity and no progression during a 9-month follow-up.[38]

Limitations of alpha-emitting particles include formation of daughter radionuclides could potentially accumulate outside of tumors, particularly in the renal cortex causing late nephrotoxicity.[38] Another difficulty involves the manufacture of these radioisotopes: for example, the half-life of [213]Bi is only 46 minutes.[39]

NEOADJUVANT PEPTIDE RECEPTOR RADIONUCLIDE THERAPIES

Several small case series and reports have described the neoadjuvant use of PRRT in patients with locally advanced or oligometastatic NETs. In 1 case series, 5 patients with inoperable pancreaticoduodenal NETs were treated with ^{177}Lu-DOTATATE concurrently with 5-fluorouracil. All 5 patients had a response on SSTR scintigraphy, and 4 had a radiologic response on cross-sectional imaging. One patient's response allowed for curative surgery.[40] There are numerous other case studies exploring the results of various neoadjuvant PRRT treatments.[41] Further data are needed to define the role of PRRT in the neoadjuvant setting.

INTRAARTERIAL ADMINISTRATION OF PEPTIDE RECEPTOR RADIONUCLIDE THERAPIES

The liver is the dominant site of metastatic disease in most well-differentiated NETs, and liver-directed therapies represent an important treatment modality. Recently, intraarterial hepatic administration of PRRT has been explored as a locoregional treatment option for patients with liver dominant metastatic disease.[42] In a preclinical rat liver model, ^{111}In-DTPA-octreotide was used and hepatic tumoral uptake was found to be twice as high after locoregional administration than after intravenous administration.[42] Similar results were noted in a clinical study of 15 patients with NET after administration of ^{68}Ga-DOTATOC, with standardized uptake values after intraarterial administration of 3.75 times the standardized uptake values found in patients with intravenous administration.[43] This finding was further explored by administering [90]Y- or ^{177}Lu-DOTATOC via the hepatic artery to 15 patients with liver disease arising from gastroenteropancreatic NETs. The objective radiologic response rate of 60% was high compared with response rates typically seen with intravenous administration.

COMBINATION THERAPIES

The combination of PRRT with potentially radiosensitizing cytotoxic drugs has been explored to improve antitumor response in the metastatic setting. Numerous studies have evaluated the combination of ^{177}Lu-DOTATATE with capecitabine as a radiosensitizing agent with promising results (ORR, 24%; median PFS not yet reached after 16 months of follow-up).[44,45] Similar results have been noted in the combination of ^{177}Lu-DOTATATE and 5-fluorouracil.[44] A particularly promising study evaluated the combination of PRRT with capecitabine and temozolomide.[46] This regimen yielded a complete response rate of 15% and partial response of 38% with a median PFS of 31 months.[46] Everolimus in combination with PRRT has been explored in a phase I trial, with an ORR of 44%.[47] Several studies have explored the combination of radionuclides by alternating ^{90}Y-DOTATOC and ^{177}Lu-DOTATATE administration over the course of 4 cycles. In a phase II study with 26 participants, a response rate of 42% was noted with a median PFS of 25 months.[48] Another study compared the combination of radionuclides to patients who received single agent ^{90}Y-DOTATOC, with results favoring combination treatment.[49]

Despite the positive results in all combination therapies mentioned, it is difficult to determine whether there is a true benefit to combination therapy versus sequential therapy. Prospective, randomized, controlled trials are required to definitively state whether or not there is an advantage to combination therapies.

RETREATMENT

Despite the durable response to PRRT, most patients experience disease progression. Several retrospective studies have reviewed the data available regarding retreatment with additional cycles of PRRT after progression and have found that retreatment is safe; however, it is associated with a lower tumor response compared with initial treatment.[9] A recent study explored the PFS and OS of patients after a first or second course of retreatment with 2 administrations of ^{177}Lu-DOTATATE. PFS and OS were similar in both the retreated and re-retreated cohorts, both with a PFS of 14 months, and an OS of 26 and 29 months, respectively. Hematologic and renal toxicities were not higher in prevalence than previously reported, indicating that salvage PRRT is a potential treatment option for patients who have an adequate response after initial treatment with PRRT.[50]

SAFETY PROFILE

PRRT is generally well-tolerated with the majority of acute side effects primarily attributable to the concurrent amino acid infusion required to prevent renal toxicity. Although arginine/lysine administrations are quite tolerable, the use of commercial amino acid formulations induce substantially higher rates of nausea and vomiting.[7] Significant acute hematologic toxicities are relatively uncommon: rates of grade 3 or 4 leukopenia and thrombocytopenia of 5% have been reported with ^{177}Lu-DOTATATE.[34] The occurrence of lymphopenia is substantially more common, but is not of clinical consequence because opportunistic infections are not observed.[9,51] Carcinoid crisis is a rare occurrence and has only been reported in less than 1% of patients who receive PRRT.[52] The known long-term adverse events associated with PRRT include renal dysfunction and leukemia/myelodysplastic syndrome.[9] Myelodysplastic syndrome or acute leukemia have been reported in approximately 2% of patients who received PRRT, typically about 3 years after treatment.[21,53] Rates of severe nephrotoxicity of nearly 10% have been reported in patients receiving ^{90}Y-DOTATOC. However, the risk of grade 3 or 4 nephrotoxicity in patients receiving ^{177}Lu-DOTATATE with amino acid prophylaxis is negligible.

FUTURE DIRECTIONS

At this time, PRRT has not been compared with an active NET treatment. The recently launched COMPETE trial randomizes patients with nonfunctioning gastroenteropancreatic NETs to receive ^{177}Lu-DOTATOC versus everolimus. This important phase III study will offer vital insight as to the appropriate positioning of PRRT within the therapeutic algorithm.

Combination studies with immunotherapy have generated interest given the potential immunostimulatory effects of radiation. However, the efficacy of immunotherapy in NETs remains uncertain.[54]

SUMMARY

PRRT has now been established as a safe and effective treatment for patients with somatostatin-receptor positive gastroenteropancreatic NETs progressing on SSAs. Future studies are needed to determine how to select the most appropriate patients for this treatment and to explore new radiolabeled SSAs as well as new modes of administration.

REFERENCES

1. Ramage JK, Davies AH, Ardill J, et al. Guidelines for the management of gastro-enteropancreatic neuroendocrine (including carcinoid) tumours. Gut 2005; 54(Suppl 4):iv1–16.
2. Cives M, Soares HP, Strosberg J. Will clinical heterogeneity of neuroendocrine tumors impact their management in the future? Lessons from recent trials. Curr Opin Oncol 2016;28(4):359–66.
3. Reubi JC, Schar JC, Waser B, et al. Affinity profiles for human somatostatin receptor subtypes SST1-SST5 of somatostatin radiotracers selected for scinti-graphic and radiotherapeutic use. Eur J Nucl Med 2000;27:273–82.
4. Chan JA, Kulke MH. Progress in the treatment of neuroendocrine tumors. Curr Oncol Rep 2009;11:193–9.
5. Hamiditabar M, Ali M, Roys J, et al. Peptide receptor radionuclide therapy with 177Lu-octreotate in patients with somatostatin receptor expressing neuroendo-crine tumors. Clin Nucl Med 2017;42(6):436–43.
6. Krenning EP, Kooij PP, Bakker WH, et al. Radiotherapy with a radiolabeled so-matostatin analogue, [111In-DTPA-D-Phe1]-octreotide. A case history. Ann N Y Acad Sci 1994;733:496–506.
7. Strosberg J, El-Haddad G, Wolin E, et al. Phase 3 trial of 177Lu-dotatate for midgut neuroendocrine tumors. N Engl J Med 2017;376(2):125–35.
8. Capello A, Krenning EP, Breeman WA, et al. Peptide receptor radionuclide ther-apy in vitro using [111In-DTPA0]octreotide. J Nucl Med 2003;44(1):98–104.
9. Cives M, Strosberg J. Radionuclide therapy for neuroendocrine tumors. Curr On-col Rep 2017;19(2):9.
10. Valkema R, De Jong M, Bakker WH, et al. Phase I study of peptide receptor radio-nuclide therapy with [In-DTPA]octreotide: the Rotterdam experience. Semin Nucl Med 2002;32:110–22.
11. Anthony LB, Woltering EA, Espenan GD, et al. Indium-111-pentetreotide prolongs survival in gastroenteropancreatic malignancies. Semin Nucl Med 2002;32: 123–32.
12. Sabet A, Biersack H-J, Ezziddin S. Advances in peptide receptor radionuclide therapy. Semin Nucl Med 2016;46(1):40–6.
13. Pool SE, Krenning EP, Koning GA, et al. Preclinical and clinical studies of peptide receptor radionuclide therapy. Semin Nucl Med 2010;40(3):209–18.
14. Kwekkeboom DJ, Kam BL, van Essen M, et al. Somatostatin-receptor-based im-aging and therapy of gastroenteropancreatic neuroendocrine tumors. Endocr Re-lat Cancer 2010;17(1):R53–73.
15. Kratochwil C, Stefanova M, Mavriopoulou E, et al. SUV of [68Ga]DOTATOC-PET/CT predicts response probability of PRRT in neuroendocrine tumors. Mol Imaging Biol 2015;17(3):313–8.
16. Kwekkeboom DJ, Teunissen JJ, Bakker WH, et al. Radiolabeled somatostatin analog [177Lu-DOTA0,Tyr3]octreotate in patients with endocrine gastroentero-pancreatic tumors. J Clin Oncol 2005;23(12):2754–62.
17. Ezziddin S, Attassi M, Yong-Hing CJ, et al. Predictors of long-term outcome in patients with well-differentiated gastroenteropancreatic neuroendocrine tumors after peptide receptor radionuclide therapy with 177Lu-octreotate. J Nucl Med 2014;55(2):183–90.

18. Bodei L, Cremonesi M, Grana CM, et al. Peptide receptor radionuclide therapy with 177Lu-DOTATATE: the IEO phase I-II study. Eur J Nucl Med Mol Imaging 2011;38(12):2125–35.
19. Delpassand ES, Samarghandi A, Zamanian S, et al. Peptide receptor radionuclide therapy with 177Lu-DOTATATE for patients with somatostatin receptor–expressing neuroendocrine tumors. Pancreas 2014;43(4):518–25.
20. Ezziddin S, Khalaf F, Vanezi M, et al. Outcome of peptide receptor radionuclide therapy with 177Lu-octreotate in advanced grade 1/2 pancreatic neuroendocrine tumours. Eur J Nucl Med Mol Imaging 2014;41(5):925–33.
21. Danthala M, Kallur KG, Prashant GR, et al. 177Lu-DOTATATE therapy in patients with neuroendocrine tumours: 5 years' experience from a tertiary cancer care centre in India. Eur J Nucl Med Mol Imaging 2014;41(7):1319–26.
22. Sabet A, Dautzenberg K, Haslerud T, et al. Specific efficacy of peptide receptor radionuclide therapy with (177)Lu-octreotate in advanced neuroendocrine tumours of the small intestine. Eur J Nucl Med Mol Imaging 2015;42(8):1238–46.
23. Brabander T, Zwan WAVD, Teunissen JJ, et al. Long-term efficacy, survival, and safety of [177 Lu-DOTA 0 ,Tyr 3]octreotate in patients with gastroenteropancreatic and bronchial neuroendocrine tumors. Clin Cancer Res 2017;23(16):4617–24.
24. Waldherr C, Pless M, Maecke HR, et al. Tumor response and clinical benefit in neuroendocrine tumors after 7.4 GBq 90Y-DOTATOC. J Nucl Med 2002;43(5):610–6.
25. Bodei L, Cremonesi M, Zoboli S, et al. Receptor-mediated radionuclide therapy with 90Y-DOTATOC in association with amino acid infusion: a phase I study. Eur J Nucl Med Mol Imaging 2003;30(2):207–16.
26. Paganelli G, Bodei L, Junak DH, et al. 90Y-DOTA-D-Phe1-Try3- octreotide in therapy of neuroendocrine malignancies. Biopolymers 2002;66(6):393–8.
27. Valkema R, Pauwels S, Kvols LK, et al. Survival and response after peptide receptor radionuclide therapy with [90Y-DOTA0, Tyr3]octreotide in patients with advanced gastroenteropancreatic neuroendocrine tumors. Semin Nucl Med 2006;36(2):147–56.
28. Bushnell DL, Odorisio TM, Odorisio MS, et al. 90Y-edotreotide for metastatic carcinoid refractory to octreotide. J Clin Oncol 2010;28(10):1652–9.
29. Cwikla JB, Sankowski A, Seklecka N, et al. Efficacy of radionuclide treatment DOTATATE Y-90 in patients with progressive metastatic gastroenteropancreatic neuroendocrine carcinomas (GEP-NETs): a phase II study. Ann Oncol 2009;21(4):787–94.
30. Imhof A, Brunner P, Marincek N, et al. Response, survival, and long-term toxicity after therapy with the radiolabeled somatostatin analogue [90Y-DOTA]-TOC in metastasized neuroendocrine cancers. J Clin Oncol 2011;29(17):2416–23.
31. Sowa-Staszczak A, Pach D, Kunikowska J, et al. Efficacy and safety of 90Y-DOTATATE therapy in neuroendocrine tumours. Endokrynol Pol 2011;62(5):392–400.
32. Savelli G, Bertagna F, Franco F, et al. Final results of a phase 2A study for the treatment of metastatic neuroendocrine tumors with a fixed activity of 90Y-DOTA-D-Phe1-Tyr3 octreotide. Cancer 2011;118(11):2915–24.
33. Vinjamuri S, Gilbert TM, Banks M, et al. Peptide receptor radionuclide therapy with 90Y-DOTATATE/90Y-DOTATOC in patients with progressive metastatic neuroendocrine tumours: assessment of response, survival and toxicity. Br J Cancer 2013;108(7):1440–8.

34. Kim S-J, Pak K, Koo PJ, et al. The efficacy of 177Lu-labelled peptide receptor radionuclide therapy in patients with neuroendocrine tumours: a meta-analysis. Eur J Nucl Med Mol Imaging 2015;42(13):1964–70.

35. Strosberg J, Wolin E, Chasen B, et al. Health-Related Quality of Life in Patients With Progressive Midgut Neuroendocrine Tumors Treated With ^{177}Lu-Dotatate in the Phase III NETTER-1 Trial. J Clin Oncol 2018. [Epub ahead of print].

36. Bison SM, Konijnenberg MW, Melis M, et al. Peptide receptor radionuclide therapy using radiolabeled somatostatin analogs: focus on future developments. Clin Transl Imaging 2014;2(1):55–66.

37. Dodson H, Wheatley SP, Morrison CG. Involvement of centrosome amplification in radiation-induced mitotic catastrophe. Cell Cycle 2007;6(3):364–70.

38. Giesel FL, Wulfert S, Zechmann CM, et al. Contrast-enhanced ultrasound monitoring of perfusion changes in hepatic neuroendocrine metastases after systemic versus selective arterial 177Lu/90Y-DOTATOC and 213Bi-DOTATOC radiopeptide therapy. Exp Oncol 2013;35(2):122–6.

39. Miederer M, Henriksen G, Alke A, et al. Preclinical evaluation of the alpha-particle generator nuclide 225Ac for somatostatin receptor radiotherapy of neuroendocrine tumors. Clin Cancer Res 2008;14(11):3555–61.

40. Barber TW, Hofman MS, Thomson BN, et al. The potential for induction peptide receptor chemoradionuclide therapy to render inoperable pancreatic and duodenal neuroendocrine tumours resectable. Eur J Surg Oncol 2012;38(1):64–71.

41. Perysinakis I, Aggeli C, Kaltsas G, et al. Neoadjuvant therapy for advanced pancreatic neuroendocrine tumors: an emerging treatment modality? Hormones (Athens) 2015. https://doi.org/10.14310/horm.2002.1636.

42. Pool SE, Kam B, Breeman WAP. Increasing intrahepatic tumour uptake of 111In-DTPA-octreotide by loco regional administration. Eur J Nucl Med Mol Imaging 2009;36:S427.

43. Kratochwil C, Giesel FL, López-Benítez R, et al. Intraindividual comparison of selective arterial versus venous 68Ga-DOTATOC PET/CT in patients with gastroenteropancreatic neuroendocrine tumors. Clin Cancer Res 2010;16(10):2899–905.

44. Claringbold PG, Brayshaw PA, Price RA, et al. Phase II study of radiopeptide 177Lu-octreotate and capecitabine therapy of progressive disseminated neuroendocrine tumours. Eur J Nucl Med Mol Imaging 2011;38(2):302–11.

45. Kong G, Thompson M, Collins M, et al. Assessment of predictors of response and long-term survival of patients with neuroendocrine tumour treated with peptide receptor chemoradionuclide therapy (PRCRT). Eur J Nucl Med Mol Imaging 2014;41(10):1831–44.

46. Claringbold PG, Price RA, Turner JH. Phase I-II study of radiopeptide 177Lu-octreotate in combination with capecitabine and temozolomide in advanced low-grade neuroendocrine tumors. Cancer Biother Radiopharm 2012;27(9):561–9.

47. Claringbold PG, Turner JH. Neuroendocrine tumor therapy with lutetium-177-octreotate and everolimus (NETTLE): a phase I study. Cancer Biother Radiopharm 2015;30(6):261–9.

48. Seregni E, Maccauro M, Chiesa C, et al. Treatment with tandem [90Y]DOTA-TATE and [177Lu]DOTA-TATE of neuroendocrine tumours refractory to conventional therapy. Eur J Nucl Med Mol Imaging 2014;41(2):223–30.

49. Kunikowska J, Królicki L, Hubalewska-Dydejczyk A, et al. Clinical results of radionuclide therapy of neuroendocrine tumours with 90Y-DOTATATE and tan- dem 90Y/177Lu-DOTATATE: which is a better therapy option? Eur J Nucl Med Mol Imaging 2011;38(10):1788–97.

50. van der Zwan W, Brabander T, Kam B, et al. PFS and OS After Salvage Peptide Receptor Radionuclide Therapy (PRRT) with 177-Lu[Dota0,Tyr3]octreotate in Patients with GastroEnteroPancreatic or Bronchial NeuroEndocrine Tumours (GEP-NETs) – The Rotterdam Cohort [284]. Pancreas 2018;47(3):332–61.

51. Bodei L, Kwekkeboom DJ, Kidd M, et al. Radiolabeled somatostatin analogue therapy of gastroenteropancreatic cancer. Semin Nucl Med 2016;46(3):225–38.

52. de Keizer B, van Aken MO, Feelders RA, et al. Hormonal crises following receptor radionuclide therapy with the radiolabeled somatostatin analogue [177Lu-DOTA0,Tyr3]octreotate. Eur J Nucl Med Mol Imaging 2008;35(4):749–55.

53. Kwekkeboom DJ, Krenning EP. Peptide receptor radionuclide therapy in the treatment of neuroendocrine tumors. Hematol Oncol Clin North Am 2016;30(1): 179–91.

54. Wu Y, Pfeifer AK, Myschetzky R, et al. Induction of anti-tumor immune responses by peptide receptor radionuclide therapy with (177)Lu-DOTATATE in a murine model of a human neuroendocrine tumor. Diagnostics (Basel) 2013;3(4):344–55.

Surgical Approaches to the Management of Neuroendocrine Liver Metastases

Andrea Frilling, MD, PhD*, Ashley Kieran Clift, BA, MBBS

KEYWORDS

- Neuroendocrine • Tumors • Neoplasm • Liver • Metastases • Surgery
- Transplantation

KEY POINTS

- Surgical treatment of hepatic metastases from neuroendocrine neoplasms may involve resection with curative intention, cytoreductive surgery, or transplantation procedures.
- Hepatic resection with microscopically clear margins represents the only modality capable of offering cure for neuroendocrine liver metastases, but patient selection criteria must be better defined.
- Cure is, however, rarely realized, as postresection recurrence is a major issue and affects most patients undergoing hepatectomy. Follow-up regimens postsurgery must be standardized and require inclusion of sensitive methods for detecting disease recurrence.
- Multimodal concepts including neoadjuvant and adjuvant therapy should be incorporated into surgical treatment of patients with neuroendocrine liver metastases, and novel biomarkers for treatment selection are required.
- Liver transplantation is a generally accepted therapeutic option in highly selected patients.

INTRODUCTION

The management of neuroendocrine (NE) liver metastases (LMs) (NELMs) occupies a critical position within the treatment of patients with NE neoplasms (NEN), as they are not only common, but their presence exerts a major impact on patient survival.[1–4] The Surveillance, Epidemiology and End Results-9 database reports a 27% rate of hepatic metastasis from NEN generally,[5] although a stronger predisposition to dissemination within the liver is recorded in cohorts treated in specialist centers (between 40% and 95%).[6,7] The incidence of hepatic metastases is arguably most marked in patients with

Disclosure Statement: The authors have no conflicts of interest to disclose.
Department of Surgery and Cancer, Imperial College London, Hammersmith Hospital Campus, Du Cane Road, London W12 0HS, UK
* Corresponding author.
E-mail address: a.frilling@imperial.ac.uk

Endocrinol Metab Clin N Am 47 (2018) 627–643
https://doi.org/10.1016/j.ecl.2018.04.001
0889-8529/18/© 2018 Elsevier Inc. All rights reserved.

small bowel NEN (67%–91%) and pancreatic NEN (28.3%–77.0%),[8,9] whereas fewer than 1% of patients with appendiceal NEN display this.[10]

The treatment of NELM may use a diverse range of therapeutic modalities incorporating surgery, medical therapies, nuclear medicine approaches, and interventional radiological techniques.[6] However, surgical intervention represents the only modality that offers potential cure. Nevertheless, there is also scope for surgical intervention with palliative intent, such as in patients symptomatic with hormonally functional tumor burden refractory to medical therapy. Here, we review the roles of surgical treatment for NELM, including radiological assessment of suitability for surgery. We discuss resection of hepatic deposits with curative intent, cytoreductive resection (or "debulking"), and transplantation approaches. Throughout, we discuss the currently available evidence for each strategy, including its limitations, provide concise recommendations regarding patient suitability for each surgical approach, and also identify avenues for further investigation and development.

RADIOLOGICAL ASSESSMENT OF NEUROENDOCRINE LIVER METASTASES

Integral concepts in surgical oncology include assessment of oncological and technical resectability, namely the appropriateness of resection given the status of an individual's malignant disease, and the feasibility of anatomic factors, respectively. In patients with NELMs considered for surgery, radiological interrogation of the number and size of LMs is crucial alongside their proximity to vascular and biliary structures, and also estimation of the resulting future liver remnant. The morphologic and functional imaging modalities for detecting and assessing the resectability of NELMs have been recently extensively reviewed elsewhere,[11] and it is notable that evaluation of the existence of extrahepatic disease is mandated when considering optimal strategies for NELM.

Three morphologic patterns of NELM growth or distribution have been described that have direct ramifications on not only patient selection, but also prognosis.[12] The "simple" type I pattern describes a single liver metastasis of any size or location; the "complex" type II pattern describes a bulk of LM in one liver lobe with smaller lesions in the other; whereas the "diffuse" type III pattern refers to disseminated multifocal spread, which represents up to 70% of cases. In the case of the latter, such patients are not eligible for curative hepatectomy, but may be candidates for liver transplantation.

Ultrasound appearances of NELMs are variable, possibly with hypo-echoic, iso-echoic, or hyper-echoic features, although a mixed type is most common, especially when compared with other hepatic secondary deposits. A central cystic appearance is typical of this tumor type, and the hypervascularity of NELMs may be elucidated on color Doppler imaging, or via arterial enhancement on contrast-enhanced ultrasound.[13] The latter does identify significantly more NELMs than conventional ultrasound, but it is not often used in clinical practice. Computed tomography (CT) is a standard morphologic modality used in oncological imaging generally, and can depict more deposits than CEUS[14]; in view of the aforementioned hypervascular nature, CT must incorporate hepatic arterial-phase examination (**Fig. 1**). MRI with hepatic arterial-phase and fat-suppressed T2-weighted images may depict the most NELMs; however, diffusion-weighted MRI possesses even higher specificity even in deposits smaller than 1 cm, and should be systematically performed.[15]

The expression of somatostatin receptors by most well-differentiated NEN may be exploited for treatment and are also a target for molecular/functional imaging with radiolabeled agonists or antagonists (**Fig. 2**). The historically universally used modality

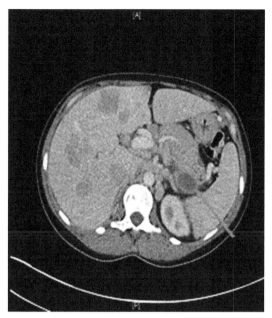

Fig. 1. CT imaging findings in a patient with bilobar multifocal type II LMs from a grade 2 NEN of the pancreas (*arrow*).

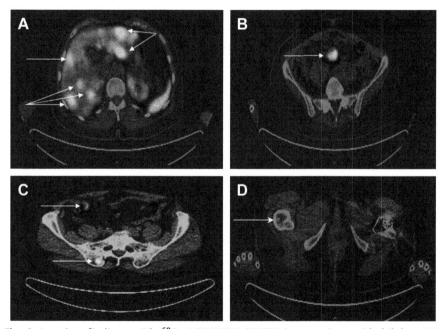

Fig. 2. Imaging findings with ^{68}Ga-DOTATATE PET/CT in a patient with bilobar LMs (*A, arrows*) from a NEN of the distal ileum (*C, arrow*). Also depicted are mesenteric lymph node metastases (*B, arrow*), a pelvic bone metastasis (*C, bottom arrow*), and a small metastatic deposit in the right femur (*D, arrow*).

of somatostatin-targeted scintigraphy with ^{111}In-octreotide has been superseded by somewhat revolutionary PET combined with CT (PET/CT) using ^{68}Ga-DOTA peptides, which may have a resolution of 5 mm.[11] Indeed, in low-grade and intermediate-grade NEN, ^{68}Ga-conjugated radiopharmaceuticals are the gold-standard imaging modality; they may detect NELM with high sensitivity (82%–100%), specificity (67%–100%), and also depict extrahepatic disease with comparable veracity (sensitivity 85%–100% and specificity 67%–90%).[16] Furthermore, PET/CT with ^{68}Ga-DOTA peptides identifies an increasingly significant number of patients to harbor bone metastases, although the oncological relevance of these deposits is not clear.[17,18] Such favorable diagnostic power may alter initially constructed treatment strategies in up to 60% of patients with NELMs, such as a modified surgical approach or deselection for surgery.[19,20]

Dual imaging with ^{68}Ga-DOTA and ^{18}F-FDG PET/CT offers further metabolic characterization of tumors, and is increasingly suggested to be performed in tandem to capture the known heterogeneity of neuroendocrine lesions and perform a more comprehensive assessment of neuroendocrine disease with prognostic relevance.[21,22]

Radiological evaluation of hepatic lesions for their amenability to resection or transplantation should ideally comprise both morphologic and functional imaging modalities. The detection and characterization of NELM is crucial for selection of appropriate treatment regardless of modality used, as is evaluation of extrahepatic disease; however, it is arguably most crucial in those considered for surgical intervention. Somatostatin receptor-targeted functional imaging, especially with ^{68}Ga-radiolabeled peptides, has significant ramifications on selection for a surgical approach, as well as identifying those suitable for alternative/additional therapies, particularly peptide receptor radionuclide therapy (PRRT).

RESECTION WITH CURATIVE INTENT

Patients with G1/G2 NEN with type 1 hepatic disease burden and selected patients with type II LM may be candidates for liver resection with curative intent. Those with predominantly hepatic and extrahepatic disease may also be candidates, provided that their extrahepatic disease is completely resectable.[6] In the case of coexistent bone metastases, these may be treated with PRRT and thus may not necessarily constitute a contraindication to curative resection. Given these restrictions, unsurprisingly only up to 20% of all patients with NELMs are eligible candidates for this approach.[3] However, a small, additional proportion of patients with primarily unresectable bilobar metastases may be rendered possibly eligible with advanced surgical procedures that focus on ensuring adequate future liver remnant function. These may include 2-step resections,[23,24] with right portal vein embolization or division with secondary left liver lobe hypertrophy.[25] Additionally, radiation lobectomy following selective internal radiotherapy using [90]Yttrium-labeled microspheres, as a bridging strategy for later resection in patients with predominant right lobar metastases and "small-for-size" left lobes, may be possible.[26]

Resection with curative intent is associated with the most favorable outcomes in patients with NELM (**Table 1**); indeed, a recent systematic review by Saxena and colleagues[27] that included 29 eligible retrospective series calculated median 1-year, 3-year, 5-year, and 10-year overall survival (OS) rates of 94% (range 79%–100%), 83% (range 63%–100%), 70.5% (range 31%–100%), and 42% (range 0%–100%), respectively. These were obtained in the context of a median rate of R0 resection of 63% (range 38%–100%), median perioperative morbidity rates of 23% (range 3%–45%), and median postoperative mortality of 0% (range 0%–9%). However, these

Table 1
Results from hepatic resection stratified on the basis of margin status from selected recent institutional series

Author and Year	Total Patients, n	N	R0/R1 Resection, OS	PFS	N	R2 Resection, OS	PFS
Fairweather et al,[28] 2017	649	58	5 y 90% 10 y 70%	NR	—	—	—
Maxwell et al,[49] 2016	228	—	—	—	108	Median 10.5 y 5 y 76.1%	Median 2.2 y 5 y 30.2%
Saxena et al,[63] 2011	74	48	Median 98 mo	Median 18 mo	26	Median 27 mo	Median 24 mo
Scigliano et al,[64] 2009	41	37	R0 88% R1 82%	R0 31% R1 9%	4	50%	0%
Frilling et al,[12] 2009	119	23	100%	96%	—	—	—
Gomez et al,[65] 2007	18	15	86%	90%	3	—	25%
Elias et al,[48] 2003	47	37	R0 74% R1 70%	R0 66% R1 46%	10	47%	30%
Sarmiento et al,[42] 2003	170	75	76%	—	95	—	9%

Abbreviations: OS, 5-year overall survival unless otherwise stated; PFS, 5-year progression-free survival unless otherwise stated; R0, microscopically clear margins; R1, microscopically invaded margins; R2, macroscopically incomplete resection.

favorable OS rates with seemingly acceptable morbidity/mortality profiles were in contrast to the reported rates of median 1-year, 3-year, 5-year, and 10-year recurrence-free survival rates of 63% (range 50%–80%), 32% (range 24%–69%), 29% (range 6%–66%), and 1% (0%–11%) only.

Several retrospective case series have compared the outcomes of hepatic resection and other liver-directed therapies. The recent single-center series of Fairweather and colleagues[28] reviewed the management of 649 patients with NELM, only 58 of whom (9%) underwent liver resection, manifesting as left or right hepatectomy, wedge resection, left lateral segmentectomy, or trisectionectomy. The median number of resected hepatic metastases per patient was 1.5 (range 1–15), with a median aggregate resected tumor size of 7 cm (range 0.4–20 cm). The median, 5-year, and 10-year OS rates for hepatic resection were 160 months, 90%, and 70%, respectively, which were significantly improved as compared with radiofrequency ablation (RFA) (123 months, 84%, 55%), chemoembolization (66 months, 55%, 28%), and systemic therapy (70 months, 58%, 31%) or just observation (38 months, 38%, 20%). However, there was no documentation of the selection criteria, nor was there any information regarding disease recurrence. Contrastingly, a larger international, multicentric series of 339 patients undergoing resection for NELM reported 5-year and 10-year OS of 75% and 51%, yet 1-year, 3-year, and 5-year recurrence-free survivals were comparatively dismal at 56.9%, 24.2%, and 5.9%, respectively.[29]

Although recurrence after resection is often anticipated, the optimal management of recurrent disease is not clear. Repeat surgery has been advocated as safe and effective for intrahepatic recurrences of hepatocellular carcinomas, colonic adenocarcinomas, and intrahepatic cholangiocarcinomas[30–32]; however, evidence is lacking in NELM. A multi-institutional analysis of 322 patients with NELM undergoing hepatic resection with curative intent identified 209 (64.9%) who subsequently developed recurrence within a median follow-up of 4.5 years.[32] Data regarding site of recurrence were available for 169 patients; in this subset, intrahepatic-only recurrence occurred in 111 (65.7%), and extrahepatic recurrence occurred in 19 (11.2%), whereas mixed intrahepatic and extrahepatic recurrence occurred in 39 (23.1%). The commonest therapeutic modalities used in recurrent LM in this study were repeat resection (36.6%) and intra-arterial therapy (21.4%), respectively. Ten-year OS for patients receiving repeat surgery or liver-directed intra-arterial therapy for recurrent NELM was 60.3% and 52.0%, respectively.

There is a fledgling body of evidence examining the role of hepatic resection in metastatic neuroendocrine carcinoma (NEC), which may be defined as poorly differentiated G3 NEN.[33] Classically, hepatic resection has not been advocated in this patient group, which may expect a median survival of just 11 months with chemotherapy,[34] with platinum-based cytotoxic agents the recommended first-line therapy.[33] This is despite there being no robust evidence to refute the utility of surgery in this patient group. In the recent case series of Galleberg and colleagues,[35] 32 patients with gastroenteropancreatic NEC underwent surgery with or without RFA (or RFA alone, n = 6). Twenty patients (62.5%) had a Ki-67 greater than 55%, with the vast majority (75%) harboring poorly differentiated tumors. OS at 3 years and 5 years postsurgery/RFA was 47% and 43%, respectively, and patients with a Ki-67 of 21% to 54% had significantly prolonged average OS compared with those with Ki-67 greater than 55% (61.6 months vs 21.2 months). Regarding recurrence, 87% of patients' disease had recurred by 5 years. Median progression-free survival (PFS) after surgery was 8.4 months, and there was an insignificant trend toward improved PFS in those with Ki-67 21% to 54% compared with those with Ki67 greater than 55%. Again, there was no clear discussion of criteria for patient selection for surgery in this retrospective analysis.

Clearly, disease recurrence after hepatic resection is a major clinical issue, which is predominantly predicated by currently available imaging techniques significantly understaging disease within the liver.[36] Given their relative indolence compared with adenocarcinomas, NEN micrometastases below the sensitivity thresholds for current morphologic and functional imaging may avoid detection and become apparent over a relatively protracted postoperative time frame. Indeed, meticulous pathologic studies of resected specimens have demonstrated that imaging fails to detect approximately 50% of lesions.[36] Neoadjuvant and adjuvant concepts are thus mandated to be offered in conjunction with hepatectomy, focusing either on control/eradication of such micrometastases (which are often miliary in nature), and/or possible downstaging of primarily unresectable disease (**Fig. 3**). Admittedly, the evidence for such concepts is scarce and mostly limited to case reports, small series, or extrapolated from trials of other therapeutic modalities.[37,38] For example, PRRT has been suggested as a suitable agent for downsizing NEN for facilitation of possible later resection, including in a Polish series of 6 patients, of whom 2 had surgical intervention facilitated by tumor size reduction predicated by PRRT.[37] The recent series of Partelli and colleagues[39] compared postoperative outcomes in patients with resectable/potentially resectable pancreatic NEN deemed at high risk of recurrence treated with or without neoadjuvant PRRT (n = 23 in each): the incidence of nodal metastases was significantly lower in the PRRT group, and the PFS in patients receiving an R0 resection was prolonged in those who underwent preoperative PRRT. Clearly, although such results require validation in larger cohorts, and specifically in the context of LMs, the limited data do suggest a role for PRRT in the neoadjuvant setting.

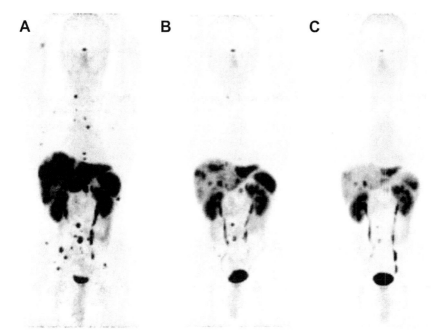

Fig. 3. Imaging findings with ^{68}Ga-DOTATATE PET/CT in a 32-year-old male patient with a metastasized insulinoma at initial diagnosis (A), and after 4 (B) and 6 (C) cycles of 177 Lutetium PRRT. Tumor downstaging with PRRT enabled later resection of LMs and the primary tumor.

Overall, complete resection of hepatic metastases does occupy a central role in the treatment of patients with NELM, but it possesses the following major limitations:

1. It is performed in an often-diminutive proportion of highly selected patients, and the selection criteria are very poorly documented in published series.
2. Candidates for surgery have lower-volume disease, and tend to be younger, with fewer comorbidities. Thus, the extent to which favorable outcomes are attributable to favorable patient or tumor-specific characteristics rather than efficacy of treatment cannot be quantified, as studies are not randomized.
3. Despite curative intention, virtually all patients develop recurrent disease. Surgical extirpation of disease is ultimately a palliative endeavor, even if complete resection is achieved.

Resection of hepatic metastases is the first-choice therapy for G1/G2 patients with low liver disease burden either with no extrahepatic disease, or resectable disease outside the liver. Small-volume bone metastases identified on ^{68}Ga-DOTA–PET/CT are not a contraindication for hepatic resection, as they may be effectively controlled by PRRT. Although R0 hepatic resection has been associated with the most favorable outcomes in patients with NELM, these results have been derived from stringently selected patients within retrospective, noncontrolled series, and recurrence is a major hindrance. To what extent the favorable outcomes are a reflection of selection bias is far from clear. As recurrence occurs in virtually all patients undergoing intended "curative" resection, this should be ultimately regarded as a palliative approach offering transient disease control, albeit for longer than other modalities. Neoadjuvant and adjuvant treatment concepts should be adopted into multimodal strategies for those undergoing hepatic resection.

DEBULKING SURGERY

Cytoreductive resection, also referred to as "debulking," may be offered to patients with G1/G2 hepatic disease burden so advanced as to render them ineligible for radical resection, or in patients with symptoms from endocrinopathy of hormone hypersecretion by bulky LMs. This also may be referred to as an R2 resection, wherein the resection margins are macroscopically incomplete. Historically, such procedures with purely palliative intent were offered to those in whom 90% extirpation of tumor burden could be attained. However, such a benchmark was derived from studies not exclusive to NEN, and the original study in NEN examined debulking as a therapeutic modality in patients with syndromic NEN before the introduction of somatostatin analog therapy.[40] Thus, the original intention of such a target was to provide a suitable threshold for symptom relief, not an oncological threshold for attaining improved survival. Nevertheless, this restrictive diktat has been persistent in the literature and may disqualify up to 90% of patients from receiving such intervention.[40–42] Recent data have suggested that a "relaxation" of selection criteria to attaining 70% disease resection may have beneficial ramifications on patient symptoms, possibly without inferior outcomes.[43–45]

In the aforementioned systematic review of hepatic resection in NELM by Saxena and colleagues,[27] the rate of R2 resection in published series was 18% (range 0%–36%). In the series of Mayo and colleagues,[29] of 339 patients undergoing surgical treatment of NELMs, 65 had an R2 margin status after the first operation; this, however, had no significant association with the risk of recurrence but was associated with decreased OS compared with R0 resection: mean survivals of 77.5 months and 156.9 months, respectively. The same article also reported superior OS with R0/R1 resection with LM from secreting NEN, whereas there was no effect of margin on OS in nonsecreting disease.

In view of the high rates of disease recurrence regardless of margin status as detailed previously, and also data from some multiple studies suggesting a lack of "penalty" on OS/PFS in terms of margins,[46–48] one may posit that all resections for NELM are in actuality cytoreductive and differ only in the duration of disease control. With skepticism surrounding the importance of microscopically versus macroscopically clear margins, accordingly, the selection of patients for debulking on the basis of anticipated percentage tumor removal requires scrutiny.

In their recent series of 42 patients with LM from pancreatic NEN undergoing 44 liver debulking procedures, Morgan and colleagues[45] examined outcomes in terms of OS and liver-specific PFS, that is, time until progression of hepatic disease (liver PFS). Five-year OS was 85%, whereas the median liver PFS was 11 months, and the estimated 5-year liver PFS was 5%. This group stratified patients on the basis of the percentage of gross hepatic metastases resected: ≥70%, ≥90%, and 100%. Interestingly, they failed to identify any significant associations between extent of debulking and rate of hepatic disease progression; the only significant predictor of disease progression within the liver was the size of the largest resected liver metastasis. Such data led the investigators to argue that expansion of criteria for debulking to a 70% threshold may be appropriate (**Fig. 4**).

This 70% threshold was also examined by the series of Maxwell and colleagues,[49] in which 108 patients with pancreatic or small-intestinal NEN underwent liver-directed surgery with parenchyma-sparing debulking techniques. Of all patients, 63.9% attained 70.0% debulking of their disease, whereas 90.0% cytoreduction was attained in only 38.9% of patients. Five-year OS with such parenchyma-sparing debulking was 72%. In patients with pancreatic NELM, PFS and OS were significantly prolonged

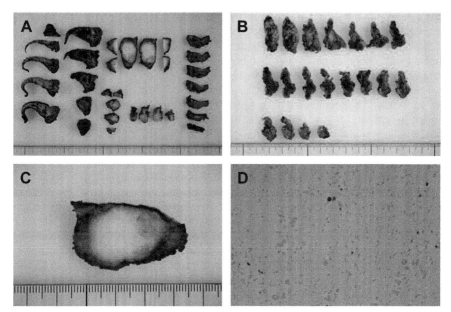

Fig. 4. Pathologic specimens of resected neuroendocrine LMs (*A–C*) with immunohistochemical staining of Ki-67 (*D*) demonstrating a proliferation index of 3%.

when greater than 70% debulking was achieved, whereas OS was not prolonged by 70% cytoreduction in patients with small-intestinal NELM. Cytoreduction of 90% was associated with improved PFS in both sets, but there was no significant effect on OS.

A final consideration regarding NELM debulking is the role for this option in the current era of multiple alternative therapeutic modalities being available, such as liver-directed intra-arterial treatments (including "bland" embolization, chemoembolization, and selective internal radiotherapy), RFA, PRRT, and medical therapies. Few studies, all of them retrospective, have compared outcomes with palliative resection and intra-arterial modalities, but that of Osborne and colleagues[50] did so in 120 symptomatic patients with NELM ineligible for resection. In this study, mean survivals with debulking and embolization were 32 months and 24 months, respectively. Of course, the classic caveat applies insofar as these data were from nonrandomized studies, and a Cochrane review stipulated that there is no evidence to support improved outcomes from cytoreductive hepatic surgery over intra-arterial therapies in NELM.[51]

Macroscopically incomplete resection (R2) has been associated with poorer survival outcomes as compared with R0/R1 resection, but the results are conflicting in this regard. Debulking surgery may be useful in symptomatic patients with incompletely resectable tumor burden, and/or hormonally active tumor bulk refractory to medical strategies. Resections of neuroendocrine LMs are all essentially cytoreductive approaches of differing fervor, rather than any being strictly curative. In light of recent advances of nonsurgical therapeutic modalities, the role for cytoreduction must be carefully considered.

ORTHOTOPIC LIVER TRANSPLANTATION

Although orthotopic liver transplantation (OLT) occupies a well-categorized and widely accepted role in the management of hepatocellular carcinoma (HCC), for which there are rigorous and validated selection criteria, indications in other primary or secondary liver tumors prove somewhat controversial. This relatively new concept of transplant oncology, however, has been increasingly applied to highly selected patients with NEN with nonresectable hepatic metastases, and experience from retrospective series suggest outcomes similar to those observed in HCC.[52–54] More than 700 patients worldwide have undergone OLT with hepatic metastases from NEN as an indication,[55] and although NENs are the indication for fewer than 0.2% of all liver transplants in the United States,[54] a recent systematic review of published registry series documented 1-year, 3-year, and 5-year OS of 89%, 69%, and 63%, respectively.[56] However, as with hepatic resection, disease recurrence is an issue, and this has ranged between 17.7% and 38.7% in the aforementioned registry series. Additional difficulties with OLT manifest as controversy regarding selection criteria. Outcomes from recent selected institutional and registry series are collated in **Table 2**.

The largest registry-based cohort reported to date is that of Le Treut and colleagues,[53] who examined outcomes in 213 European patients undergoing liver transplantation (LT) between 1982 and 2009. Overall, 3-month postoperative mortality was 10%, and OS and disease-free survival post-LT was 52% and 30%, respectively. In a subanalysis of patients undergoing transplantation after 2000, the 5-year OS attained was 59%. Of this cohort, 24 (11.3%) underwent major resection in addition to LT. Hepatomegaly, patient age older than 45 years, and any concurrent resection were all associated with poorer outcomes in patients undergoing transplantation after 2000; however, it is not clear what proportion of the detriment in survival in patients is attributable to the morbidity of a concomitant resection, or actual tumor biology. The investigators devised a 4-point scoring system based on the presence of the aforementioned parameters (ie, scores of 0–3): patients with a score of ≤ 1 and ≥ 2 demonstrated 5-year OS and disease-free survival of 79% and 57%, versus 35% and 19%, respectively.

There are data to suggest that several other clinicopathological factors may be associated with poorer long-term outcomes post-OLT, including greater than 50% liver involvement, higher proliferative index as measured by Ki-67%, and the organ site of the primary tumor,[56] which may merit their inclusion in selection criteria. Other factors, including patient age, have been included in suggested selection criteria by some centers; however, their validity have been contradicted in other reports.[57] In patients undergoing OLT for NEN since the implementation of the Model for End-Stage Liver Disease in the United States, higher bilirubin and lower albumin in the recipient,

Table 2
Results with orthotopic liver transplantation from selected institutional series

Author and Year	Patients, n	OS 1 y	OS 3 y	OS 5 y	OS 10 y	DFS 1 y	DFS 3 y	DFS 5 y	DFS 10 y
Mazzaferro et al,[59] 2016	42	—	—	97.2%	88.8%	—	—	86.9%	86.9%
Bonaccorsi-Riani et al,[66] 2010	9	88%	77%	33%	—	67%	33%	11%	—
Olausson et al,[57] 2007	15[a]	—	—	90%	—	—	70%	20%	—
Marín et al,[67] 2007	10	86%	57%	—	—	—	38%	—	—
van Vilsteren et al,[68] 2006	19	88%	—	—	—	80%	—	—	—
Frilling et al,[69] 2006	15[b]	78.3%	—	67.2%	—	69.4%	—	48.3%	—

Abbreviations: DFS, disease-free survival; OS, overall survival.
[a] Includes 5 patients undergoing multivisceral transplantation.
[b] Includes 1 patient undergoing multivisceral transplantation.

as well as higher creatinine in the donor, have been associated with poorer survival.[54] However, these parameters act as prognosticators in patients undergoing OLT for any indication, that is, they are not NEN-specific.

The Milan criteria as adapted for NEN patient selection by Mazzaferro and colleagues[58] ardently stipulate the following for selection for OLT: patients must have low-grade neuroendocrine tumor (NET) (with or without clinical syndrome), drainage of the primary tumor must be by the portal venous system, and patients must be aged ≤55 years, have ≤50% liver involvement, have complete resection of primary tumor and any extrahepatic disease before OLT, and display at least 6 months of disease response or stable disease before transplantation. Such a restrictive approach has been associated with 5-year, and 10-year survivals of 97.2% and 88.8%, respectively.[59] In their most recent institutional report, Mazzaferro and colleagues[59] evaluated 280 patients referred for consideration of NELM. Ultimately, 88 were eligible, and 42 of these actually underwent OLT. Those undergoing OLT had significantly lower tumor stages, had lower tumor grade, were younger, received more locoregional therapies such as trans-arterial chemoembolisation, and received less somatostatin analog therapy than those who did not receive a transplant but were eligible (n = 46). However, the 2 subgroups were not statistically different in terms of extent of hepatic disease burden, the grade of disease differentiation, nor the site of the primary tumor. Five-year and 10-year OS rates in the transplanted and nontransplanted groups were 97.2% and 88.8%, versus 50.9% and 22.4%. Rates of disease recurrence at 5 years and 10 years were 13.1% and 13.1%, versus 83.5% and 89%, respectively. Last, this group calculated that the magnitude of benefit from OLT increased over time; in multivariate analyses, the gain in survival duration in favor of transplantation was 6.82 months at 5 years, but 38.43 months at 10 years. Such impressive results must of course be interpreted in the context of inherent selection bias; for example, younger patients with fewer comorbidities and lower-grade NEN undergoing OLT, and without treatment randomization. Additionally, many of the transplanted patients had hepatic disease burden low enough to be likely treated with resection in other centers. Clearly, the plausibility of randomized trials of OLT in NEN is hindered by stark logistical challenges.

Despite these appealing results, there are no universally accepted optimal selection criteria for LT in NELM. The necessity of such a strictly selective process is possibly debatable when results from Scandinavian centers are analyzed; for example, in their study of 15 patients undergoing either OLT (n = 10) or multivisceral transplantation (n = 5), Olausson and colleagues[57] treated patients who were up to 64 years of age, 12 of 15 patients had greater than 50% hepatic involvement, and tumor proliferation rates (Ki-67) were up to 10% (ie, G2 tumors). Despite this, the Scandinavian group reported a 5-year OS of 90% for OLT, and found no significant association among age, hepatic involvement, or Ki-67 on outcomes. One-year recurrence-free survival rate was 70% for the entire cohort. Clearly, these data come with the caveats of smaller sample size, and a divergence in the aggression of primary tumor–directed management within the setting of multivisceral transplantation.

There is essentially no quality evidence regarding the use of neoadjuvant and adjuvant therapies in the setting of OLT. Indeed, many patients underwent OLT before the development/availability of novel targeted therapies and immunosuppressive protocols, including agents with antiproliferative effects. Last, the optimal time point in the patient journey for OLT needs to be defined; OLT should not be used as an *ultima ratio* option after all other therapies have failed, and the use of a 6-month period to observe for disease stability or response before transplantation may be useful.[55]

LT is a generally accepted therapeutic option in patients with NELM. The best reported outcomes from surgical NELM treatment appear to be observed in patients undergoing OLT according to Milan selection criteria. Patients must be stringently selected; however, the optimal selection methodology is yet to be elucidated. Literature-derived contraindications for OLT in NEN comprise higher tumor grade, nonportal tumor drainage, extrahepatic metastases (excepting resectable perihilar deposits), and advanced carcinoid heart disease. Innovative approaches to adjuvant and neoadjuvant strategies to reduce posttransplant disease recurrence are needed. An additional unmet need in this area is the development of patient-specific biomarkers that are capable of predicting which patients may derive the most benefit from OLT, especially in the context of increased demand on deceased donor organ availability and low use of living-donor LT in most countries.

MULTIVISCERAL TRANSPLANTATION

Despite the development of multiple advanced surgical techniques that may render "classically" unresectable NEN amenable to resection, some tumors remain nonresectable, such as small bowel NEN with lymph node metastases encasing the mesenteric root with retroperitoneal extension either posterior or superior to the pancreas, or large infiltrating pancreatic head tumors. Bulky intra-abdominal metastatic burden may lead to obstruction and/or threaten bowel ischemia by encasement of the mesenteric vessels. Multivisceral transplantation (MVT) typically includes exenteration and thereafter replacement with an allograft of the stomach, small bowel, and pancreas, with or without the liver (modified MVT [MMVT], in the latter).[60] A very small number of patients with metastatic NEN have undergone such surgical procedures. In the report of Olausson and colleagues,[57] 5 patients with NEN within the pancreatic head underwent MVT in Gothenburg; none had symptoms of hormone hypersecretion, but all had greater than 50% liver tumor burden. Two patients died within 4 months of surgery due to MVT-associated morbidity, specifically lymphoproliferative disease and bleeding secondary to arteritis, whereas one other died at 27 months of recurrent disease, one was alive with recurrent disease at 66 months, and the last was alive without disease at 12 months. Of 6 patients undergoing MVT for pancreatic NEN within Norway and Sweden, a 2-year OS of 67% was reported, which was interestingly not inferior to that observed for intestinal failure.[61] Such observations have been echoed in reviews of the United Network for Organ Sharing database, which have demonstrated comparable outcomes in OLT versus MVT.[52]

As with OLT, there is limited evidence for the possible roles of neoadjuvant or adjuvant therapies in MVT/MMVT. There is evidence from case reports from our own center that the use of neoadjuvant PRRT before MMVT may be implemented,[62] and this should be further evaluated.

Multivisceral transplantation has been used in very few patients with metastatic NEN, mostly with pancreatic primary tumors. Validated selection tools are not possible to formulate at present, and possible evaluation for MVT or MMVT should occur only in specialist transplantation centers.

SUMMARY

Surgical treatment for NELM comprises hepatic resection with curative intent, palliative surgery with the intent of debulking tumor burden, combination of resection with RFA, and transplantation approaches. Although radical surgery possesses the possibility of cure, this is rarely attained and regardless of margin status with resection, disease recurrence should be not only anticipated but actively expected. Repeat resection for recurrent NELM is justified in view of the low morbidity and mortality of the procedure. In the setting of recurrence rates approaching 95%, the introduction of neoadjuvant and adjuvant concepts to complement hepatic resection is urgently needed within the field to protect against this Achilles heel by reducing recurrence rates and thus improving long-term survival and reducing costs for treatment of recurrent disease.

The traditional 90% target for cytoreduction is outdated, and patients in whom 70% (or perhaps less) cytoreduction can be attained could still benefit from debulking procedures. Meticulously selected patients with NELM may be eligible for LT and may expect excellent overall and disease-free survivals. However, the optimal selection criteria are not apparent, and expanded use of this therapy is hindered by the already considerable demands on donor organs. Consensus on selection criteria, as well as novel tools capable of predicting those most likely to benefit from surgery, will be clinically useful. Tumor ablation modalities may be offered in conjunction with surgery as part of efforts for disease control. Overall, surgery should be discussed for all patients during the initial evaluation process for treatment planning; if surgery is selected as an option, then this should be embedded within a multimodal treatment approach with multidisciplinary team input.

REFERENCES

1. Pape U-F, Berndt U, Müller-Nordhorn J, et al. Prognostic factors of long-term outcome in gastroenteropancreatic neuroendocrine tumours. Endocr Relat Cancer 2008;15:1083–97.
2. Ahmed A, Turner G, King B, et al. Midgut neuroendocrine tumours with liver metastases: results of the UKINETS study. Endocr Relat Cancer 2009;16:885–94.
3. Frilling A, Modlin IM, Kidd M, et al. Recommendations for management of patients with neuroendocrine liver metastases. Lancet Oncol 2014;15:e8–21.
4. Dasari A, Shen C, Halperin D, et al. Trends in the incidence, prevalence, and survival outcomes in patients with neuroendocrine tumors in the United States. JAMA Oncol 2017;3:1335.
5. Yao JC, Hassan M, Phan A, et al. One hundred years after "carcinoid": epidemiology of and prognostic factors for neuroendocrine tumors in 35,825 cases in the United States. J Clin Oncol 2008;26:3063–72.
6. Frilling A, Clift AK. Therapeutic strategies for neuroendocrine liver metastases. Cancer 2015;121. https://doi.org/10.1002/cncr.28760.
7. Riihimäki M, Hemminki A, Sundquist K, et al. The epidemiology of metastases in neuroendocrine tumors. Int J Cancer 2016;15(139):2679–86.
8. Panzuto F, Boninsegna L, Fazio N, et al. Metastatic and locally advanced pancreatic endocrine carcinomas: analysis of factors associated with disease progression. J Clin Oncol 2011;29:2372–7.
9. Pavel M, O'Toole D, Costa F, et al. ENETS consensus guidelines update for the management of distant metastatic disease of intestinal, pancreatic, bronchial neuroendocrine neoplasms (NEN) and NEN of unknown primary site. Neuroendocrinology 2016;103:172–85.
10. Pawa N, Clift AK, Osmani H, et al. Surgical management of patients with neuroendocrine neoplasms of the appendix: appendectomy or more? Neuroendocrinology 2017. https://doi.org/10.1159/000478742.
11. Ronot M, Clift AK, Vilgrain V, et al. Functional imaging in liver tumours. J Hepatol 2016;65. https://doi.org/10.1016/j.jhep.2016.06.024.
12. Frilling A, Li J, Malamutmann E, et al. Treatment of liver metastases from neuroendocrine tumours in relation to the extent of hepatic disease. Br J Surg 2009; 96:175–84.

13. Mörk H, Ignee A, Schuessler G, et al. Analysis of neuroendocrine tumour metastases in the liver using contrast enhanced ultrasonography. Scand J Gastroenterol 2007;42:652–62.

14. d'Assignies G, Fina P, Bruno O, et al. High sensitivity of diffusion-weighted MR imaging for the detection of liver metastases from neuroendocrine tumors: comparison with T2-weighted and dynamic gadolinium-enhanced MR imaging. Radiology 2013;268:390–9.

15. Vilgrain V, Esvan M, Ronot M, et al. A meta-analysis of diffusion-weighted and gadoxetic acid-enhanced MR imaging for the detection of colorectal liver metastases. Eur Radiol 2016;26(12):4595–615.

16. Breeman WAP, de Blois E, Sze Chan H, et al. (68)Ga-labeled DOTA-peptides and (68)Ga-labeled radiopharmaceuticals for positron emission tomography: current status of research, clinical applications, and future perspectives. Semin Nucl Med 2011;41:314–21.

17. Carreras C, Kulkarni HR, Baum RP. Rare metastases detected by 68Ga-somatostatin receptor PET/CT in patients with neuroendocrine tumors. Recent Results Cancer Res 2013;194:379–84.

18. Van Loon K, Zhang L, Keiser J, et al. Bone metastases and skeletal-related events from neuroendocrine tumors. Endocr Connect 2015;4:9–17.

19. Frilling A, Sotiropoulos GC, Radtke A, et al. The impact of 68Ga-DOTATOC positron emission tomography/computed tomography on the multimodal management of patients with neuroendocrine tumors. Ann Surg 2010;252:850–6.

20. Ruf J, Heuck F, Schiefer J, et al. Impact of multiphase 68Ga-DOTATOC-PET/CT on therapy management in patients with neuroendocrine tumors. Neuroendocrinology 2010;91:101–9.

21. Kayani I, Bomanji JB, Groves A, et al. Functional imaging of neuroendocrine tumors with combined PET/CT using 68Ga-DOTATATE (DOTA-DPhe1,Tyr3-octreotate) and 18F-FDG. Cancer 2008;112:2447–55.

22. Chan DL, Pavlakis N, Schembri GP, et al. Dual somatostatin receptor/FDG PET/CT imaging in metastatic neuroendocrine tumours: proposal for a novel grading scheme with prognostic significance. Theranostics 2017;7:1149–58.

23. Kianmanesh R, Sauvanet A, Hentic O, et al. Two-step surgery for synchronous bilobar liver metastases from digestive endocrine tumors: a safe approach for radical resection. Ann Surg 2008;247:659–65.

24. Schnitzbauer AA, Lang SA, Goessmann H, et al. Right portal vein ligation combined with in situ splitting induces rapid left lateral liver lobe hypertrophy enabling 2-staged extended right hepatic resection in small-for-size settings. Ann Surg 2012;255:405–14.

25. Jaeck D, Oussoultzoglou E, Bachellier P, et al. Hepatic metastases of gastroenteropancreatic neuroendocrine tumors: safe hepatic surgery. World J Surg 2001; 25:689–92.

26. Vouche M, Lewandowski RJ, Atassi R, et al. Radiation lobectomy: time-dependent analysis of future liver remnant volume in unresectable liver cancer as a bridge to resection. J Hepatol 2013;59:1029–36.

27. Saxena A, Chua TC, Perera M, et al. Surgical resection of hepatic metastases from neuroendocrine neoplasms: a systematic review. Surg Oncol 2012;21: e131–41.

28. Fairweather M, Swanson R, Wang J, et al. Management of neuroendocrine tumor liver metastases: long-term outcomes and prognostic factors from a large prospective database. Ann Surg Oncol 2017;24:2319–25.

29. Mayo SC, de Jong MC, Pulitano C, et al. Surgical management of hepatic neuro-endocrine tumor metastasis: results from an international multi-institutional analysis. Ann Surg Oncol 2010;17:3129–36.

30. de Jong MC, Mayo SC, Pulitano C, et al. Repeat curative intent liver surgery is safe and effective for recurrent colorectal liver metastasis: results from an international multi-institutional analysis. J Gastrointest Surg 2009;13:2141–51.

31. Kneuertz PJ, Cosgrove DP, Cameron AM, et al. Multidisciplinary management of recurrent hepatocellular carcinoma following liver transplantation. J Gastrointest Surg 2012;16:874–81.

32. Spolverato G, Bagante F, Aldrighetti L, et al. Management and outcomes of patients with recurrent neuroendocrine liver metastasis after curative surgery: an international multi-institutional analysis. J Surg Oncol 2017;116:298–306.

33. Garcia-Carbonero R, Sorbye H, Baudin E, et al. ENETS consensus guidelines ENETS consensus guidelines for high-grade gastroenteropancreatic neuroendocrine tumors and neuroendocrine carcinomas. Neuroendocrinology 2016;103:186–94.

34. Sorbye H, Welin S, Langer SW, et al. Predictive and prognostic factors for treatment and survival in 305 patients with advanced gastrointestinal neuroendocrine carcinoma (WHO G3): the NORDIC NEC study. Ann Oncol 2013;24:152–60.

35. Galleberg RB, Knigge U, Tiensuu Janson E, et al. Results after surgical treatment of liver metastases in patients with high-grade gastroenteropancreatic neuroendocrine carcinomas. Eur J Surg Oncol 2017;43:1682–9.

36. Elias D, Lefevre JH, Duvillard P, et al. Hepatic metastases from neuroendocrine tumors with a "thin slice" pathological examination: they are many more than you think. Ann Surg 2010;251:307–10.

37. Sowa-Staszczak A, Pach D, Chrzan R, et al. Peptide receptor radionuclide therapy as a potential tool for neoadjuvant therapy in patients with inoperable neuroendocrine tumours (NETs). Eur J Nucl Med Mol Imaging 2011;38:1669–74.

38. Dumont F, Goudard Y, Caramella C, et al. Therapeutic strategies for advanced pancreatic neuroendocrine tumors with segmental portal hypertension. World J Surg 2015;39:1974–80.

39. Partelli S, Bertani E, Bartolomei M, et al. Peptide receptor radionuclide therapy as neoadjuvant therapy for resectable or potentially resectable pancreatic neuroendocrine neoplasms. Surgery 2017. https://doi.org/10.1016/j.surg.2017.11.007.

40. McEntee GP, Nagorney DM, Kvols LK, et al. Cytoreductive hepatic surgery for neuroendocrine tumors. Surgery 1990;108:1091–6.

41. Frilling A, Al-Nahhas A, Clift AK. Transplantation and debulking procedures for neuroendocrine tumors. Front Horm Res 2015;44:164–76.

42. Sarmiento JM, Heywood G, Rubin J, et al. Surgical treatment of neuroendocrine metastases to the liver: a plea for resection to increase survival. J Am Coll Surg 2003;197:29–37.

43. Chamberlain RS, Canes D, Brown KT, et al. Hepatic neuroendocrine metastases: does intervention alter outcomes? J Am Coll Surg 2000;190:432–45.

44. Graff-Baker AN, Sauer DA, Pommier SJ, et al. Expanded criteria for carcinoid liver debulking: maintaining survival and increasing the number of eligible patients. Surgery 2014;156:1369–77.

45. Morgan RE, Pommier SJ, Pommier RF. Expanded criteria for debulking of liver metastasis also apply to pancreatic neuroendocrine tumors. Surgery 2018;163:218–25.

46. Glazer ES, Tseng JF, Al-Refaie W, et al. Long-term survival after surgical management of neuroendocrine hepatic metastases. HPB (Oxford) 2010;12:427–33.

47. Que FG, Nagorney DM, Batts KP, et al. Hepatic resection for metastatic neuroendocrine carcinomas. Am J Surg 1995;169:36–42 [discussion: 42–3].

48. Elias D, Lasser P, Ducreux M, et al. Liver resection (and associated extrahepatic resections) for metastatic well-differentiated endocrine tumors: a 15-year single center prospective study. Surgery 2003;133:375–82.

49. Maxwell JE, Sherman SK, O'Dorisio TM, et al. Liver-directed surgery of neuroendocrine metastases: what is the optimal strategy? Surgery 2016;159:320–35.

50. Osborne DA, Zervos EE, Strosberg J, et al. Improved outcome with cytoreduction versus embolization for symptomatic hepatic metastases of carcinoid and neuroendocrine tumors. Ann Surg Oncol 2006;13:572–81.

51. Gurusamy KS, Pamecha V, Sharma D, et al. Palliative cytoreductive surgery versus other palliative treatments in patients with unresectable liver metastases from gastro-entero-pancreatic neuroendocrine tumours. Cochrane Database Syst Rev 2009;(1):CD007118.

52. Gedaly R, Daily MF, Davenport D, et al. Liver transplantation for the treatment of liver metastases from neuroendocrine tumors: an analysis of the UNOS database. Arch Surg 2011;146:953–8.

53. Le Treut YP, Grégoire E, Klempnauer J, et al. Liver transplantation for neuroendocrine tumors in Europe—results and trends in patient selection: a 213-case European liver transplant registry study. Ann Surg 2013;257:807–15.

54. Nguyen NTT, Harring TR, Goss JA, et al. Neuroendocrine liver metastases and orthotopic liver transplantation: the US experience. Int J Hepatol 2011;2011: 742890.

55. Fan ST, Le Treut YP, Mazzaferro V, et al. Liver transplantation for neuroendocrine tumour liver metastases. HPB (Oxford) 2015;17:23–8.

56. Moris D, Tsilimigras DI, Ntanasis-Stathopoulos I, et al. Liver transplantation in patients with liver metastases from neuroendocrine tumors: a systematic review. Surgery 2017;162:525–36.

57. Olausson M, Friman S, Herlenius G, et al. Orthotopic liver or multivisceral transplantation as treatment of metastatic neuroendocrine tumors. Liver Transpl 2007; 13:327–33.

58. Mazzaferro V, Pulvirenti A, Coppa J. Neuroendocrine tumors metastatic to the liver: how to select patients for liver transplantation? J Hepatol 2007;47:460–6.

59. Mazzaferro V, Sposito C, Coppa J, et al. The long-term benefit of liver transplantation for hepatic metastases from neuroendocrine tumors. Am J Transplant 2016; 16:2892–902.

60. Abu-Elmagd KM. The small bowel contained allografts: existing and proposed nomenclature. Am J Transplant 2011;11:184–5.

61. Varkey J, Simrén M, Bosaeus I, et al. Survival of patients evaluated for intestinal and multivisceral transplantation—the Scandinavian experience. Scand J Gastroenterol 2013;48:702–11.

62. Frilling A, Giele H, Vrakas G, et al. Modified liver-free multivisceral transplantation for a metastatic small bowel neuroendocrine tumor: a case report. Transplant Proc 2015;47:858–62.

63. Saxena A, Chua TC, Sarkar A, et al. Progression and survival results after radical hepatic metastasectomy of indolent advanced neuroendocrine neoplasms (NENs) supports an aggressive surgical approach. Surgery 2011;149:209–20.

64. Scigliano S, Lebtahi R, Maire F, et al. Clinical and imaging follow-up after exhaustive liver resection of endocrine metastases: a 15-year monocentric experience. Endocr Relat Cancer 2009;16:977–90.

65. Gomez D, Malik HZ, Al-Mukthar A, et al. Hepatic resection for metastatic gastrointestinal and pancreatic neuroendocrine tumours: outcome and prognostic predictors. HPB (Oxford) 2007;9:345–51.
66. Bonaccorsi-Riani E, Apestegui C, Jouret-Mourin A, et al. Liver transplantation and neuroendocrine tumors: lessons from a single centre experience and from the literature review. Transpl Int 2010;23:668–78.
67. Marín C, Robles R, Fernández JA, et al. Role of liver transplantation in the management of unresectable neuroendocrine liver metastases. Transplant Proc 2007; 39:2302–3.
68. van Vilsteren FGI, Baskin-Bey ES, Nagorney DM, et al. Liver transplantation for gastroenteropancreatic neuroendocrine cancers: defining selection criteria to improve survival. Liver Transpl 2006;12:448–56.
69. Frilling A, Malago M, Weber F, et al. Livor transplantation for patients with metastatic endocrine tumors: single-center experience with 15 patients. Liver Transpl 2006;12:1089–96.

Gastric Carcinoids

Simona Grozinsky-Glasberg, MD[a], Krystallenia I. Alexandraki, MD[b],
Anna Angelousi, MD[b], Eleftherios Chatzellis, MD[b], Stavros Sougioultzis, MD[c],
Gregory Kaltsas, MD, FRCP[b,*]

KEYWORDS

- Carcinoids • Neuroendocrine • Gastrin • Atrophic gastritis • Endoscopic ultrasound

KEY POINTS

- Gastric carcinoids are derived from enterochromaffin cells and are increasingly recognized.
- They are divided into the relatively indolent types I and II lesions that are usually multiple and gastrin-related and type III lesions not related to gastrin that metastasize.
- Small (1–2 cm), not invading the muscularis propria, grade 1, types I and II lesions, can be locally excised.
- Multiple and/or recurrent lesions may respond to gastrin-reducing medical or surgical treatments.
- Type III lesions are aggressive and should be treated as adenocarcinoma of the stomach.

INTRODUCTION

Gastrointestinal (GI) neuroendocrine neoplasms (NENs), known as GI carcinoids, were originally regarded as rare but over the past decades their incidence has increased.[1–4] They are currently diagnosed with an incidence of 2 cases/100,000/y to 5 cases/100,000/y[2,3] but may be even more common.[5–7] GI carcinoids can secrete bioactive substances and cause distinct clinical syndromes (functioning tumors) and/or symptoms due to mass effects (nonfunctioning tumors). The recent use of validated classification systems has made it possible to stratify tumors according to their malignant potential and prognosis and direct treatment accordingly. Based on their proliferation rate, GI carcinoids are divided in 3 groups, grade (G)1, G2, and G3, with increasing malignant potential (**Table 1**). In addition, these tumors are now preferably called NENs.[4]

Disclosure: The authors have nothing to disclose.
[a] Neuroendocrine Tumor Unit, Department of Endocrinology, Hadassah-Hebrew University Medical Center, P.O.B. 12000, Jerusalem 91120, Israel; [b] 1st Department of Propaedeutic Internal Medicine, National and Kapodistrian University of Athens, Mikras Asias 75, Athens 11527, Greece; [c] Department of Pathophysiology, National and Kapodistrian University of Athens, Mikras Asias 75, Athens 11527, Greece
* Corresponding author. 1st Department of Propaedeutic Internal Medicine, National and Kapodistrian University of Athens, Mikras Asias 75, Athens 11527, Greece.
E-mail address: gkaltsas@med.uoa.gr

Endocrinol Metab Clin N Am 47 (2018) 645–660
https://doi.org/10.1016/j.ecl.2018.04.013
0889-8529/18/© 2018 Elsevier Inc. All rights reserved.

Table 1		
Grading system for gastrointestinal neuroendocrine neoplasms		
Grade (G)	**Mitotic Count (10 High-Power Fields)[a]**	**Ki-67 Index (%)[b]**
G1	<2	<3
G2	2–20	3–20
G3[c]	>20	>20

[a] 10 High-power Fields—2 mm³, at least 40 fields (at ×40 magnification) evaluated in areas of highest mitotic density.
[b] MIBI antibody: % of 2000 tumor cells in areas of highest nuclear labeling.
[c] G3: according to morphology G3 tumors are divided in well-differentiated neuroendocrine tumors and poorly differentiated neuroendocrine carcinomas.

Gastric carcinoids (GCs) were previously considered to represent a small percentage of GI-NENs, but recent data have shown that their incidence has increased 7-fold to 10-fold.[2,8,9] GCs are divided in 3 distinct types; types I and II: are originating from enterochromaffin like (ECL) cells (formally named ECLomas).[10] The former develop from continuously elevated gastrin levels, mainly in the context of chronic autoimmune gastritis (CAG), and the latter in the context of gastrinomas that may be a part of the multiple endocrine neoplasia (MEN1) syndrome; both types I and type II tumors develop from prodromal ECL-hyperplastic lesions[10,11] (**Figs. 1** and **2**). A great majority

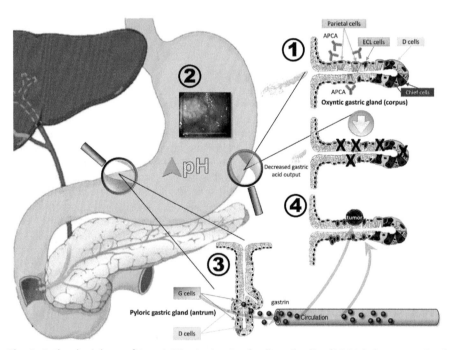

Fig. 1. Pathophysiology of type I GCs. Antiparietal cell antibodies (APCAs) destroy parietal cells diminishing gastric acid output at the stomach corpus (1). Gastric mucosa atrophies (2). High pH gastric content stimulates G cells to secrete increased amounts of gastrin (3). Gastrin reaches corpus gastric glands and causes ECL-cell hyperplasia (4), which can then lead to neuroendocrine tumors (GC type I). GCs: gastric carcinoids.

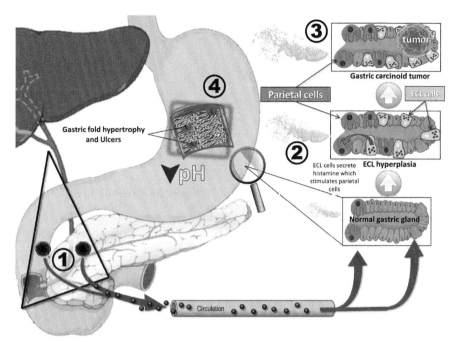

Fig. 2. Pathophysiology of type II GCs. Gastrinomas usually located inside the gastrinoma triangle (duodenum or pancreas) secrete excess amount of gastrin (1). Gastrin stimulates parietal cells to secrete gastric acid (2). Gastrin also stimulates mucosal growth in the stomach causing ECL-cell hyperplasia (3), which can then lead to the formation of a neuroendocrine tumor (GC type II). Increased gastric acid production is associated with multiple gastric and duodenal ulcer formation (4). ECL hyperplasia, enterochromaffin like hyperplasia; GCs, gastric carcinoids.

are well differentiated, exerting low proliferation rates, and only a minority develop metastases.[10,11] In contrast, type III GCs are not derived from any underlying gastric pathology and are not related to gastrin secretion (**Table 2**). These tumors can be well differentiated, albeit with higher proliferative rates, although a subset may be highly aggressive, resembling large cell or small cell carcinomas.[11,12] Rarely, GCs may become functioning producing an atypical carcinoid syndrome.[8,11] Hypergastrinemia found in types I and II carcinoids may also be related to the development of other dysplastic and/or malignant lesions in the stomach.[6,9,13]

In this article, current and evolving knowledge regarding the epidemiology, pathogenesis, diagnosis, and treatment of GCs is reviewed to provide evidence of the natural course of these tumors and identify lesions at high risk for an aggressive course, necessitating prompt diagnosis and treatment.

EPIDEMIOLOGY

Recent epidemiologic evidence suggests that the incidence of gastric NENs varies between 6.9% and 8.7% of all GI-NENs[14–18] and 0.3% to 1.8% of all gastric tumors.[2,11] This increase in incidence is attributed to the increased number of endoscopic and diagnostic procedures performed.[9,11] In a prospective study, however, that evaluated all new NENs diagnosed during a period of a year, gastric NENs accounted for 23% of all NENs.[17] This finding calls for prospective multicenter studies to evaluate their true incidence and potential differences among ethnic groups.

Table 2
Specific characteristics of the different types of gastric carcinoids

	Type I	Type II	Type III
Prevalence (%) among gastric NENs	70%–80%	5%–10%	15%–20%
Background	Chronic atrophic gastritis	Gastrinomas	Normal mucosa
Number of lesions	Multiple	Multiple	Single
Serum gastrin levels	↑–↑↑	↑–↑↑↑	Normal
Gastric pH	↑	↓	Normal
Underlying mucosa	Atrophic	Hypertrophic	Normal
Histopathology	ECL hyperplasia	ECL hyperplasia	Normal gastric mucosa
Size	1–2 cm	1 cm	>2 cm
Invasion	Muscularis mucosa or submucosa	Muscularis mucosa or submucosa	Any depth
Mitotic count	<2/10 HPF	<2/10 HPF	2–20/10 HPF or >20/10 HPF
Grade	G1	G1	G2/3
Metastases			
Lymph nodes	5%–10%	10%–20% (duodenal tumors)	50%–100%
Liver	2%–5%	10%	22%–75%
Prognosis	Excellent	Very good	Similar to gastric adenocarcinoma
Other syndromes	Autoimmune polyglandular syndrome	MEN1 syndrome	—

Abbreviations: ↑, increased; ECL hyperplasia, enterochromaffin like hyperplasia; G, grade; HPF, High-power Fields; NENs, neuroendocrine neoplasms.

Type I tumors are the most common GCs, accounting for 75% to 80% of cases and arise in atrophic body gastritis in the presence of achlorydria.[19] In general, GCs are more common in women and tend to occur after the fifth decade of life, although they are increasingly diagnosed at younger ages.[20,21] The prevalence of type I GCs in patients with CAG ranges between 1.5% and 12.5%, reflecting patient and referral bias. Although there seems to be a relation with the duration and the age at diagnosis, other factors besides hypergastrinemia are also involved in the transformation of the hyperplastic ECL cells.[1,11] Type II lesions (ECLomas in the context of Zollinger-Ellison syndrome [ZES]) account for 5% to 6% of GCs and are often seen in patients with the MEN1 syndrome in approximately 23% to 29% of cases.[22–24] In contrast, in patients with sporadic gastrinomas, they are present in only 1% to 3%, confirming the role of the MEN1 gene in their pathogenesis.[25,26] Type III lesions are solitary and occur mostly in men over the age of 50 years[10,20,22] (see **Table 2**).

CLINICAL PRESENTATION
Type I Gastric Neuroendocrine Neoplasms

Type I gastric NENs are usually diagnosed incidentally during endoscopic procedures performed for dyspepsia or investigation of anemia and are rarely functioning.[3,11,20]

Symptoms may be related to slow gastric emptying and progressive diminishing gastric acid production, leading to impairment of vitamin B_{12} and iron absorption.[27] They present mostly as gastric fundus polyps without ulceration on an atrophic mucosa but can be identified only in biopsies in 22.2% of patients and are named microcarcinoids; in approximately 65% of cases, lesions are multiple and their mean diameter is 5 mm.[28] Most are of very low malignant potential confined to the mucosa/submucosa, although occasionally they may metastasize.[29] In a recent study, 20 of 254 patients had metastases (12 regional and 8 hepatic); mean tumor diameter was 20.1 mm ± 10.8 mm and mean Ki-67 index 6.8% ± 11.2%.[30] During a follow-up period of 83 months, 3 patients developed progressive liver lesions, whereas all remained alive.[30] Similar results were also produced in a study of 984 patients, where tumor size and depth of invasion predicted the presence of lymph node metastases.[31]

Type II Gastric Neuroendocrine Neoplasms

Type II ZES-associated lesions are also derived from ECL cells and are multiple, of small (<1 cm) size, located in the fundus and antrum of the stomach[3] (see **Fig. 2**). Clinical presentation is caused by gastrin-induced excessive acid production, leading to nausea, vomiting, peptic ulcer disease, and diarrhea, secondary to low pH fluid entering to the intestine.[32] The behavior of type II GCs is more aggressive than type I, and, although their metastatic rate is reported to be higher (3%–12%), short-term survival seems similar.[32] Their long-term prognosis, however, is dominated by the behavior of the gastrinoma, better for duodenal than pancreatic lesions.[1] When gastrinomas occur in the context of the MEN1 syndrome, the clinical manifestations from other organ involvement may be evident or need to be looked for.[33]

Type III Gastric Neuroendocrine Neoplasms

Type III GCs are usually single lesions that do not develop in the context of ECL hyperplasia and occur on an apparently normal-looking gastric mucosa. Gastrin levels are not raised and the pH of the stomach is normal, whereas their size often exceeds 2 cm.[1,3,4,12] Their clinical presentation resembles that of adenocarcinoma of the stomach with symptoms, such as anorexia, weight loss, anemia, and the development of metastases. A majority are nonfunctioning but occasionally an atypical carcinoid syndrome may develop.[12] This is secondary to the production of mainly histamine from ECL cells and is characterized by prolonged cutaneous flushing, headache, lacrimation, itching, and bronchospasm. It can occur spontaneous or after the ingestion of foods high in tyramine.[8]

PATHOGENESIS—GENETICS

GCs are mostly derived from histamine-secreting ECL cells and, rarely, serotonin-secreting ECL cells, somatostatin, or ghrelin cells.[9] In response to food, antral G cells secrete gastrin that binds to cholecystokinin (CCK)-B receptors, located on the membrane of ECL cells, leading to histamine release that after binding to H_2 receptors on parietal cells stimulates gastric acid secretion.[34,35] In addition, gastrin controls the maturation of parietal cells and stimulates the production of growth factors, such as epidermal growth factor, transforming growth factor α, and amphiregulin, which increase the proliferation of cells in the epithelium. In patients with prolonged increases in plasma gastrin, as in CAG, there is a tendency for ECL cell hyperplasia that may result in the development of type I GCs from dysplastic changes. This notion is reinforced further by findings in animal models; the mastomys (*Praomys natalensis*) is a rodent that develops GCs in 20% to 50% as a result of constitutive activation of the CCK-B receptor.[9] Although germ-line mutations of the MENIN gene are not found, loss of heterozygosity has been noted.[36] In transgenic mouse lines, conditional MEN1 deletion, in the absence of somatostatin expression, led to the development of GCs within 2 years, whereas omeprazole accelerated their development to 6 months; tumors were associated with hypergastrinemia and correlated with increased CCK-B receptor expression and nuclear export of p27[Kip118].[37] Although CAG is a well-known predisposing factor for type I GCs, in approximately 50% of cases no such underlying pathology is found.[29] This finding suggests that other causes, such as inflammatory/infective states, may also be involved.[38] Chronic inflammation with *Helicobacter pylori* is linked to CAG and hypergastrinemia that leads to ECL hyperplasia and the development of type I GCs.[39,40] It has recently been shown that CAG is more prevalent in *H pylori*–positive compared with *H pylori*–negative subjects,[41] whereas in the mastomys model, the development of type I GCs is accelerated by concomitant *H pylori* infection.[42,43]

Like type I lesions, type II tumors exhibit the same spectrum of hyperplasia, dysplasia, and neoplasia. They consist of ECL cells, and loss of *MENIN* heterozygosity is found in the vast majority (75%) of ZES-MEN1 tumors.[44] Type II lesions are more common in the ZES-MEN1 compared with sporadic ZES, supporting the view that the genetic changes in MEN1 patients render ECL cells more sensitive to the proliferative effect of gastrin.[45] Although *H pylori* infection and associated hypergastrinemia are linked to the development of type I GCs, this does not seem the case in patients with ZES and concomitant *H pylori* infection, because its eradication does not affect the degree of ECL hyperplasia/dysplasia.[46]

Type III lesions are composed of different sporadically grown endocrine cells, not related to gastrin hypersecretion in a normal-looking gastric mucosa.[47] A majority exhibit deep wall invasion involving the muscular layers and lympho-angioinvasion and develop regional/distant metastases in 50% to 70% of well-differentiated and almost 100% of poorly differentiated lesions.[34,48] Although they do not develop in MEN1 patients, there is loss of heterozygosity at the MEN1 gene locus in approximately 25%.[49]

DIAGNOSIS
Endoscopic, Histopathologic, and Biochemical Diagnosis

Upper GI endoscopy is the main means of identifying GCs in the relevant clinical setting. Biopsy samples should be taken from the antrum and body/fundus in addition to biopsies of the largest lesions in all types I and II lesions.[50] In patients with larger lesions (>1 cm), endoscopic ultrasonography (EUS) is the best mean to determine the depth of tumor invasion of the gastric wall and the presence of regional lymph nodes[3,28] (**Fig. 3**). The optimal size of lesions that need to be investigated with EUS, however, needs to be defined by prospective studies.

Type I GCs develop in patients with CAG on a background of ECL-cell hyperplastic/dysplastic lesions (see **Fig. 1**). ECL-cell hyperplasia can be diffuse, linear, nodular, or adenomatoid. The presence of ECL hyperplasia confers a 26-fold increase in the risk of developing ECLomas, mainly in dysplastic adenomatoid (150–500 μm) lesions.[50] Adenomatoid lesions form multiple membrane bound micronodules that can be either intramucosal carcinoids (>500 μm) with or without infiltrating the submucosa; most type I GCs have a Ki-67 index of $1.9 \pm 2.4\%$.[35,51]

In type II GCs, the gastric mucosa is normal or mildly inflamed whereas the fundic mucosa is often hypertrophic with no significant inflammation; ECL-cell hyperplasia

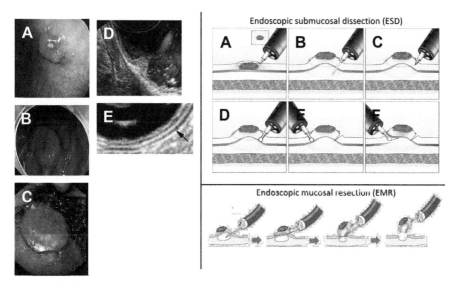

Fig. 3. Role of endoscopy. (*Left*) (*A*) Endoscopic appearance of a GC type I (notice the surrounding mucosal atrophy); (*B*) endoscopic appearance of a GC type II (notice the surrounding mucosal hypertrophy with eminent gastric folds); (*C*) endoscopic appearance of a GC type III; (*D*) EUS image of a GC type I restricted to mucosa; and (*E*) normal gastric wall layers as seen with EUS (*black arrow*). (*Right*) ESD. (*A*) Markings with knife or argon plasma coagulation probe around the edge of the lesions; (*B*) submucosal injection around the edge of the lesions; (*C*) incision hole with a needle-knife or hook knife; (*D*) margin cutting with insulated-tip knife at the incision hole; (*E*) circumferential margin cutting; and (*F*) submucosal dissection with IT knife beneath the muscularis mucosa. The technique of EMR involves the injection of a specialized solution into the submucosa just below where the polyp is attached. This lifts the polyp up and can be safely snared off either in 1 or many pieces, until it has been completely removed. EUS, endoscopic ultrasound; GC, gastric carcinoid.

is found in 92% to 100% of cases.[45] These figures are also similar to findings in sporadic ZES, in which 80% to 100% show some ECL cell changes; in a majority of ZES-MEN1 patients, the ECL cell changes are advanced.[23,24,26]

Type III GCs are usually large (>2 cm) solitary lesions arising in normal gastric mucosa; they may have an ulcerated appearance and can cause significant hemorrhage.[4,12] There is no associated gastric atrophy or peptic ulcers and these lesions are commonly associated with *H pylori*–related gastritis.[12] Type III tumors vary in histologic grade and differentiation although G3 tumors are common. Invasion beyond the submucosa is common; concurrent gastric adenocarcinoma can occur in 5% to 10% of cases.[10,52]

Gastrin levels are invariably elevated in patients with type I carcinoids, whereas chromogranin A (CgA) levels are increased in greater than 90%, being directly related to the size and number of the neoplasms.[53] Because many cases are associated with CAG, antiparietal cell and anti-intrinsic factor antibodies along with B12 levels should be measured.[3,53] In cases of negative antibodies, the *H pylori* status needs to be defined.[12,28] Thyroid function tests and autoantibody status are also measured because many patients have concomitant autoimmune thyroid disease (AITD) and/or hypothyroidism.[53] In patients with type II tumors and the ZES, investigations are limited to serum CgA and gastrin measurements,[23–25] along with investigations for the MEN1 syndrome.[54] In patients with type III lesions that are independent of gastrin,

CgA and neuron-specific enolase levels are measured in well-differentiated tumors.[12] In the presence of an atypical carcinoid syndrome, the histamine metabolite methyl-imidazoleacetic acid in the urine can be measured.[8]

Imaging and Nuclear Medicine

Imaging studies, including CT scan and MRI, are not routinely performed in small types I and II lesions to detect residual or metastatic disease.[3,4] In a study of 111 patients in whom morphologic (CT/MRI) and functional imaging studies (^{111}In-octreotide scintig-raphy or ^{68}Ga-DOTATOC PET-CT) were performed, conventional imaging identified extensive disease in 2 high-risk patients, whereas in all other cases findings were already identified with EUS.[53] Functional imaging conveyed no further information than conventional imaging. It was suggested that these modalities are mostly needed in patients with extensive disease and in patients with type III lesions for staging purposes.[3,4]

ASSOCIATED DISEASES
Gastric Carcinoma

There are concerns regarding the role of long-standing hypergastrinemia and the pu-tative relation with gastric adenocarcinomas besides carcinoids.[13,55] In animal models (*Sigmoid hispidus*), spontaneous hypergastrinemia and hypoacidity can lead to the development of adenocarcinomas that arise from ECL cells also exhibiting a neuroen-docrine component.[9,56] In a recent epidemiologic study, gastrin levels in the higher upper quad rum (Q4) compared with those in the lower (Q1) were associated with a 1.92 overall risk (95% CI, 1.21–3.05) of developing gastric adenocarcinoma.[6]

The 2 main reasons leading to the development of gastric carcinoma are gastric at-rophy and intestinal metaplasia.[57,58] Previous epidemiologic data suggested that the pooled gastric cancer incidence rate in pernicious anemia is 0.27% per person-years with an estimated 7-fold relative risk.[59] Not all patients with *H pylori*–induced gastritis develop GCs, and chances are higher when as CgA-positive strains are present.[60] Eradication of *H pylori* in patients with known precancerous lesions has not signifi-cantly lowered the incidence of GCs.[61]

Primary Hypothyroidism and Other Autoimmune Endocrine Disorders

Pernicious anemia affects almost 0.1% of the population and 2% of those over the age of 60 years.[58] Approximately one-third of patients with AITD and 6% to 10% of pa-tients with type 1 diabetes mellitus have concurrent autoimmune CAG.[62,63] A study that evaluated the risk patients with AITD had in developing GCs found that of the 33% of patients who had CAG, 17.5% had concomitant ECL hyperplasia that devel-oped into a carcinoid tumor in 1 (2.5%).[64] Other autoimmune conditions that can co-occur with autoimmune CAG include vitiligo, Addison disease, myasthenia gravis, and perioral cutaneous autoimmune conditions.[11,58] Familial cases of pernicious anemia have been described, including those in twins, suggesting a genetic component of the disease.[58] Rare cases of coexistence of 2 inherited disorders (familial cases of per-nicious anemia) and hereditary hemochromatosis have also been described.[65]

Primary Hyperparathyroidism

Non–MEN1-related primary hyperparathyroidism is common in patients with type I GCs. It was biochemically diagnosed in 4 of 26 (15%) patients with histologically proved GCs; 3 were operated and were found to harbor an adenoma.[66] Further studies have consistently revealed this association that was most probably attributed to the stimulatory effect of elevated gastrin levels to the parathyroid gland.[11]

Several studies have also shown that patients with type I lesions are at increased risk of developing diabetes mellitus, hypertension, thyroid carcinomas, adrenal adenomas, and hypertension.[8,40,64]

TREATMENT AND FOLLOW-UP
Localized Disease

Type I gastric carcinoids

Small ($\leq$1 cm) lesions not infiltrating the muscularis propria and without evidence of angioinvasion follow an indolent course, do not metastasize, and should be endoscopically resected during annual endoscopic surveillance[3,51,67,68] (**Fig. 4**). Endoscopic mucosal resection (EMR) is used to maximize complete resection rates, particularly in larger lesions.[67,69] Endoscopic submucosal dissection (ESD) is safe for larger lesions and those not amenable to EMR, with high en bloc complete resection.[4,12] Endoscopic resection of nonmetastatic localized lesions less than 2 cm and/or less than or equal to 6 lesions is as effective as surgical resection if there is no muscularis propria invasion.[11,12] Recurrence after presumed successful treatment is common because hypergastrinemia and underlying ECL-hyperplastic/dysplastic changes persist, as high as 65% within a year after initial treatment.[51,53] For lesions greater than 1 cm, with EUS-assessed involvement of the muscularis propria and/or local lymph nodes, surgical resection is indicated.[3,11,12] Surgical oncological resection is also considered for endoscopically resected lesions with positive resection margins, those >2 cm, multiple lesions (particularly if >6 and recurrent several lesions >1 cm), and atypical pathology (Ki-67 >2%).[12]

Although antrectomy has been used in the past, wedge resection or localized excision is mainly used for single or multiple lesions adjacent to each other.[1,3] Antrectomy is used in patients with multifocal (>6 lesions, 3–4 lesions >1 cm, or 1 lesion >2 cm), invasive, or recurrent disease because in approximately 70% to 80% of cases it induces regression of the tumors and ECL-cell hyperplastic lesions.[12] In some cases, however, lesions may recur due to established genomic changes in residual ECL cells that have undergone hyperplasia.[70] Because type I carcinoids are relatively indolent, long-acting somatostatin analogs (SSAs) can be used as they inhibit gastrin secretion from G cells and have a direct effect on the ECL cells acting on somatostatin receptors on their surface.[11] Several studies have shown that the administration of these agents reduces significantly/normalizes gastrin and CgA levels and induces regression of type I lesions in a majority of treated patients.[40,53,71] Treatment is well tolerated but a significant number of successfully treated lesions recur with cessation of treatment.[12] Although the precise indications and duration of such treatment have not been defined, it may present an alternative treatment of patients with multiple and highly recurrent tumors not amenable to surgical treatment.[11]

Type II gastric carcinoids

All type II lesions should be resected, because there is a greater risk of lymph node involvement and metastases than type I along with the primary tumor(s). Endoscopic resection is performed for all localized lesions and surgery for those with invasive or metastatic features; multiple lesions can be managed with both endoscopy and surgery.[12,45] Annual endoscopic surveillance is advocated for recurrence, particularly if ZES persists from an in situ gastrinoma. Acid-hypersecretion in ZES should be controlled to prevent complications.[72] High-dose proton pump inhibitor therapy is the preferred choice to control acid secretion, although long-acting SSAs have also been used.[32]

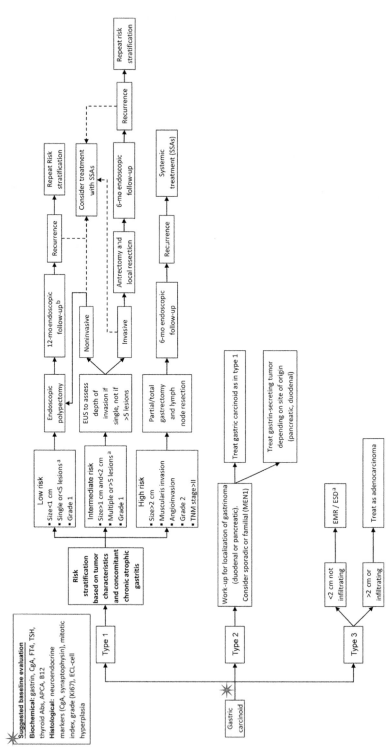

Fig. 4. Proposed algorithm for treatment and follow-up of patients with GCs. [a] Suggested approach, insufficient evidence. [b] The duration of follow-up can be extended (every 2–3 years depending on findings of consequent endoscopies (ie, no recurrence) or patient characteristics (elderly). Abs, antibodies; APCA, antiparietal cell antibodies; B12, vitamin B12; CgA, chromogranin A; EMR, endoscopic mucosal resection; ESD, endoscopic submucosal dissection; MEN1, multiple endocrine neoplasia 1; mo, months; SSAs, somatostatin analogs.

Type III gastric carcinoids

Type III GCs can vary in histologic grade and differentiation, although G3 tumors are common. The prognosis is overall much worse than types I and II tumors, with mortality rates of 22% to 30%[73]; concurrent gastric adenocarcinoma can be present in 5% to 10%.[3,12] The decision to resect type III GCs follows the guidelines for gastric adenocarcinomas; partial or total gastrectomy with local lymph node resection is often performed.[3,12] In a recent study of 119 patients with type III tumors, 50 patients with lesions less than 2 cm and no evidence of lymphovascular invasion underwent treatment with EMR/ESD that proved adequate because there was no recurrence.[47] Surveillance with CT and endoscopy after a resection of a type III tumor mirrors that of gastric adenocarcinoma.

Treatment of Hypergastrinemia

Gastrin increases the proliferation of epithelial cells in the stomach. Besides SSAs, immuno-neutralization of circulating gastrin or administration of CCK-B receptor antagonists inhibits gastric acid responses to food.

An orally administered CCK-B receptor antagonist (netazepide-YF476) was shown efficacious for GCs in patients with hypergastrinemia.[74,75] In a single-arm, phase-2 study, 8 patients with multiple type I carcinoids received netazepide, 50 mg orally, for 12 weeks.[74] After 12 weeks, all patients had a reduction in the number of lesions and a significant reduction of CgA values at 3 weeks.[74] In a subsequent study, 13 patients took netazepide for 52 weeks leading to resolution of all tumors in 5 patients, reduction of the number and size of tumors in the other patients, and normalization of CgA in all patients. Treatment should be continuous, however, because tumors regrow if stopped.[76]

An immune-neutralization strategy using a vaccine that promotes the development of antibodies directly to the N-terminus of gastrin-17, 17-Gly is being explored in patients with pancreatic cancer. This strategy has also been applied in 3 patients with type I GCs and CAG who were followed-up for a mean of 36-month. After vaccination, carcinoid regression was observed in 2 of the 3 patients and in 1 led to disappearance of ECL hyperplasia.[77] Since then, however, no further studies have been reported.

Treatment of Advanced Disease

In rare cases of patients with type I tumors and advanced disease not amenable to surgical treatment, long-acting SSAs can be administered because a majority have a Ki-67 index less than 10%.[78] Although there are not enough data, it seems that even in the presence of metastatic disease, such patients may still have a favorable prognosis.[11,30] Patients with types I and II lesions that progress can receive further treatment with molecular targeted therapies, interferon α, radiopeptides, and/or temozolomide based chemotherapy.[4,11,12] Patients with well-differentiated G2 type III lesions are treated similarly to patients with types I and II lesions and advanced disease, although the sequence of treatments administered may differ. Patients with G3 type III are treated exclusively with chemotherapy, although the scheme may differ according to their morphology according to the recent newly introduced grading system.[79]

SUMMARY

GCs are currently increasingly recognized, most probably due to the increased number of the endoscopic procedures performed. This increment mostly refers to type I tumors that develop in the context of autoimmune or nonautoimmune CAG as a result of the effect of prolonged hypergastrinemia to ECL cells that undergo neoplastic transformation. A vast majority of these lesions have an indolent course, metastasize rarely, and are mainly treated with endoscopic resection, although antrectomy and long-acting SSAs can be used for multiple and frequently recurring lesions. Type II carcinoids develop in patients with ZES, more commonly in the context of the MEN1-syndrome and, although more aggressive than type I tumors, are dealt in a similar manner along with treatment of the gastrin-secreting tumor. The precise indications regarding the tumor size cutoffs that can be endoscopically resected are still evolving. Endoscopic ultrasound is a powerful tool in identifying high-risk patients with types I and II tumors and direct treatment accordingly. Type III carcinoids are not gastrin related and behave like adenocarcinomas. Although the molecular profile in types I and III lesions has not been delineated, several candidate genes have recently been proposed. The long-term squeal of hypergastrinemia and associated comorbidities are currently being addressed and several therapeutic options are under investigation.

REFERENCES

1. O'Toole D, Delle FG, Jensen RT. Gastric and duodenal neuroendocrine tumours. Best Pract Res Clin Gastroenterol 2012;26:719–35.
2. Modlin IM, Oberg K, Chung DC, et al. Gastroenteropancreatic neuroendocrine tumours. Lancet Oncol 2008;9:61–72.
3. Delle FG, Kwekkeboom DJ, Van CE, et al. ENETS consensus guidelines for the management of patients with gastroduodenal neoplasms. Neuroendocrinology 2012;95:74–87.
4. Delle FG, O'Toole D, Sundin A, et al. ENETS consensus guidelines update for gastroduodenal neuroendocrine neoplasms. Neuroendocrinology 2016;103: 119–24.
5. Dasari A, Shen C, Halperin D, et al. Trends in the incidence, prevalence, and survival outcomes in patients with neuroendocrine tumors in the United States. JAMA Oncol 2017;3:1335–42.
6. Murphy G, Abnet CC, Choo-Wosoba H, et al. Serum gastrin and cholecystokinin are associated with subsequent development of gastric cancer in a prospective cohort of Finnish smokers. Int J Epidemiol 2017;46:914–23.
7. Broder MS, Cai B, Chang E, et al. Epidemiology of gastrointestinal neuroendocrine tumors in a U.S. commercially insured population. Endocr Pract 2017;23: 1210–6.
8. Kaltsas GA, Besser GM, Grossman AB. The diagnosis and medical management of advanced neuroendocrine tumors. Endocr Rev 2004;25:458–511.
9. Kidd M, Gustafsson B, Modlin IM. Gastric carcinoids (neuroendocrine neoplasms). Gastroenterol Clin North Am 2013;42:381–97.
10. Rindi G, Luinetti O, Cornaggia M, et al. Three subtypes of gastric argyrophil carcinoid and the gastric neuroendocrine carcinoma: a clinicopathologic study. Gastroenterology 1993;104:994–1006.
11. Kaltsas G, Grozinsky-Glasberg S, Alexandraki KI, et al. Current concepts in the diagnosis and management of type 1 gastric neuroendocrine neoplasms. Clin Endocrinol (Oxf) 2014;81:157–68.
12. Basuroy R, Srirajaskanthan R, Prachalias A, et al. Review article: the investigation and management of gastric neuroendocrine tumours. Aliment Pharmacol Ther 2014;39:1071–84.
13. Hayakawa Y, Chang W, Jin G, et al. Gastrin and upper GI cancers. Curr Opin Pharmacol 2016;31:31–7.

14. O'Connor JM, Marmissolle F, Bestani C, et al. Observational study of patients with gastroenteropancreatic and bronchial neuroendocrine tumors in Argentina: results from the large database of a multidisciplinary group clinical multicenter study. Mol Clin Oncol 2014;2:673–84.

15. Hallet J, Law CH, Cukier M, et al. Exploring the rising incidence of neuroendocrine tumors: a population-based analysis of epidemiology, metastatic presentation, and outcomes. Cancer 2015;121:589–97.

16. Yao JC, Hassan M, Phan A, et al. One hundred years after "carcinoid": epidemiology of and prognostic factors for neuroendocrine tumors in 35,825 cases in the United States. J Clin Oncol 2008;26:3063–72.

17. Niederle MB, Hackl M, Kaserer K, et al. Gastroenteropancreatic neuroendocrine tumours: the current incidence and staging based on the WHO and European Neuroendocrine Tumour Society classification: an analysis based on prospectively collected parameters. Endocr Relat Cancer 2010;17:909–18.

18. Modlin IM, Lye KD, Kidd M. A 50-year analysis of 562 gastric carcinoids: small tumor or larger problem? Am J Gastroenterol 2004;99:23–32.

19. Vannella L, Sbrozzi-Vanni A, Lahner E, et al. Development of type I gastric carcinoid in patients with chronic atrophic gastritis. Aliment Pharmacol Ther 2011;33: 1361–9.

20. Modlin IM, Lye KD, Kidd M. Carcinoid tumors of the stomach. Surg Oncol 2003; 12:153–72.

21. Ruszniewski P, Delle FG, Cadiot G, et al. Well-differentiated gastric tumors/carcinomas. Neuroendocrinology 2006;84:158–64.

22. Rindi G, Bordi C, Rappel S, et al. Gastric carcinoids and neuroendocrine carcinomas: pathogenesis, pathology, and behavior. World J Surg 1996;20: 168–72.

23. Lehy T, Cadiot G, Mignon M, et al. Influence of multiple endocrine neoplasia type 1 on gastric endocrine cells in patients with the Zollinger-Ellison syndrome. Gut 1992;33:1275–9.

24. Cadiot G, Laurent-Puig P, Thuille B, et al. Is the multiple endocrine neoplasia type 1 gene a suppressor for fundic argyrophil tumors in the Zollinger-Ellison syndrome? Gastroenterology 1993;105:579–82.

25. Cadiot G, Lehy T, Mignon M. Gastric endocrine cell proliferation and fundic argyrophil carcinoid tumors in patients with the Zollinger-Ellison syndrome. Acta Oncol 1993;32:135–40.

26. Norton JA, Melcher ML, Gibril F, et al. Gastric carcinoid tumors in multiple endocrine neoplasia-1 patients with Zollinger-Ellison syndrome can be symptomatic, demonstrate aggressive growth, and require surgical treatment. Surgery 2004; 136:1267–74.

27. Marignani M, Delle FG, Mecarocci S, et al. High prevalence of atrophic body gastritis in patients with unexplained microcytic and macrocytic anemia: a prospective screening study. Am J Gastroenterol 1999;94:766–72.

28. Merola E, Sbrozzi-Vanni A, Panzuto F, et al. Type I gastric carcinoids: a prospective study on endoscopic management and recurrence rate. Neuroendocrinology 2012;95:207–13.

29. La RS, Inzani F, Vanoli A, et al. Histologic characterization and improved prognostic evaluation of 209 gastric neuroendocrine neoplasms. Hum Pathol 2011; 42:1373–84.

30. Grozinsky-Glasberg S, Thomas D, Strosberg JR, et al. Metastatic type 1 gastric carcinoid: a real threat or just a myth? World J Gastroenterol 2013; 19:8687–95.

31. Saund MS, Al Natour RH, Sharma AM, et al. Tumor size and depth predict rate of lymph node metastasis and utilization of lymph node sampling in surgically managed gastric carcinoids. Ann Surg Oncol 2011;18:2826–32.

32. Ito T, Igarashi H, Jensen RT. Zollinger-Ellison syndrome: recent advances and controversies. Curr Opin Gastroenterol 2013;29:650–61.

33. Newey PJ, Thakker RV. Role of multiple endocrine neoplasia type 1 mutational analysis in clinical practice. Endocr Pract 2011;17(Suppl 3):8–17.

34. Burkitt MD, Pritchard DM. Review article: pathogenesis and management of gastric carcinoid tumours. Aliment Pharmacol Ther 2006;24:1305–20.

35. Cockburn AN, Morgan CJ, Genta RM. Neuroendocrine proliferations of the stomach: a pragmatic approach for the perplexed pathologist. Adv Anat Pathol 2013; 20:148–57.

36. D'Adda T, Keller G, Bordi C, et al. Loss of heterozygosity in 11q13-14 regions in gastric neuroendocrine tumors not associated with multiple endocrine neoplasia type 1 syndrome. Lab Invest 1999;79:671–7.

37. Sundaresan S, Kang AJ, Hayes MM, et al. Deletion of Men1 and somatostatin induces hypergastrinemia and gastric carcinoids. Gut 2017;66:1012–21.

38. Annibale B, Lahner E, Fave GD. Diagnosis and management of pernicious anemia. Curr Gastroenterol Rep 2011;13:518–24.

39. Annibale B, Di GE, Caruana P, et al. The long-term effects of cure of Helicobacter pylori infection on patients with atrophic body gastritis. Aliment Pharmacol Ther 2002;16:1723–31.

40. Borch K, Ahren B, Ahlman H, et al. Gastric carcinoids: biologic behavior and prognosis after differentiated treatment in relation to type. Ann Surg 2005;242: 64–73.

41. Rugge M, Correa P, Dixon MF, et al. Gastric mucosal atrophy: interobserver consistency using new criteria for classification and grading. Aliment Pharmacol Ther 2002;16:1249–59.

42. Kidd M, Modlin IM, Eick GN, et al. Role of CCN2/CTGF in the proliferation of Mastomys enterochromaffin-like cells and gastric carcinoid development. Am J Physiol Gastrointest Liver Physiol 2007;292:G191–200.

43. Schaffer K, McBride EW, Beinborn M, et al. Interspecies polymorphisms confer constitutive activity to the Mastomys cholecystokinin-B/gastrin receptor. J Biol Chem 1998;273:28779–84.

44. Debelenko LV, Emmert-Buck MR, Manickam P, et al. Haplotype analysis defines a minimal interval for the multiple endocrine neoplasia type 1 (MEN1) gene. Cancer Res 1997;57:1039–42.

45. Berna MJ, Annibale B, Marignani M, et al. A prospective study of gastric carcinoids and enterochromaffin-like cell changes in multiple endocrine neoplasia type 1 and Zollinger-Ellison syndrome: identification of risk factors. J Clin Endocrinol Metab 2008;93:1582–91.

46. Hirschowitz BI, Haber MM. Helicobacter pylori effects on gastritis, gastrin and enterochromaffin-like cells in Zollinger-Ellison syndrome and non-Zollinger-Ellison syndrome acid hypersecretors treated long-term with lansoprazole. Aliment Pharmacol Ther 2001;15:87–103.

47. Kwon YH, Jeon SW, Kim GH, et al. Long-term follow up of endoscopic resection for type 3 gastric NET. World J Gastroenterol 2013;19:8703–8.

48. Rindi G, Azzoni C, La RS, et al. ECL cell tumor and poorly differentiated endocrine carcinoma of the stomach: prognostic evaluation by pathological analysis. Gastroenterology 1999;116:532–42.

49. Zikusoka MN, Kidd M, Eick G, et al. The molecular genetics of gastroentero-pancreatic neuroendocrine tumors. Cancer 2005;104:2292–309.

50. Annibale B, Azzoni C, Corleto VD, et al. Atrophic body gastritis patients with enterochromaffin-like cell dysplasia are at increased risk for the development of type I gastric carcinoid. Eur J Gastroenterol Hepatol 2001;13:1449–56.

51. Crosby DA, Donohoe CL, Fitzgerald L, et al. Gastric neuroendocrine tumours. Dig Surg 2012;29:331–48.

52. Gough DB, Thompson GB, Crotty TB, et al. Diverse clinical and pathologic features of gastric carcinoid and the relevance of hypergastrinemia. World J Surg 1994;18:473–9.

53. Thomas D, Tsolakis AV, Grozinsky-Glasberg S, et al. Long-term follow-up of a large series of patients with type 1 gastric carcinoid tumors: data from a multicenter study. Eur J Endocrinol 2013;168:185–93.

54. Thakker RV, Newey PJ, Walls GV, et al. Clinical practice guidelines for multiple endocrine neoplasia type 1 (MEN1). J Clin Endocrinol Metab 2012;97: 2990–3011.

55. Smith AM, Watson SA, Caplin M, et al. Gastric carcinoid expresses the gastrin autocrine pathway. Br J Surg 1998;85:1285–9.

56. Martinsen TC, Kawase S, Hakanson R, et al. Spontaneous ECL cell carcinomas in cotton rats: natural course and prevention by a gastrin receptor antagonist. Carcinogenesis 2003;24:1887–96.

57. Spence AD, Cardwell CR, McMenamin UC, et al. Adenocarcinoma risk in gastric atrophy and intestinal metaplasia: a systematic review. BMC Gastroenterol 2017; 17:157.

58. Minalyan A, Benhammou JN, Artashesyan A, et al. Autoimmune atrophic gastritis: current perspectives. Clin Exp Gastroenterol 2017;10:19–27.

59. Toh BH. Diagnosis and classification of autoimmune gastritis. Autoimmun Rev 2014;13:459–62.

60. Yamaoka Y. Mechanisms of disease: helicobacter pylori virulence factors. Nat Rev Gastroenterol Hepatol 2010;7:629–41.

61. Wong BC, Lam SK, Wong WM, et al. Helicobacter pylori eradication to prevent gastric cancer in a high-risk region of China: a randomized controlled trial. JAMA 2004;291:187–94.

62. Centanni M, Marignani M, Gargano L, et al. Atrophic body gastritis in patients with autoimmune thyroid disease: an underdiagnosed association. Arch Intern Med 1999;159:1726–30.

63. De Block CE, De Leeuw IH, Van Gaal LF. Autoimmune gastritis in type 1 diabetes: a clinically oriented review. J Clin Endocrinol Metab 2008;93:363–71.

64. Alexandraki KI, Nikolaou A, Thomas D, et al. Are patients with autoimmune thyroid disease and autoimmune gastritis at risk of gastric neuroendocrine neoplasms type 1? Clin Endocrinol (Oxf) 2014;80:685–90.

65. Bonafoux B, Henry L, Delfour C, et al. Association of familial pernicious anaemia and hereditary haemochromatosis. Acta Haematol 2008;119:12–4.

66. Thomas D, Alexandraki K, Nikolaou A, et al. Primary hyperparathyroidism in patients with gastric carcinoid tumors type 1: an unusual coexistence. Neuroendocrinology 2010;92:252–8.

67. Scherübl H, Jensen RT, Cadiot G, et al. Management of early gastrointestinal neuroendocrine neoplasms. World J Gastrointest Endosc 2011;3:133–9.

68. Vannella L, Lahner E, Annibale B. Risk for gastric neoplasias in patients with chronic atrophic gastritis: a critical reappraisal. World J Gastroenterol 2012;18:1279–85.

69. Ichikawa J, Tanabe S, Koizumi W, et al. Endoscopic mucosal resection in the management of gastric carcinoid tumors. Endoscopy 2003;35:203–6.
70. Wangberg B, Grimelius L, Granerus G, et al. The role of gastric resection in the management of multicentric argyrophil gastric carcinoids. Surgery 1990;108: 851–7.
71. Zatelli MC, Torta M, Leon A, et al. Chromogranin A as a marker of neuroendocrine neoplasia: an Italian Multicenter Study. Endocr Relat Cancer 2007;14:473–82.
72. Jensen RT, Cadiot G, Brandi ML, et al. ENETS consensus guidelines for the management of patients with digestive neuroendocrine neoplasms: functional pancreatic endocrine tumor syndromes. Neuroendocrinology 2012;95:98–119.
73. Rappel S, Altendorf-Hofmann A, Stolte M. Prognosis of gastric carcinoid tumours. Digestion 1995;56:455–62.
74. Fossmark R, Sordal O, Jianu CS, et al. Treatment of gastric carcinoids type 1 with the gastrin receptor antagonist netazepide (YF476) results in regression of tumours and normalisation of serum chromogranin A. Aliment Pharmacol Ther 2012;36:1067–75.
75. Boyce M, David O, Darwin K, et al. Single oral doses of netazepide (YF476), a gastrin receptor antagonist, cause dose-dependent, sustained increases in gastric pH compared with placebo and ranitidine in healthy subjects. Aliment Pharmacol Ther 2012;36:181–9.
76. Sundaresan S, Kang AJ, Merchant JL. Pathophysiology of gastric NETs: role of gastrin and menin. Curr Gastroenterol Rep 2017;19:32.
77. Cavallo F, De GC, Nanni P, et al. 2011: the immune hallmarks of cancer. Cancer Immunol Immunother 2011;60:319–26.
78. Pavel M, O'Toole D, Costa F, et al. ENETS consensus guidelines update for the management of distant metastatic disease of intestinal, pancreatic, bronchial neuroendocrine neoplasms (NEN) and NEN of unknown primary site. Neuroendocrinology 2016;103:172–85.
79. Garcia-Carbonero R, Sorbye H, Baudin E, et al. ENETS consensus guidelines for high-grade gastroenteropancreatic neuroendocrine tumors and neuroendocrine carcinomas. Neuroendocrinology 2016;103:186–94.

The Problem of Appendiceal Carcinoids

Michail Galanopoulos, MD[a], Christos Toumpanakis, MD, PhD, FRCP, FEBGH[b],*

KEYWORDS

- Appendiceal carcinoid • Carcinoid of the appendix
- Appendiceal neuroendocrine tumors • Right hemicolectomy

KEY POINTS

- Because the vast majority of appendiceal neuroendocrine neoplasms' reported series are heterogeneous, the real incidence/risk of distant metastases remains unclear.
- The current neuroendocrine biomarkers, especially chromogranin-A and 5-hydroxyindoleacetic acid, are not valid for the diagnosis and follow-up of the majority of appendiceal neuroendocrine neoplasms.
- Appendectomy alone is almost always an adequate treatment for tumors measuring less than 1 cm, and a prophylactic right hemicolectomy is mandatory in tumors greater than 2 cm.
- There remains controversy regarding the factors that identify the risk of metastases and, therefore, the need for prophylactic right hemicolectomy in tumors measuring between 1 and 2 cm.
- The importance of regional lymph node metastases for the prediction of subsequent development of distant metastases and overall disease prognosis is unknown.

INTRODUCTION AND EPIDEMIOLOGY

Neuroendocrine neoplasms (NEN) of the gastroenteropancreatic (GEP) tract represent approximately 1.5% of all tumors of the gastrointestinal system, demonstrating a wide spectrum of clinical presentation as well as a diversity in malignancy predisposition and prognosis.[1]

Regarding the epidemiology of appendiceal NEN (ANEN), there remain some gray zones owing to inconsistencies in some registries and national databases. Particularly,

Disclosure Statement: Dr M. Galanopoulos has no conflicts of interest with any commercial company. Dr C. Toumpanakis has received honoraria for lectures and Educational Grants for Royal Free Hospital Neuroendocrine Tumor Unit from IPSEN, Novartis, LEXICON, and AAA.
[a] Department of Gastroenterology, Evangelismos Hospital, 45-47 Ipsilantou Street, Athens 105 52, Greece; [b] Neuroendocrine Tumour Unit, ENETS Centre of Excellence, Royal Free Hospital, 8 South, Pond Street, London NW3 2QG, UK
* Corresponding author.
E-mail address: c.toumpanakis@ucl.ac.uk

Endocrinol Metab Clin N Am 47 (2018) 661–669
https://doi.org/10.1016/j.ecl.2018.04.004   endo.theclinics.com
0889-8529/18/Crown Copyright © 2018 Published by Elsevier Inc. All rights reserved.

in many previous studies goblet cell tumors of the appendix were included arbitrarily as ANEN, as well as ANEN being considered in some registries as part of colonic NEN. Moreover, the incidence rates of ANEN exhibit a significant variety in different countries. For example, although ANEN comprises 3.5% to 5.0% of all NEN in the Surveillance, Epidemiology, and End Results database and especially in many countries in the East, there are European countries (ie, Spain and UK) where, according to studies of Alsina and colleagues[2] and Ellis and colleagues,[3] respectively, ANEN frequency, among all NEN, is as high as 38%.

Even though an ANEN represents a substantial proportion of GEP-NEN, it is still considered a rare entity, with an estimated incidence rate of 0.15 to 0.60 per 100,000 per year.[4] There are many studies showing, however, that the reported incidence has increased recently. During the early 1970s, the incidence rate of ANEN was around 0.4 in Europe and Australia, based on studies of Hauso and colleagues,[5] Luke and colleagues,[6] and Hemminki and colleagues.[7] Over the same period in UK, the rate was even lower, whereas nowadays there is a tremendous increase (10-fold in both sexes), partly owing to the inclusion of benign neoplasms in recent registries.[3]

ANEN is still judged as a condition associated with a young age, because different studies have shown a mean age ranging between 31 and 51 years.[8–10] According to studies from Europe and the United States, there is a female preponderance, which may be due to a higher proportion of operations (appendicectomies and gynecologic surgery) in women.[3,9] As far as racial differences are concerned, a study by Yao and colleagues[11] that included 35,825 patients with neuroendocrine tumor showed that there was no diversity between whites and blacks. Nevertheless, high-grade tumors are believed to present commonly in Caucasians.[8]

Another ANEN gray area is thought to be the prognosis of these tumors, because there is a substantial inconsistency when reviewing the current literature. Although there are many studies supporting an excellent prognosis in terms of 5-year survival rates, other investigators state that significantly lower rates may be due to the inclusion of goblet cell tumors or mixed adenoneuroendocrine carcinomas, as shown in the study by Hauso and colleagues.[5] Yet, ANEN of low TNM stages demonstrate a 5-year survival rates of nearly 100%, mainly because of their incidental identification during appendectomy, which is curative for most ANEN.[12–14]

Nonetheless, ANEN are no longer considered completely indolent lesions, given that 25% to 50% exhibit lymph node dissemination, and subsequently distant metastases are present in up to 10% of cases.[15,16]

METHODS

An electronic literature search of the PubMed database was performed using the following search terms: appendiceal carcinoid, carcinoid of the appendix, appendiceal neuroendocrine tumors, and right hemicolectomy (RHC) for appendiceal neuroendocrine tumors. Only full articles published in peer-reviewed journals and in English were included.

DIAGNOSIS OF APPENDICEAL NEUROENDOCRINE NEOPLASMS
Clinical Presentation

As noted, ANEN are almost always discovered incidentally in postappendectomy specimens, with an incidence of 0.1% to 2.5%,[17] making any correlation between ANEN and possible preoperative symptomatology difficult to prove. Also, because ANEN are usually located at the tip of the appendix and usually measure less than 1 cm, the notion that ANEN may cause acute appendicitis or bowel obstruction seems to be unrealistic.[8] It has been stated that, in rare cases of ANEN-associated distant metastases,[16] symptoms may occur owing to their localization, either directly (ie, liver lesions causing discomfort/pain) or indirectly presenting with the "carcinoid syndrome," although the latter entity is mainly present in advanced small intestinal NEN.[18]

Biomarkers

Another interesting area in which ANEN seem to be different from other GEP-NEN is the biochemical testing. Although 5-hydroxyindoleacetic acid (5-HIAA) excretion is considered as a standard tool for the diagnostic workup for small intestinal NEN, in ANEN 5-HIAA might be helpful only when the extremely rare condition of a carcinoid syndrome is suspected.[19] The same notion is believed for the role of chromogranin A (CgA). Owing to the small size of ANENs at diagnosis, CgA levels often remain within the normal range, hampering its use as a screening or diagnostic tool.[20] Nevertheless, Modlin and colleagues[21] demonstrated an overexpression of tissue CgA and NALP1 in ANEN when compared with goblet cell tumors, where there was a decrease of NALP1 gene expression. Thus, this study suggests a possible differentiation tool between these 2 types of neuroendocrine tumors, and at the same time introduces gene expression (ie, NALP1, MTA1, MAGE-D2) as a candidate marker to distinguish ANEN from other malignant and mixed types of appendiceal neuroendocrine tumors. Last, although CgA and 5-HIAA are nondiagnostic tools for the follow-up of the largest proportion of ANEN, Grozinsky-Glasberg and colleagues[22] showed in their study that patients with a primary neoplasm size of greater than 2 cm and progressive disease during their follow-up had elevated levels of CgA and 5-HIAA, respectively. Because no definitive conclusions can be made, the real usefulness of these biomarkers needs to be clarified via larger studies.

Last but not least, there has been recently a great interest in discovering novel biomarkers for GEP-NEN to overtake the low sensitivity and specificity of current monoanalyte blood-based biomarker (CgA). According to Modlin and colleagues,[23] the analysis of blood-based multianalyte NET gene transcript of well-differentiated GEP-NEN seems to be more accurate than CgA. Finally, a fascinating approach to provide innovative and more sensitive biomarkers is the metabonomic analysis of some subgroups of NEN, which may show a specific metabolic phenotype.[24]

Imaging

Owing to the indolent nature of ANENs and their de novo treatment by appendectomy, there have been no validated studies to specify the ideal imaging algorithm for the diagnosis, postoperative staging, and follow-up of these patients. Although the cross-sectional imaging studies and somatostatin receptor scintigraphy studies applied to small intestinal NEN are considered as valid for ANEN as well, those studies can be all normal in diminutive tumors.[25] Endoscopy seems to have no role in tumor detection, and in terms of transabdominal ultrasound imaging, the guidelines of the European Neuroendocrine Tumor Society (ENETS) suggest a role in ANEN detection owing to its noninvasive nature, although no validated data have confirmed this.[8] The latter is in keeping with the study of Degnan and colleagues,[26] who showed, in a cohort of 7,691 surgical appendectomy samples from a pediatric pathology department, of the 36 patients in whom ANEN was diagnosed, none demonstrated any finding on CT/US during the preappendectomy period.

SURGICAL MANAGEMENT OF APPENDICEAL NEUROENDOCRINE NEOPLASMS

During the last 10 years, a great dichotomy has been demonstrated among scientists regarding the exact criteria by which a patient would be considered as a candidate for an extensive surgical approach for ANEN disease control. This was made more than clear with the ENETS guidelines in 2012, where RHC was clearly suggested for tumors greater than 2 cm, and only in tumors 1 to 2 cm with positive or unclear margins or with deep mesoappendiceal invasion (MAI), higher proliferation rate (G2), and/or angioinvasion.[27] Especially for the latter group (1–2 cm ANEN), G2 and angioinvasion were considered as less studied criteria and with no strong evidence to support them unequivocally. In line with this consideration, a retrospective study by Volante and colleagues[28] claimed that some factors, namely size, vascular invasion, and tumor grade, should be reevaluated with regard to RHC criteria, because the ENETS 2012 guidelines produced an overestimation and subsequently led to patients' overtreatment. In contrast, Grozinsky-Glasberg and colleagues[22] showed that in patients with a ANEN size of 1 cm or less and less than 2 cm, the risk of residual/locoregional disease, when considering RHC criteria according to the ENETS 2012 guidelines, may be as high as 18%. Furthermore, the authors suggested that MAI of any size as a critical factor harboring potential tumor aggressiveness. Owing to these conflicting data, it was suggested that many patients were overtreated, whereas others may have been undergone incomplete resection of tumor load. To face those inconsistencies, an update of ENETS consensus guidelines of the ANEN was published in 2016. According to these recommendations, tumor size is deemed the cornerstone factor influencing surgical strategy.

APPENDICEAL NEUROENDOCRINE NEOPLASMS WITH A SIZE OF GREATER THAN 2 CM

Currently, it is well-recognized that for ANEN size of greater than 2 cm, oncological RHC is the gold standard practice.[8] In keeping with this finding is the study by Goede and colleagues,[29] where the authors showed that, although metastatic dissemination of ANEN is a rare phenomenon, it is more common in ANENs with a size of greater than 2 cm. The same notion is reflected in the UK and Ireland Neuroendocrine Tumour Society Guidelines in 2012, where participants agreed on a more extensive surgical approach for that kind of tumor.[30] Other studies include that of Bamboat and Berger,[31] who claimed that simple appendectomy was effective for ANEN with size greater than 2 cm, taking into account their benign prognosis, whereas only in young patients does RHC need to be considered. In line with the latter study, Moertel and colleagues,[32] who interestingly were the pioneers of size cutoff of 2 cm, demonstrated that oncological RHC was justified only for young individuals in whom the surgical morbidity and mortality were low. Nevertheless, based on a substantial number of cohorts, ANEN greater than 2 cm exhibit locoregional spread in up to 80% of patients, rendering RHC as the appropriate therapy strategy for all those tumors.[16,33]

APPENDICEAL NEUROENDOCRINE NEOPLASMS WITH A SIZE OF LESS THAN 1 CM

In terms of ANEN with a size of less than 1 cm, there seems to be a unanimous acceptance regarding the treatment modality of these ANEN subgroup, that is, simple appendectomy.[16,26–28] This finding is clarified by the recent study from Raoof and collagues,[34] who demonstrated in the largest study to date to evaluate the significance of mesenteric lymphadenectomy in ANENs, that owing to the rarity of node metastases of ANEN size of less than 1 cm (2.8%), simple appendectomy is the only necessary curative approach for such lesions. Yet, ENETS guidelines in 2016, include following the quote: "The exception that proves the rule," and set some exclusion criteria in performing a simple appendectomy, namely incomplete surgical margins, ANEN located at the base, and an MAI of greater than 3 mm.[8] It is well-known that ANENs are situated at base of appendix in up to 10% of cases, and although this is considered as a rare phenomenon, it is linked with an increased odds of incomplete ANEN resection during simple appendectomy.[8] Thus, there is the potential for disease recurrence, yet the cohorts or guidelines have not elucidated the exact significance of the base location in correlation with survival.[8,27]

APPENDICEAL NEUROENDOCRINE NEOPLASMS WITH A SIZE OF GREATER THAN 1 CM TO LESS THAN 2 CM

For ANEN with size of greater than 1 cm to less than 2 cm, other factors are taken into account to identify patients who may need a prophylactic RHC.

The significance of MAI is highlighted clearly, based on ENETS 2012 consensus guidelines,[27] the study of Mullen and Savarese,[16] as well as the one from Goede and colleagues.[29] However, a substantial number of studies have reported no recurrence dependent exclusively on MAI, followed a simple appendectomy for ANENs measuring 1 to 2 cm. Interestingly, Syracuse and colleagues,[35] who were the pioneers of introducing MAI as a prognosticator of metastatic disease, showed that MAI, only when correlated with tumor size, was responsible for a worse outcome. In keeping with this finding, other long-term studies demonstrated that MAI was not a prerequisite for lymph node dissemination.[26,32,36] Furthermore, the problematic nature of MAI as a poor prognostic factor was seen clearly in paediatric population studies where, according to Moertel and colleagues,[37] Corpron and colleagues,[38] and Prommegger and colleagues,[39] no metachronous nodal dissemination was revealed in patients with MAI who underwent an appendectomy. The follow-up period in those series was 26 years, 1.5 - 30 years and 10 years, respectively. Finally, there is a gray zone regarding the true correlation between tumor size and the depth of MAI, especially for ANEN 1 to 2 cm in size. A study in 2013 documented that 38% of patients with ANEN measured 1 to 2 cm who exhibiting MAI of less than 3 mm had locoregional metastatic nodal disease at RHC.[22] Thus, questions have arisen regarding the arbitrary definition of 3 mm in MAI, as suggested in the ENETS guidelines in 2012.[27]

Apart from MAI as a critical pathologic factor contributing to treatment choice for ANEN at a size of 1 to 2 cm, the presence of angioinvasion should be taken into consideration when we are to judge our patient as a further surgical candidate. As has been shown by Stinner and Rothmund,[33] approximately 30% of such cases harbor lymph node metastases. Although this finding has been clearly mentioned in the ENETS guidelines since 2012, available data were scarce as to whether this has been validated for tumors smaller than 2 cm.[8,27] This matter was the focus of the recent study from Kleiman and colleagues,[40] who were the first to show that, even for tumors measured of less than 2 cm, there is an increased incidence of lymph node dissemination when angioinvasion was present, independent of the existence of other worrisome pathologic features. More studies are needed to clarify whether this is applicable for ANEN smaller than 1 cm.

Finally, the Ki-67 index, which determines the ANEN grading according to the World Health Organization classification, is believed to play an important role in the risk of recurrence and/or metastasis, according to European guidelines.[8] Nevertheless, conflicting data exist in this area as well, revealing an additional problem in ANEN approaches. Liu and colleagues[41] demonstrated a clear association of the Ki-67 index with decreased survival, even though it was not correlated with the existence of metastatic disease. This discrepancy, in addition to the diminutive number of patients presenting with a Ki-67 of greater than 2%, justifies the need for more studies to be carried out. In contrast, a well-designed study from Italy including 138 cases of ANEN (according to the World Health Organization's 2010 guidelines) showed that the grading system is not the appropriate prognosticator of poor prognosis of clinically aggressive cases in this cohort.[28] Interestingly, the authors of the study ended up questioning the adequacy of the Ki-67 cutoff levels in ANEN, distancing their position from the study of Strosberg and colleagues,[42] who delineated a strong relationship between the tumor grading and overall survival.

FOLLOW-UP

The majority of clinicians agree that follow-up for ANEN of less than 2 cm without risk factors is not needed, because appendectomy alone is considered as curative. In the rare scenario of distant metastases associated with ANEN, long-term follow-up is mandatory and needs to be similar of patients with advanced small bowel NEN.

For other groups, such as patients who, for some reason, underwent appendectomy despite the presence of risk factors, or patients who had RHC because of any risk factors but without lymph node metastases, and patients who had RHC because of any risk factors and were found to have lymph node metastases in the resected specimen, the decision for follow-up is based on the presumed importance of each risk factor and the association of regional lymph node metastasis with the disease outcome and overall prognosis.

Based on the current ENET guidelines, no follow-up is needed in patients who did not have lymph node invasion at the time of RHC.[8] However, the long-term risks of local/distal disease recurrence in that group, and whether the absence of regional lymph node invasion excludes the subsequent development of distant metastases, remain unclear. The guidelines suggest that all patients with documented lymph node metastases will need to be followed up. However, the duration of follow-up and the appropriate follow-up modalities are still not entirely clear. As noted, the usefulness of the established NEN biomarkers that are routinely used in small bowel NEN have not been validated. 5-HIAA would be normal in the absence of carcinoid syndrome and CgA may be still within normal limits, even in the presence of locoregional metastases, especially if the tumor load is low.

The decision for imaging modalities needs to be adapted to patient age and comorbidities. Patients with ANEN are often diagnosed at a young age and recurrence may occur after a long period of time. In low-risk groups and with young age, radiation should be avoided, rendering ultrasound examination and MRI the preferred methods. Somatostatin receptor scintigraphy imaging should be reserved for patients with known focal lesions. In older patients and patients with high-risk or distant metastases, computed tomography scanning or MRI together with somatostatin receptor scintigraphy imaging are the methods of choice.

SUMMARY AND FUTURE DEVELOPMENTS

Good quality studies need to be designed, because they may resolve the gray areas discussed herein. For example, a multicenter, large, retrospective trial could include all patients who underwent a prophylactic RHC (or a limited ileocecal resection) for any of the known risk factors, addressed in the existing guidelines. The presence of lymph node metastases, after RHC, could then help to identify the predictive role of each risk factor. Also, taking into account that patients with lymph node metastases would have been followed up by the vast majority of the NEN units, information could be obtained with regard to the real risk of disease recurrence in those patients. It would be interesting also to answer the following questions: (a) What should be the standard approach of lymphadenectomy during the prophylactic operation? and (b) Is a more limited ileocecal resection, rather than an oncological RHC, sufficient in some patients?

Furthermore, as mentioned, novel circulating biomarkers such as circulating transcripts or other "-omics" and molecular markers such as tissue expression of NAP1LI, MAGE-D2, and MTA1 may provide more information in the future with regard to the identification of residual disease after appendectomy and for overall disease prognosis.

The resolution of controversies in ANEN is mandatory, because many of patients are young and some of them may be overtreated through an additional prophylactic operation. Although RHC is not a technically challenging procedure nowadays and may be performed laparoscopically; however, its morbidity and mortality cannot be ignored. Therefore, all decisions ideally should be individualized, well-supported, and balanced between the risks and benefits.

REFERENCES

1. Lepage C, Bouvier AM, Faivre J. Endocrine tumours: epidemiology of malignant digestive neuroendocrine tumours. Eur J Endocrinol 2013;168:R77–83.
2. Alsina M, Marcos-Gragera R, Capdevila J, et al. Neuroendocrine tumors: a population-based study of incidence and survival in Girona province, 1994–2004. Cancer Epidemiol 2011;35:e49–54.
3. Ellis L, Shale MJ, Coleman MP. Carcinoid tumors of the gastrointestinal tract: trends in incidence in England since 1971. Am J Gastroenterol 2010;105:2563–9.
4. Lawrence B, Gustafsson BI, Chan A, et al. The epidemiology of gastroenteropancreatic neuroendocrine tumors. Endocrinol Metab Clin North Am 2011;40:1–18, vii.
5. Hauso O, Gustafsson BI, Kidd M, et al. Neuroendocrine tumor epidemiology: contrasting Norway and North America. Cancer 2008;113:2655–64.
6. Luke C, Price T, Townsend A, et al. Epidemiology of neuroendocrine cancers in an Australian population. Cancer Causes Control 2010;21:931–8.
7. Hemminki K, Li X. Incidence trends and risk factors of carcinoid tumors: a nationwide epidemiologic study from Sweden. Cancer 2001;92:2204–10.
8. Pape U-F, Niederle B, Costa F, et al. ENETS consensus guidelines for neuroendocrine neoplasms of the appendix (excluding goblet cell carcinomas). Neuroendocrinology 2016;103:144–52.
9. Modlin IM, Lye KD, Kidd M. A 5-decade analysis of 13,715 carcinoid tumors. Cancer 2003;97:934–59.
10. Tsikitis VL, Wertheim BC, Guerrero MA. Trends of incidence and survival of gastrointestinal neuroendocrine tumors in the United States: a SEER analysis. J Cancer 2012;3:292–302.
11. Yao JC, Hassan M, Phan A, et al. One hundred years after 'carcinoid': epidemiology of and prognostic factors for neuroendocrine tumors in 35,825 cases in the United States. J Clin Oncol 2008;26:3063–72.
12. Hsu C, Rashid A, Xing Y, et al. Varying malignant potential of appendiceal neuroendocrine tumors: importance of histologic subtype. J Surg Oncol 2013;107:136–43.
13. Scott A, Upadhyay V. Carcinoid tumors of the appendix in children in Auckland, New Zealand: 1965–2008. N Z Med J 2011;124:56–60.

14. Kulkarni KP, Sergi C. Appendix carcinoids in childhood: long-term experience at a single institution in Western Canada and systematic review. Pediatr Int 2013;55: 157–62.

15. Landry CS, Woodall C, Scoggins CR, et al. Analysis of 900 appendiceal carcinoid tumors for a proposed predictive staging system. Arch Surg 2008;143:664–70 [discussion: 670].

16. Mullen JT, Savarese DMF. Carcinoid tumors of the appendix: a population-based study. J Surg Oncol 2011;104:41–4.

17. Amr B, Froghi F, Edmond M, et al. Management and outcomes of appendicular neuroendocrine tumours: retrospective review with 5-year follow-up. Eur J Surg Oncol 2015;41:1243–6.

18. Clift AK, Faiz O, Al-Nahhas A, et al. Role of staging in patients with small intestinal neuroendocrine tumours. J Gastrointest Surg 2016;20:180–8 [discussion: 188].

19. Alexandraki KI, Kaltsas GA, Grozinsky-Glasberg S, et al. Appendiceal neuroendocrine neoplasms: diagnosis and management. Endocr Relat Cancer 2016; 23:R27–41.

20. de Herder WW. Biochemistry of neuroendocrine tumours. Best Pract Res Clin Endocrinol Metab 2007;21:33–41.

21. Modlin IM, Kidd M, Latich I, et al. Genetic differentiation of appendiceal tumor malignancy: a guide for the perplexed. Ann Surg 2006;244:52–60.

22. Grozinsky-Glasberg S, Alexandraki KI, Barak D, et al. Current size criteria for the management of neuroendocrine tumors of the appendix: are they valid? Clinical experience and review of the literature. Neuroendocrinology 2013;98:31–7.

23. Modlin IM, Kidd M, Bodei L, et al. The clinical utility of a novel blood-based multitranscriptome assay for the diagnosis of neuroendocrine tumors of the gastrointestinal tract. Am J Gastroenterol 2015;110(8):1223–32.

24. Kinross JM, Drymousis P, Jimenez B, et al. Metabonomic profiling: a novel approach in neuroendocrine neoplasias. Surgery 2013;154:1185–92.

25. Coursey CA, Nelson RC, Moreno RD, et al. Carcinoid tumors of the appendix: are these tumors identifiable prospectively on preoperative CT? Am Surg 2010;76: 273–5.

26. Degnan AJ, Tocchio S, Kurtom W, et al. Pediatric neuroendocrine carcinoid tumors: management, pathology, and imaging findings in a pediatric referral center. Pediatr Blood Cancer 2017;64(9):1–9.

27. Pape UF, Perren A, Niederle B, et al. ENETS consensus guidelines for the management of patients with neuroendocrine neoplasms from the jejuno-ileum and the appendix including goblet cell carcinomas. Neuroendocrinology 2012;95: 135–56.

28. Volante M, Daniele L, Asioli F, et al. Tumor staging but not grading is associated with adverse clinical outcome in neuroendocrine tumors of the appendix. Am J Surg Pathol 2013;37:606–12.

29. Goede AC, Caplin ME, Winslet MC. Carcinoid tumour of the appendix. Br J Surg 2003;90:1317–22.

30. Ramage JK, Ahmed A, Ardill J, et al. Guidelines for the management of gastroenteropancreatic neuroendocrine (including carcinoid) tumours (NETs). Gut 2012;61:6–32.

31. Bamboat ZM, Berger DL. Is right hemicolectomy for 2.0-cm appendiceal carcinoids justified? Arch Surg 2006;141:349–52 [discussion: 352].

32. Moertel CG, Weiland LH, Nagorney DM, et al. Carcinoid tumor of the appendix: treatment and prognosis. N Engl J Med 1987;317:1699–701.

33. Stinner B, Rothmund M. Neuroendocrine tumours (carcinoids) of the appendix. Best Pract Res Clin Gastroenterol 2005;19:729–38.
34. Raoof M, Dumitra S, O'Leary MP, et al. Mesenteric lymphadenectomy in well differentiated appendiceal neuroendocrine tumors. Dis Colon Rectum 2017;60: 674–81.
35. Syracuse DC, Perzin KH, Price JB, et al. Carcinoid tumors of the appendix: mesoappendiceal extension and nodal metastases. Ann Surg 1979;190:58–63.
36. Svendsen LB, Bülow S. Carcinoid tumours of the appendix in young patients. Acta Chir Scand 1980;146:137–9.
37. Moertel CL, Weiland LH, Telander RL. Carcinoid tumor of the appendix in the first two decades of life. J Pediatr Surg 1990;25:1073–5.
38. Corpron CA, Black CT, Herzog CE, et al. A half century of experience with carcinoid tumors in children. Am J Surg 1995;170:606–8.
39. Prommegger R, Obrist P, Ensinger C, et al. Retrospective evaluation of carcinoid tumors of the appendix in children. World J Surg 2002;26:1489–92.
40. Kleiman DA, Finnerty B, Beninato T, et al. Features associated with metastases among well-differentiated neuroendocrine (Carcinoid) tumors of the appendix: the significance of small vessel invasion in addition to size. Dis Colon Rectum 2015;58:1137–43.
41. Liu E, Telem DA, Hwang J, et al. The clinical utility of Ki-67 in assessing tumor biology and aggressiveness in patients with appendiceal carcinoids. J Surg Oncol 2010;102:338–41.
42. Strosberg J, Nasir A, Coppola D, et al. Correlation between grade and prognosis in metastatic gastroenteropancreatic neuroendocrine tumors. Hum Pathol 2009; 40:1262–8.

Carcinoid Heart Disease
A Review

Aimee R. Hayes, BSc (Med), MMed (Clin Epi), FRACP[a], Joseph Davar, MRCP, MD, PhD[b], Martyn E. Caplin, DM, FRCP[a],*

KEYWORDS

• Carcinoid heart disease • Carcinoid syndrome • Neuroendocrine tumor

KEY POINTS

- Carcinoid heart disease remains a major cause of morbidity and mortality among patients with carcinoid syndrome and metastatic neuroendocrine tumours.
- Screening of all patients with NT-proBNP and transthoracic echocardiogram is critical for early detection as early symptoms and signs have low sensitivity for the disease.
- Cardiac surgery, in appropriate cases, is the only definitive therapy for advanced carcinoid heart disease and it improves patient symptoms and survival.
- Management of carcinoid heart disease is complex and multidisciplinary assessment of cardiac status, hormonal syndrome and tumour burden is critical in guiding optimal timing of surgery.

INTRODUCTION

Although progress in the medical and surgical management of patients with metastatic neuroendocrine tumors (NETs) has resulted in improved symptoms and survival, carcinoid heart disease (CHD) remains a major cause of morbidity and mortality among patients with carcinoid syndrome. CHD has been previously described in up to 50% of patients with carcinoid syndrome,[1,2] although recent studies suggest the prevalence has fallen to approximately 20%,[3,4] perhaps secondary to the more widespread use of somatostatin analog therapy. It is reported to occur most frequently in patients with primary small bowel NETs (72%), followed by NETs arising from the lung, large bowel, pancreas, appendix, and ovaries.[1] A slight male predominance has been reported (approximately 60%), with a mean age at diagnosis 59 ($\pm$ 11) years.[1]

Disclosure: The authors maintain they have no conflicts of interest for this article. No external funding or grants were used.
[a] Neuroendocrine Tumour Unit, Royal Free Hospital, Pond Street, London NW3 2QG, UK;
[b] Carcinoid Heart Disease Clinic, Department of Cardiology, Royal Free Hospital, Pond Street, London NW3 2QG, UK
* Corresponding author.
E-mail address: m.caplin@ucl.ac.uk

Endocrinol Metab Clin N Am 47 (2018) 671–682
https://doi.org/10.1016/j.ecl.2018.04.012
0889-8529/18/© 2018 Elsevier Inc. All rights reserved.

Without treatment, the prognosis of CHD is poor, with 3-year survival as low as 31% (compared with 68% in patients with NETs but without CHD).[1] CHD with advanced symptoms (New York Heart Association [NYHA] functional class III or IV) carries a particularly poor prognosis, with median survival only 11 months.[5] Over the past few decades, however, the prognosis of patients with CHD has improved. In a retrospective series of 200 patients with carcinoid syndrome and CHD,[6] the median survival improved from 1.5 years in the 1980s to 4.4 years in the late 1990s, with the data suggesting this improvement is related to increased rates of cardiac surgery and the use of somatostatin analogs.

PATHOPHYSIOLOGY

The pathogenesis of CHD is thought to be multifactorial and is not completely understood. A variety of vasoactive substances secreted by the tumor, including serotonin, prostaglandins, histamine, bradykinin, and other substances with fibroblast proliferative properties, such as tachykinins (substance P, neurokinin A, neuropeptide K) or transforming growth factor-beta, are thought to be involved in the disease pathogenesis.[7]

The Role of Serotonin

There is a growing body of evidence that suggests serotonin plays a major role in the pathogenesis of CHD. It is well known that urinary 5-hydroxyindoleacetic acid (5-HIAA), the serotonin metabolite, is significantly higher in patients with CHD compared with those without cardiac involvement.[1,2,8,9] Other support for the pathophysiological role of serotonin arises from the observation that serotoninergic drugs, such as the ergot-alkaloid derivatives (eg, ergotamine and methysergide used for treatment of migraine; pergolide and cabergoline used for treatment of Parkinson disease) or the anorectic drugs (eg, fenfluramine, alone or in combination with phentermine, and dexfenfluramine), cause valvular fibrosis similar to that seen in CHD.[10,11] These agents are full or partial 5-HT2B receptor agonists, suggesting that activation of this receptor is involved in the pathologic process that leads to plaque development.[12,13] Furthermore, in cell culture studies, serotonin has been shown to promote cell proliferation in valvular subendocardial cells,[14] and human heart valves have been demonstrated to express the serotonin receptors 5-HT1B, 1D, 2A, and 2B.[13,15] In addition, preliminary animal studies, using Sprague-Dawley rats and cynomolgus monkeys, have demonstrated that long-term exposure to elevated levels of serotonin induces carcinoid-like plaques on cardiac valves, as well as echocardiogram findings similar to those seen in humans with CHD.[16–18] Furthermore, the concomitant administration of the ergoline terguride (transdihydrolisuride), a 5-HT2B/2C receptor antagonist, inhibited these changes.[19] Nevertheless, despite the growing evidence that serotonin plays a major role in the development of CHD, it is likely that other biochemical mediators are also significant and may act as cofactors in the fibrotic process.[20–22]

Pathologic Findings

CHD is characterized by plaque-like deposits on the endocardium of valvular cusps, leaflets, chordae, and papillary muscles and cardiac chambers, and occasionally within the intima of the pulmonary arteries or aorta.[23–25] The deposits are composed of myofibroblasts and smooth muscle cells surrounded by extracellular matrix components (collagen and myxoid matrix) and covered by an endothelial cell layer.[23,26] The valves and endocardium of the right side of the heart are most frequently affected and this is usually due to the presence of hepatic metastases that secrete large quantities of vasoactive peptides that subsequently reach the right heart without being inactivated.[27,28] The plaque is usually deposited on the ventricular aspect of the tricuspid valve leaflet and the pulmonary arterial aspect of the pulmonary valve cusps.[24,29] In the pulmonary valve, this leads to adherence of the leaflets to the pulmonary artery endothelium with consequent regurgitation, stenosis, or both. In contrast, regurgitation tends to predominate with tricuspid valve disease due to retraction of leaflets.

The left-sided valves are less commonly affected, and it is hypothesized that they are spared because of inactivation of the vasoactive hormones by the pulmonary circulation.[1,30] Involvement of the left-sided valves is usually associated with a patent foramen ovale and right-to-left atrial shunt allowing serotonin-rich blood to enter the left heart chambers without passing through the pulmonary circulation.[1,4,29] In a study by Bhattacharyya and colleagues,[4] 52 (21%) of 252 patients with carcinoid syndrome were found to have CHD. Of those patients with CHD, 15 (29%) had left-sided carcinoid valve involvement and of those patients with left-sided involvement, 13 (87%) of 15 had a patent foramen ovale. Left-sided valve disease can also occur in patients with bronchial carcinoids and in patients with high levels of circulating serotonin due to severe, refractory carcinoid syndrome.[31] CHD affecting the aortic or mitral valve usually manifests as valve regurgitation rather than valve stenosis.[4,23,30]

Intramyocardial metastases from carcinoid tumors are rare and are seen in approximately 4% of patients.[4,31]

CLINICAL MANIFESTATIONS
Symptoms

Early valvular changes of CHD can be well tolerated for protracted periods, and hence the initial clinical manifestations can be subtle or absent leading to delay in diagnosis. Early symptoms of isolated, severe tricuspid regurgitation include fatigue and exertional dyspnea due to low cardiac output.[32] Peripheral edema with hepatic congestion and consequent anorexia can also occur with elevated right atrial pressure.[32] Atrial arrhythmias also are common in the setting of right atrial enlargement. Without treatment, progressive right heart failure typically ensues with ascites and anasarca.[32]

Physical Examination

The earliest finding of severe tricuspid regurgitation is often jugular venous distension with prominent systolic "v" wave, although its presence varies between 35% and 75% of patients.[33–35] Other findings may include a palpable right ventricular impulse and murmurs of tricuspid and pulmonary regurgitation. Less frequently, a systolic murmur of pulmonary stenosis or a diastolic murmur of tricuspid stenosis may be audible, although findings on auscultation may be subtle due to the low pressure in the pulmonary circulation.[36] As the valvular disease progresses, and right ventricular enlargement and dysfunction develop, peripheral edema, ascites, and pulsatile hepatomegaly may become evident.

It should be noted, however, that early symptoms and physical signs have low sensitivity for the presence of CHD, and screening with N-terminal pro-B-type natriuretic peptide (NT-proBNP), even in those patients who are asymptomatic, is paramount for early CHD detection (**Fig. 1**). In a series by Bhattacharyya and colleagues,[3] 8 (27%) of 30 patients with CHD had moderate to severe carcinoid valve disease but were in NYHA functional class I, whilst 11 patients (37%) had no physical signs.

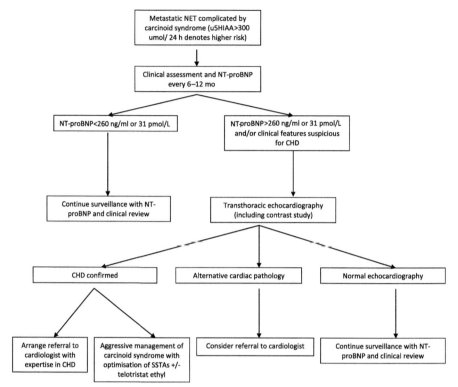

Fig. 1. Screening and evaluation of CHD. u5HIAA, urinary 5-hydroxyindoleacetic. (*Adapted from* Davar J, Connolly HM, Caplin ME, et al. Diagnosing and managing carcinoid heart disease in patients with neuroendocrine tumours. J Am Coll Cardiol 2017;69(10):1296; with permission.)

Biomarkers

Urinary 5- hydroxyindoleacetic acid

Patients with neuroendocrine tumors and CHD have been shown to have significantly higher (two-fold to four-fold) levels of serum serotonin, platelet serotonin, and urinary 5-HIAA compared with those without CHD.[8] In addition, elevated urinary 5-HIAA levels have been demonstrated to positively correlate with progression of CHD.[9,37–39] In a retrospective series of 71 patients with carcinoid syndrome who underwent serial echocardiographic studies performed more than 1 year apart, peak urinary 5-HIAA levels were significantly higher (median 265 mg/24 hours vs 189 mg/24 hours; $P = .004$) in patients with progressive CHD and in patients with severe symptomatic disease who were referred directly for cardiac surgery.[38]

Chromogranin A

Chromogranin A is a secretory protein found in the large dense-core vesicles of neuroendocrine cells. Despite a number of limitations, it remains a valuable tumor marker, usually of neuroendocrine tumor burden. Chromogranin A is also a sensitive biomarker for CHD but is not specific for the detection of severe CHD (specificity 0.30).[40]

N-terminal pro-B-type natriuretic peptide

Natriuretic peptides belong to the neurohormone family and are produced primarily within the heart and released into the circulation due to increased wall stress.[41] In a study of 200 patients with carcinoid syndrome,[42] NT-proBNP was found to be significantly higher in those with CHD (1149 pg/mL) compared with those without CHD (101 pg/mL, $P<.001$). At a cutoff level of 260 pg/mL for detection of CHD, the sensitivity and specificity of NT-proBNP was 0.92 and 0.91, respectively. It was also found to positively correlate with severity of carcinoid symptoms ($r = 0.81$, $P<.001$) and NYHA functional class ($P<.001$). The negative and positive predictive values were 98% and 71%, respectively. The high negative predictive value allows NT-proBNP to serve as a good screening test for CHD in the NET population.

The role of NT-proBNP paired with chromogranin A to predict prognosis has also been studied. In a retrospective study by Korse and colleagues[40] ($n = 102$), levels of chromogranin A and NT-proBNP were independently associated with CHD and overall mortality. Five-year survival was 81% in patients with normal chromogranin A levels, 11% in those with elevated chromogranin A but normal NT-proBNP, and 16% in those with elevations of both chromogranin A and NT-proBNP.

Activin A

Plasma activin A, a growth factor with fibrogenic properties and a cytokine member of the transforming growth factor-beta superfamily, has also been demonstrated to be an independent predictor for the presence of CHD in patients with NETs. Plasma activin A levels were found to be significantly higher in patients with NETs and CHD compared with those patients without CHD ($P = .005$), and a positive correlation was also found between plasma activin A and urinary 5-HIAA ($r = 0.31$, $P = .02$).[22] A cutoff value of 0.34 ng/mL for activin A had a high negative predictive value (94%) but a weak positive predictive value (sensitivity 87%, specificity 57%) and is another potential biomarker that may serve as a screening test for CHD in the NET population.[22] Interestingly, in contrast to NT-proBNP, activin A was found to be elevated in patients with early CHD but without right heart dilatation.[22]

Imaging Modalities

Echocardiography is the gold standard for the diagnosis of CHD and reveals a wide spectrum of CHD findings.[4] A multimodality approach, including 2-dimensional (2D) transthoracic echocardiography (TTE), 3-dimensional (3D) TTE, transoesophageal echocardiography (TOE), cardiac computed tomography (CT) and MRI can help to comprehensively assess different aspects of CHD (eg, valve pathology, presence of patent foramen ovale, ventricular and atrial volumes, coronary anatomy, presence of cardiac metastases and their relationship to coronary arteries).[4,43]

Echocardiography

TTE is the main modality to diagnose and evaluate CHD, as it allows assessment of valvular disease as well as right heart chamber size and function. Advanced techniques including 3D TTE and 3D TOE may help diagnose and assess valve pathology, especially in the tricuspid and pulmonary valves, as all leaflets may not be visualized on 2D TTE. Moreover, 3D echocardiography allows detailed assessment of the subvalvular apparatus and assessment of the relationship between valve leaflets to each other and surrounding structures. Agitated saline contrast echocardiography (*bubble study*) should also be performed at the time of initial echocardiogram to assess for a patent foramen ovale.

Typical echocardiographic appearances of advanced tricuspid valve involvement include thickening and retraction of the leaflets that are fixed and do not coapt.[4] This is typically associated with severe tricuspid regurgitation, a "dagger-shaped" doppler profile and mild to moderate tricuspid stenosis.[4]

Early tricuspid valve carcinoid involvement includes thickening of the valve leaflets and subvalvular apparatus leading to loss of the normal concave curvature of the leaflets and a stiffer "board-like" dynamic motion during diastole rather than the normal undulating motion.[4] Only trivial or mild, centrally directed tricuspid regurgitation is noted at this stage. Thickening of the valve leaflets may be associated with thickening of the chordae and papillary muscles, which results in greater retraction and reduction excursion of the valve cusps.[4]

Pulmonary valve carcinoid disease has a similar appearance to that of tricuspid valve pathology. Mild involvement produces diffusely thickened valve cusps, which causes them to become straightened.[4] As the disease progresses, varying degrees of retraction and reduction in excursion of the valve cusps occurs, and in severe cases valves appear fixed, retracted, and thickened and are associated with severe pulmonary regurgitation.[4] In severe disease, pulmonary annular constriction may also occur, resulting in predominant outflow obstruction and pulmonary stenosis.[4]

Cardiac MRI and computed tomography

Cardiac CT or MRI can complement echocardiography when incomplete data are obtained or when structures (eg, the pulmonary valve) are poorly visualized. CT or MRI allows delineation of valve pathology, assessment of valve regurgitation and stenosis, and may be particularly helpful for quantification of ventricular volumes.[4] MRI also allows assessment of myocardial metastases, including measurement of size and extracardiac invasion that cannot be assessed on echocardiography.[4] Furthermore, cardiac CT can delineate coronary artery anatomy and the relationship to myocardial metastases if present.

[68]Gallium DOTA-somatostatin analog PET/computed tomography

[68]Gallium DOTA-somatostatin analog PET/CT is more specific than CT or MRI in detecting metastatic, well-differentiated NETs[44] and may enhance the detection of rare intramyocardial metastases.

MANAGEMENT
Management Approach

The management of patients with metastatic NETs complicated by carcinoid syndrome and CHD is complex and referral to a specialist center and multidisciplinary team with CHD experience is critical.

Medical Management of Right Heart Failure

Loop diuretic therapy, fluid and salt restriction, and compression stockings may provide temporary relief by reducing symptoms of edema; however, they must be used judiciously, as depletion of intravascular volume may further reduce cardiac output and, in turn, lead to worsening fatigue and breathlessness.[36] In selected cases, ultrafiltration could be useful.

Control of Carcinoid Syndrome

Given the strong body of evidence that suggest serotonin, or its metabolites, plays a major role in the pathogenesis of CHD, it is likely that somatostatin analogs, telotristat ethyl (a novel serotonin synthesis inhibitor), liver-directed or cytoreductive therapies, and systemic therapies (eg, peptide receptor radionuclide therapy) that reduce circulating levels of serotonin may reduce the risk of developing CHD. Optimal doses of somatostatin analogs to appropriately reduce urinary 5-HIAA levels may be of importance. In an observational cohort study by Bhattacharyya and colleagues,[39] urinary 5-HIAA levels greater than 300 μmol/24 hours conferred a two-fold to three-fold risk for the development or progression of CHD and reducing urinary 5-HIAA to below this level may be an important therapeutic strategy. There is no evidence, however, that reducing urinary 5-HIAA can reverse established carcinoid valvular lesions.

Telotristat ethyl is a peripheral tryptophan hydroxylase inhibitor and reduces the production of serotonin. It has recently been approved in the United States and Europe, in combination with somatostatin analog therapy, for control of diarrhea associated with refractory carcinoid syndrome. In a post hoc analysis of a phase III study (n = 135),[45] telotristat ethyl reduced urinary 5-HIAA levels by ≥30% in 78% (n = 25) and 87% (n = 26) of patients in the 250 mg and 500 mg (3 times a day) treatment arms, respectively, compared with 10% (n = 3) in the placebo group. It may be reasonable to consider telotristat therapy in patients at higher risk of CHD (eg, urinary 5-HIAA >300 μmol/24 hours despite optimal doses of somatostatin analogs); however, as yet, there is no evidence that telotristat ethyl can prevent the development or progression of CHD.

Surgical Valve Replacement

Cardiac valve replacement is the only definitive therapy for advanced CHD, and it improves patient symptoms and survival.[6,46] CHD may progress rapidly[39] and, therefore, early diagnosis and careful cardiac monitoring are pivotal to identify those patients likely to benefit from surgery.

In the largest retrospective series to date of surgical patients with CHD (n = 195), symptomatic improvement was seen in 69 (75%) of 92 patients with significant preoperative symptoms (NYHA functional class III or IV).[46] Survival for the entire cohort at 1, 5, and 10 years was 69%, 35%, and 24%, respectively,[46] which is a marked improvement compared with medically managed historical control subjects with NYHA functional class symptoms greater than II, only 10% of whom survive 2.5 years.[5,6]

All patients with severe tricuspid valve regurgitation should be carefully considered for valve replacement surgery. In the past, patients with pulmonary valve disease underwent pulmonary valvectomy with outflow tract enlargement, given that many patients tolerate some degree of pulmonary regurgitation.[46] However, severe pulmonary valve regurgitation, which can occur after valvectomy, has been demonstrated to adversely impair right ventricular remodeling[47] and replacement of the pulmonary valve when involved by CHD is now preferred. In addition, homografts are sometimes used to replace the pulmonary valve, although some centers report premature valve dysfunction related to constriction of the homograft and, alternatively, prefer placement of a large stented bioprosthesis facilitated with patch enlargement of the pulmonary valve annulus and right ventricular outflow tract.[46] When the mitral and/or aortic valves are affected, valve repair or replacement may be performed depending on the severity of carcinoid involvement.[48] Other procedures may include closure of a patent foramen ovale and, rarely, excision of intramyocardial metastases in selected cases.[48]

Timing of Surgery

The most optimal time for valve replacement surgery in CHD has not been determined, but generally patients with well-controlled carcinoid syndrome and a life expectancy of at least 12 months are referred once they develop progressive symptoms and right-sided heart failure or asymptomatic/minimally symptomatic patients who develop progressive right ventricular dilatation or dysfunction.[46,48] Rarely, asymptomatic patients with CHD and increased right atrial pressure require valve replacement surgery to enable cytoreductive hepatic resection.[32]

Due to the previous high perioperative mortality risk, valve replacement surgery has historically been performed relatively late in the natural history of the disease and on patients with advanced right-sided heart failure.[49,50] However, more recent series demonstrate a significant improvement in perioperative outcomes, probably secondary to a combination of improved patient selection, experience of the multidisciplinary team, improved perioperative management of carcinoid syndrome, and possible advances in surgical and valve technology.[46] In 1995, Connolly and colleagues[5] published on the initial Mayo Clinic experience and reported an overall early perioperative mortality of 35%. In a recent update, however, the overall 30-day mortality rate was 10%.[46] Furthermore, the surgical deaths were not equally distributed over the 27 year study period. Of the 20 perioperative deaths, 12 occurred in the first 71 patients (before 2000; 17%). Since 2000, 8 (6%) perioperative deaths occurred in 124 patients: 7 (7.2%) of 97 occurred between 2000 to 2009 and 1 (3.7%) of 27 occurred between 2010 and 2012. On multivariate analysis, perioperative mortality was not only independently related to the era of operation but also the need for preoperative intravenous diuretic therapy, suggesting that patients with advanced right heart failure have worse perioperative survival.

The significant improvement in perioperative outcomes and survival will likely impact surgical referral patterns in the imminent future. Further data, however, are needed to determine if there is survival benefit with presymptomatic surgical intervention. Based on current data, presymptomatic intervention is not associated with late survival benefit.[46]

Choice of Valve Prosthesis

The choice of valve prosthesis remains controversial, as the literature is limited to retrospective, non-randomized studies. Historically, mechanical valve prostheses were preferred for tricuspid valve replacement due to the risk of premature degeneration of bioprostheses secondary to persistent circulating vasoactive peptides.[51] However, the literature has progressively supported the use of bioprostheses because of (1) the improved management of carcinoid syndrome, (2) the low rates of carcinoid involvement in recent pathologic series of explanted bioprostheses, (3) the favorable short-term outcomes, (4) the likelihood that the longevity of newer generation bioprosthetic valves will succeed the medium to long-term survival of the patient, (5) the inherent bleeding risk in patients with liver metastases and hepatic dysfunction, and (6) the likelihood of oncological surgery or chemotherapy in the future for which long-term anticoagulation may represent additional risk.[46] Furthermore, the recent development of transcutaneous therapies could facilitate "valve-in-valve" replacement in patients with implanted bioprostheses.

In the Mayo Clinic series,[46] tricuspid valve replacement involved bioprostheses in 159 patients and mechanical valves in 36 patients. Of note, there was no significant difference in survival or reoperation rate in relation to type of prosthesis. Pathologic review of explanted bioprostheses demonstrated carcinoid involvement in only one explanted valve, with thrombus being the most frequent alternative cause of tricuspid bioprosthesis dysfunction. For this reason, vitamin K antagonist anticoagulation is recommended for 3 to 6 months after bioprostheses insertion, followed by serial echocardiography thereafter. Importantly, the reversal of bioprosthesis dysfunction has been reported with reinitiation of vitamin K antagonist anticoagulation.

Anesthesia Management

Patients with carcinoid syndrome represent a high-risk surgical cohort because of potentially life-threatening carcinoid crisis that can cause hemodynamic lability characterized by profound peripheral vasodilation and hypotension, tachycardia, arrhythmias, and bronchoconstriction.[32,48] Carcinoid crisis can be precipitated directly by the surgery or when receiving anesthetic and other perioperative pharmacologic agents, including vasopressors and opioids.[48]

Meticulous preoperative planning and perioperative care are required. In the perioperative setting, continuous intravenous somatostatin analog (octreotide) infusion should be commenced at least 12 hours before surgery and continued for 48 hours afterwards, with slow tapering of the infusion before discontinuation (commenced at 50–100 μg/h and titrated up to 200 μg/h should signs or symptoms occur).[7,48]

SUMMARY AND RECOMMENDATIONS

- CHD remains a major cause of morbidity and mortality among patients with carcinoid syndrome.
- Recent studies suggest the prevalence of CHD among patients with carcinoid syndrome to be approximately 20%.
- CHD with advanced symptoms of right heart failure carries a particularly poor prognosis with median survival of only 11 months.
- Early symptoms and physical signs have low sensitivity for the presence of CHD, and screening, even in those patients who are asymptomatic, is critical for early CHD detection. NT-proBNP appears to be the best biomarker for CHD screening to date.
- Transthoracic echocardiography is the gold standard for the diagnosis of CHD and should be performed in all patients with suspicious symptoms or elevated NT-proBNP and/or urinary 5-HIAA.
- Measurement of urinary 5-HIAA is important in all patients with NETs and a level greater than 300 μmol/24 hours may denote increased risk of developing CHD.
- It is essential to aggressively treat patients at every stage of CHD. Optimal doses of somatostatin analogs to appropriately reduce urinary 5-HIAA levels may be of importance.
- Cardiac surgery, in appropriate cases, is the only definitive therapy for advanced, symptomatic CHD and it improves patient symptoms and survival.
- In recent decades, there has been significant improvement in perioperative outcomes and survival of patients with CHD.
- The most optimal time for valve replacement surgery in CHD has not been determined. Patients with well-controlled carcinoid syndrome and a life expectancy of at least 12 months are often referred once they develop progressive symptoms of right-sided heart failure or asymptomatic/minimally symptomatic patients who develop progressive right ventricular dilatation or dysfunction.
- The management of patients with metastatic NETs complicated by carcinoid syndrome and CHD is complex, and comprehensive multidisciplinary assessment of cardiac status, hormonal syndrome, and tumor burden is critical in guiding optimal timing of surgery.

REFERENCES

1. Pellikka PA, Tajik AJ, Khandheria BK, et al. Carcinoid heart disease. Clinical and echocardiographic spectrum in 74 patients. Circulation 1993;87(4): 1188–96.
2. Lundin L, Norheim I, Landelius J, et al. Carcinoid heart disease: relationship of circulating vasoactive substances to ultrasound-detectable cardiac abnormalities. Circulation 1988;77(2):264–9.

3. Bhattacharyya S, Toumpanakis C, Caplin ME, et al. Analysis of 150 patients with carcinoid syndrome seen in a single year at one institution in the first decade of the twenty-first century. Am J Cardiol 2008;101(3):378–81.

4. Bhattacharyya S, Toumpanakis C, Burke M, et al. Features of carcinoid heart disease identified by two- and three-dimensional echocardiography and cardiac magnetic resonance imaging. Circ Cardiovasc Imaging 2010;3(1):103–11.

5. Connolly HM, Nishimura RA, Smith HC, et al. Outcome of cardiac surgery for carcinoid heart disease. J Am Coll Cardiol 1995;25(2):410–6.

6. Møller JE, Pellikka PA, Bernheim AM, et al. Prognosis of carcinoid heart disease. Circulation 2005;112(21):3320–7.

7. Grozinsky-Glasberg S, Grossman AB, Gross DJ. Carcinoid heart disease: from pathophysiology to treatment-'Something in the way it moves'. Neuroendocrinology 2015;101(4):263–73.

8. Robiolio P, Rigolin V, Wilson J, et al. Carcinoid heart disease. Correlation of high serotonin levels with valvular abnormalities detected by cardiac catheterization and echocardiography. Circulation 1995;92(4):790.

9. Denney WD, Kemp WE, Anthony LB, et al. Echocardiographic and biochemical evaluation of the development and progression of carcinoid heart disease. J Am Coll Cardiol 1998;32(4):1017–22.

10. Connolly HM, Crary JL, McGoon MD, et al. Valvular heart disease associated with fenfluramine–phentermine. N Engl J Med 1997;337(9):581–8.

11. Khan MA, Herzog CA, St. Peter JV, et al. The prevalence of cardiac valvular insufficiency assessed by transthoracic echocardiography in obese patients treated with appetite-suppressant drugs. N Engl J Med 1998;339(11):713–8.

12. Rothman RB, Baumann MH, Savage JE, et al. Evidence for possible involvement of 5-HT 2B receptors in the cardiac valvulopathy associated with fenfluramine and other serotonergic medications. Circulation 2000;102(23):2836–41.

13. Fitzgerald LW, Burn TC, Brown BS, et al. Possible role of valvular serotonin 5-HT2B receptors in the cardiopathy associated with fenfluramine. Mol Pharmacol 2000;57(1):75–81.

14. Rajamannan N, Caplice N, Anthikad F, et al. Cell proliferation in carcinoid valve disease: a mechanism for serotonin effects. J Heart Valve Dis 2001;10(6):827–31.

15. Roy A, Brand N, Yacoub M. Expression of 5-hydroxytryptamine receptor subtype messenger RNA in interstitial cells from human heart valves. J Heart Valve Dis 2000;9(2):256–60 [discussion: 260–1].

16. Elangbam CS, Lightfoot RM, Yoon LW, et al. 5-Hydroxytryptamine (5HT) receptors in the heart valves of cynomolgus monkeys and Sprague-Dawley rats. J Histochem Cytochem 2005;53(5):671–7.

17. Elangbam CS, Job LE, Zadrozny LM, et al. 5-hydroxytryptamine (5HT)-induced valvulopathy: compositional valvular alterations are associated with 5HT2B receptor and 5HT transporter transcript changes in Sprague-Dawley rats. Exp Toxicol Pathol 2008;60(4):253–62.

18. Gustafsson BI, Tømmerås K, Nordrum I, et al. Long-term serotonin administration induces heart valve disease in rats. Circulation 2005;111(12):1517–22.

19. Hauso Ø, Gustafsson BI, Loennechen JP, et al. Long-term serotonin effects in the rat are prevented by terguride. Regul Pept 2007;143(1):39–46.

20. Walker GA, Masters KS, Shah DN, et al. Valvular myofibroblast activation by transforming growth factor-β. Circ Res 2004;95(3):253–60.

21. Modlin IM, Shapiro MD, Kidd M. Carcinoid tumors and fibrosis: an association with no explanation. Am J Gastroenterol 2004;99(12):2466.

22. Bergestuen DS, Edvardsen T, Aakhus S, et al. Activin A in carcinoid disease: a possible role in diagnosis and pathogenesis. Neuroendocrinology 2010;92(3):168–77.
23. Simula DV, Edwards WD, Tazelaar HD, et al. Surgical pathology of carcinoid heart disease: a study of 139 valves from 75 patients spanning 20 years. Mayo Clin Proc 2002;77(2):139–47.
24. Pandya UH, Pellikka PA, Enriquez-Sarano M, et al. Metastatic carcinoid tumor to the heart: echocardiographic-pathologic study of 11 patients. J Am Coll Cardiol 2002;40(7):1328–32.
25. Roberts WC, Sjoerdsma A. The cardiac disease associated with the carcinoid syndrome (carcinoid heart disease). Am J Med 1964;36(1):5–34.
26. Ferrans VJ, Roberts WC. The carcinoid endocardial plaque: an ultrastructural study. Hum Pathol 1976;7(4):387–409.
27. Moertel CG. Treatment of the carcinoid tumor and the malignant carcinoid syndrome. J Clin Oncol 1983;1(11):727–40.
28. Ross EM, Roberts WC. The carcinoid syndrome: comparison of 21 necropsy subjects with carcinoid heart disease to 15 necropsy subjects without carcinoid heart disease. Am J Med 1985;79(3):339–54.
29. Roberts WC. A unique heart disease associated with a unique cancer: carcinoid heart disease. Am J Cardiol 1997;80(2):251–6.
30. Connolly HM, Schaff HV, Mullany CJ, et al. Surgical management of left-sided carcinoid heart disease. Circulation 2001;104(suppl 1):I36–40.
31. Bhattacharyya S, Davar J, Dreyfus G, et al. Carcinoid heart disease. Circulation 2007;116(24):2860–5.
32. Bruce CJ, Connolly HM. Right-sided valve disease deserves a little more respect. Circulation 2009;119(20):2726–34.
33. Sepulveda G, Lukas DS. The diagnosis of tricuspid insufficiency. Circulation 1955;11(4):552–63.
34. Salazar E, Levine HD. Rheumatic tricuspid regurgitation: the clinical spectrum. Am J Med 1962;33(1):111–29.
35. Müller O, Shillingford J. Tricuspid incompetence. Br Heart J 1954;16(2):195–207.
36. Bernheim AM, Connolly HM, Hobday TJ, et al. Carcinoid heart disease. Prog Cardiovasc Dis 2007;49(6):439–51.
37. Zuetenhorst J, Bonfrer J, Korse C, et al. Carcinoid heart disease: the role of urinary 5-hydroxyindoleacetic acid excretion and plasma levels of atrial natriuretic peptide, transforming growth factor-beta and fibroblast growth factor. Cancer 2003;97(7):1609.
38. Møller JE, Connolly HM, Rubin J, et al. Factors associated with progression of carcinoid heart disease. N Engl J Med 2003;348(11):1005–15.
39. Bhattacharyya S, Toumpanakis C, Chilkunda D, et al. Risk factors for the development and progression of carcinoid heart disease. Am J Cardiol 2011;107(8): 1221–6.
40. Korse CM, Taal BG, de Groot CA, et al. Chromogranin-A and N-terminal pro-brain natriuretic peptide: an excellent pair of biomarkers for diagnostics in patients with neuroendocrine tumor. J Clin Oncol 2009;27(26):4293–9.
41. Kinnunen P, Vuolteenaho O, Ruskoaho H. Mechanisms of atrial and brain natriuretic peptide release from rat ventricular myocardium: effect of stretching. Endocrinology 1993;132(5):1961–70.
42. Bhattacharyya S, Toumpanakis C, Caplin ME, et al. Usefulness of N-terminal pro–brain natriuretic peptide as a biomarker of the presence of carcinoid heart disease. Am J Cardiol 2008;102(7):938–42.

43. Bhattacharyya S, Burke M, Caplin ME, et al. Utility of 3D transoesophageal echo-cardiography for the assessment of tricuspid and pulmonary valves in carcinoid heart disease. Eur J Echocardiogr 2011;12(1):E4.

44. Sundin A, Arnold R, Baudin E, et al. ENETS consensus guidelines for the standards of care in neuroendocrine tumors: radiological, nuclear medicine and hybrid imaging. Neuroendocrinology 2017;105(2):212–44.

45. Kulke M, Hörsch D, Caplin M, et al. Telotristat ethyl, a tryptophan hydroxylase inhibitor for the treatment of carcinoid syndrome. J Clin Oncol 2017;35(1):14–23.

46. Connolly HM, Schaff HV, Abel MD, et al. Early and late outcomes of surgical treatment in carcinoid heart disease. J Am Coll Cardiol 2015;66(20):2189–96.

47. Connolly HM, Schaff HV, Mullany CJ, et al. Carcinoid heart disease: impact of pulmonary valve replacement in right ventricular function and remodeling. Circulation 2002;106(12 suppl 1):I51–6.

48. Davar J, Connolly HM, Caplin ME, et al. Diagnosing and managing carcinoid heart disease in patients with neuroendocrine tumours. J Am Coll Cardiol 2017; 69(10):1288–304.

49. Nishimura RA, Otto CM, Bonow RO, et al. 2014 AHA/ACC guideline for the management of patients with valvular heart disease: a report of the American College of Cardiology/American Heart Association task force on practice guidelines. J Am Coll Cardiol 2014;63:e57–185 [Erratum appears in J Am Coll Cardiol 2014;63: 2489].

50. Lee R, Li S, Rankin JS, et al. Society of Thoracic Surgeons adult cardiac surgical database. Fifteen-year outcome trends for valve surgery in North America. Ann Thorac Surg 2011;91(3):677–84.

51. Schoen F, Hausner R, Howell J, et al. Porcine heterograft valve replacement in carcinoid heart disease. J Thorac Cardiovasc Surg 1981;81(1):100–5.

The Problem of High-Grade Gastroenteropancreatic Neuroendocrine Neoplasms

Well-Differentiated Neuroendocrine Tumors, Neuroendocrine Carcinomas, and Beyond

Halfdan Sorbye, MD[a,b,*], Eric Baudin, MD[c], Aurel Perren, MD[d]

KEYWORDS

- Neuroendocrine • Neoplasms • Carcinoma • Digestive • Gastroenteropancreatic
- NET G3 • NEC

KEY POINTS

- Gastroenteropancreatic high-grade neuroendocrine neoplasms have 2 major subgroups: neuroendocrine tumors and neuroendocrine carcinoma.
- Diagnosis and treatment of high-grade gastroenteropancreatic neuroendocrine neoplasms is challenging owing to the lack of high-quality data.
- Diagnosis of high-grade gastroenteropancreatic neuroendocrine neoplasms depends on extensive pathology workup, including genetic data, because the morphologic criteria for defining well-differentiated versus poorly differentiated are not clear in all cases.
- Treatment of high-grade gastroenteropancreatic neuroendocrine neoplasms should separate between neuroendocrine tumors and neuroendocrine carcinoma and depends further on primary tumor site, stage, proliferation rate, and the clinical course.
- Future study reports on high-grade gastroenteropancreatic neuroendocrine neoplasms should give separate data for neuroendocrine carcinoma, neuroendocrine tumors, uncertain neuroendocrine neoplasms (uncertain differentiation), and mixed neuroendocrine-non-neuroendocrine neoplasm, as well as specifications of organ of origin, TNM and Ki-67.

Disclosure Statement: H. Sorbye: Honoraria and research funding: Novartis, Ipsen. A. Perren: Honoraria: Novartis, Ipsen.
[a] Department of Oncology, Haukeland University Hospital, Jonas Lies vei 65, Bergen 5021, Norway; [b] Department of Clinical Science, Haukeland University Hospital, Jonas Lies vei 65, Bergen 5021, Norway; [c] Endocrine Oncology, Gustave Roussy, rue Édouard-Vaillant 114, Villejuif 94800, France; [d] Department of Pathology, University of Bern, Murtenstrasse 31, Bern 3008, Switzerland
* Corresponding author. Department of Oncology, Haukeland University Hospital, Jonas Lies vei 65, Bergen 5021, Norway.
E-mail address: halfdan.sorbye@helse-bergen.no

BACKGROUND

The 2010 World Health Organization (WHO) classification of gastroenteropancreatic (GEP) neuroendocrine neoplasms (NEN) introduced morphology and grade with proliferation rate as the main determinant of NEN behavior. It defined NEN as either well-differentiated low-grade (G1-G2) neuroendocrine tumors (NET) or poorly differentiated high-grade (G3) neuroendocrine carcinomas (NEC).[1] The 2017 WHO classification of pancreatic NETs defined a new group of well-differentiated G3 pancreatic tumors (NET G3).[2] The NET category is now only used for well-differentiated tumors regardless of their proliferation index (G1-G3), whereas the NEC category is used for poorly differentiated G3 NEC. The terminology of NEN G3 relates to all G3 (Ki-67 >20%) neuroendocrine malignancies; that is, both NET G3 and NEC (**Table 1**). The separation of NET G3 and NEC depends on the different genetic backgrounds of the 2 groups and resulting different biology. NET G3 has been formally only been implemented for pancreatic NEN; however, an expansion to other GEP NEN entities seems likely. Although the WHO classification for NEN G3 has been validated for its prognostic relevance, several problems remain and different morphologic, molecular, clinical, and prognostic entities were recently highlighted.[3–8] The robustness of histomorphologic criteria for defining well-differentiated versus poorly differentiated is questioned even among expert pathologists. Finally, its relevance for predictive benefits of therapy is even more problematic, although lower response rates to cisplatin-based chemotherapy in NETG3 was evident very early.[9,10] Currently, the NEN G3 category has been considered a single entity in most studies, making a final understanding of the benefit of various therapeutic options for NET or NEC category of patients uncertain. In this article, we address the problem of how to diagnose and treat GEP NEN G3, with a specific focus on NET G3 versus NEC, and we propose a new NEN G3 category.

DIAGNOSING WELL-DIFFERENTIATED NEUROENDOCRINE NEOPLASMS: FROM A SINGLE ENTITY TO A HIGH-GRADE NEUROENDOCRINE TUMOR OR NEUROENDOCRINE CARCINOMA CATEGORIZATION
Epidemiology, and Diagnostic and Prognostic Characteristics

Epidemiologic data on NET G3 compared with NEC are very scarce, and the numbers of NET G3 cases reported in studies are very few. Both NET G3 and NEC are more common in male patients. The main primary tumor sites in NEC are quite similar, distributed between the colon, rectum, pancreas, stomach, and esophagus.[11–14] In contrast, NET G3 are mainly located in the pancreas, with other primary sites of like

Table 1 Nomenclature for GEP NEN G3		
	Used for	
NEN G3	Addressing both NET G3 and NEC	If differentiation is uncertain
NET G3	Well-differentiated, Ki-67 >20%	
NEC	Poorly differentiated, Ki-67 >20%	
MiNEN	Neoplasms with both >30% neuroendocrine and gland-forming component	

Abbreviations: G3, high grade; GEP, gastroenteropancreatic; MiNEN, mixed neuroendocrine-non-neuroendocrine neoplasm; NEN, neuroendocrine neoplasm.
Data from Klöppel G, Couvelard A, Hruban RH, et al. Introduction to chapter 6 neoplasms of the neuroendocrine pancreas. In: Lloyd RV, Osamura RY, Klöppel G, et al, editors. WHO classification of tumors of endocrine organs. 4th edition. Lyon (France): IARC; 2017. p. 211–4.

NEC[4,9,10] (**Table 2**). In 1 study, 11 of 24 NET G3 cases (46%) were located in the pancreas.[4] In other studies, 65% of NET G3 cases had their primary neoplasm in the pancreas, whereas 20% to 25% of GEP NEC cases were located in the pancreas.[10,14] In initial reports, GEP NET G3 constitute about 15% to 20% of the GEP NEN G3 group; however, among the non–small cell subgroup, it may consist of 30% to 40% of the cases.[4,9,10,15] In 2 large studies on 204 and 136 GEP NEN G3 cases, 18% and 17% were identified as NET G3, respectively.[4,10] In a surgical report on pancreatic NEN G3, 17% of cases were well-differentiated.[16] A higher proportion was seen in 2 other studies; among 49 and 70 pancreatic NEN G3, 30% and 36% were classified as NET G3, respectively.[17,18] No difference among pancreatic NEN has been seen concerning location at head versus body/tail and tumor size.[17] Given their aggressive nature, most patients with GEP NEC (60%–80%) have metastatic disease at the time of presentation.[4,10,12,14,19] The scarce data available for NET G3 suggest also a high percentage of metastatic disease (62%–70%) at diagnosis.[4,10,17] All these studies are hampered by a center bias, operability, and resulting availability of histologic materials; therefore, all studies show a bias toward resected tumors. Functioning syndromes can be present in NET G3 patients as compared with NET, whereas this is extremely rare in NEC.[9,10,18] The presence of functioning syndromes such as carcinoid, insulinoma or gastrinoma, or inherited syndrome would favor the diagnosis of NET G3 rather than NEC.

In the Surveillance, Epidemiology, and End Results database, the median survival for GEP NEN G3 was 34 months with localized disease, 14 to 16 months with regional disease, and 5 months with distant disease.[3,12] The 5-year survival was 42% in localized disease, 26% in regional disease and, 5% with advanced disease, depending on primary tumor site, and seemed to be better for large cell GEP NEN G3.[12,20] Survival of patients with GEP NET G3 is significantly better than of patients with GEP NEC.[4,9,10,21] The median survival for metastatic patients was 41 months for GEP NET G3 versus

Table 2
Clinical characteristics of gastroenteropancreatic NET G3 versus NEC

	NET G3[a]	NEC
Primary tumor location	50%–60% in pancreas	25% in pancreas
Proportion among GEP NEN	17%–18%	82%–83%
Proportion among pancreatic NEN G3	30%–36%	
Stage IV at diagnosis	60%–70%	60%–80%
Functioning tumors	14%–25%	4%–6%
Hypervascularity on CT scan	33%	5%
High uptake on SRI	88%	40%–50%
High uptake on FDG-PET	75%	92%
Response to platinum based chemotherapy	0%–5%	30%–40%
Progression-free survival	2.4 - ? mo	4–6 mo
Median survival	41–99 mo[b]	8–13 mo

Abbreviations: CT, computed tomography; FDG-PET, positron emission tomography with 18F-fluorodexyglucose; G3, high grade; GEP, gastroenteropancreatic; MiNEN, mixed neuroendocrine–nonneuroendocrine neoplasm; NEC, neuroendocrine carcinoma; NEN, neuroendocrine neoplasm; SRI, somatostatin receptor imaging.
[a] Based on a very low number of cases.
[b] Stage mixture in most studies, but mainly stage 4.
Data from Refs.[3,4,9–22]

17 months for non–small cell GEP NEC.[9] Other studies, unfortunately, do not separate according to stage, and present overall survival data combining all stages although the majorities are stage IV patients. In 1 study, survival for GEP NET G3 was 99 months versus 19 months for GEP NEC.[10] For pancreatic NET G3 primaries, the median overall survival was 42 to 75 months compared with pancreatic NEC, with a median overall survival of 8.5 to 13 months.[7,16,17,22] A recent proposal not included in the 2017 WHO classification was to separate the NEN G3 into 3 groups based on morphology and Ki-67.[4] In a G3 GEP-NEN population of 136 patients, the median survival was best for 24 cases of NET G3 (43.6 months), intermediate for 30 cases NEC with a Ki-67 of 21% to 55% (24.5 months), and only 5.3 months for 82 NEC cases with a Ki-67 55% or greater.

Pathology

The terms G3 NEN and poorly differentiated NEC have been used synonymously, and the 2010 WHO classification on digestive tumors presumed that all G3 NEN tumors were poorly differentiated. All small cell NEN are by definition considered poorly differentiated. Since 2010, a large heterogeneity of this group of G3 NEN emerged: although all poorly differentiated cancers have a high proliferation rate, not all G3 large cell neoplasms are poorly differentiated. A subset of patients with large cell NEN that seem to be histologically well-differentiated have a Ki-67 of greater than 20%, usually in the 20% to 50% range.[9,10,17,21] In the WHO 2017 classification for pancreatic NEN, these tumors are defined as NET G3. Although the present WHO 2010 classification for digestive tumors do not mention NET G3, it seems reasonable at present also to use the term NET G3 in digestive GEP-NEN so further data can be collected and the relevance of NET G3 outside the pancreas can be determined.

The European Neuroendocrine Tumor Society recommend that a pathology report on GEP NEN G3 should report morphology concerning both differentiation (well-differentiated or poorly differentiated) and small cell versus large cell, as well as proliferation rate as an absolute Ki-67 value in hot spots.[23] Unfortunately, the Ki-67 value alone cannot distinguish between NET G3 and NEC, because the Ki-67 value overlaps among NET G3 and NEC, especially in the area of 30% to 50%, although a Ki-67 of greater than 60% is rare for NET G3[7,10,14] (Fig. 1). The median Ki-67 for GEP NET G3 is 30% compared with 70% to 80% for GEP NEC.[10,14] For pancreatic primaries, the median Ki-67 has been reported in pancreatic NET G3 to be 29% to 47% (range, 21%–80%), compared with pancreatic NEC with a median Ki-67 of 70% to 80% (range, 21%–100%)[7,17,18] (Table 3). Furthermore, the diagnosis requires histologic immunohistochemical examination for chromogranin A and synaptophysin.[2,23] Chromogranin A staining may be lacking; in 2 studies chromogranin A staining was present in 91% to 100% of NET G3 cases compared with 75% to 89% NEC cases.[10,17] Among NEC, there is a small cell histologic preponderance in the squamous cell parts (esophagus and anus) and a large cell carcinoma in the glandular parts in the gastrointestinal tract.[12] There seems to be a dominance of large cell carcinoma in GEP NEC: an estimate is 60% large cell versus 40% small cell.[10,14] If the neoplasm consists of a neuroendocrine component and a gland-forming component both exceeding 30%, the new 2017 WHO classification defines it as a mixed neuroendocrine–non-NEN (MiNEN).[2,24,25] A frequent limitation of pathology in NEN G3 is the small size of specimen in a significant number of cases.

By histomorphology, well-differentiated NET G3 show minimal to moderate atypia, with organoid growth pattern with apposition of capillary vessels to tumor cells lacking geographic necrosis (Fig. 2). Poorly differentiated NEC show highly atypical small cells

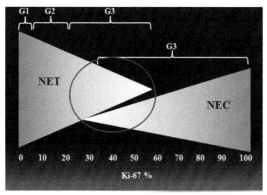

Fig. 1. Neuroendocrine neoplasms separation according to grade, Ki-67, and morphology. Red circle is showing the overlap in Ki-67 index between NET G3 and NEC.

or intermediate to large cells with a solid growth pattern lacking organoid features, but showing rosette formation and palisading (**Fig. 3**). Geographic necrosis might be found. Minor components of an adenocarcinoma might be present in NEC; components of a NET G1/G2 indicate a well-differentiated NET. Classification based on morphologic differentiation alone is challenging in a highly specialized NET center, NET pathologists could not agree or were uncertain of the morphologic classification on reviewing 1 histologic slide in 61% of pancreatic NEN G3.[7] In the ambiguous group (n = 20), examining additional slides showed the presence of low-grade NET in 7 cases, 7 additional cases were classified as NET G3 based on loss of DAXX or ATRX expression, and 5 tumors were established as NEC based on abnormal expression of p53 and/or Rb1. In total, in the setting of resection specimens, 19 of 21 NET G3 cases had a G1/G2 NET component either in another tumor section within the same neoplasm or a prior pathologic diagnosis of G1/G2 NET. Ductal adenocarcinoma was present in 4 of 12 NEC; the others were homogeneous throughout. These results indicate that NET G3 may develop from an initial NET G1-G2 in contrast with NEC.

Table 3
Pathologic characteristics of gastroenteropancreatic NET G3 versus NEC

	NET G3[a]	NEC
Morphology	Well-differentiated	Poorly differentiated
Ki-67	Median, 29%–47% (range 21%–80%)	Median, 70%–80% (range 21%–100%)
Chromogranin A staining	91%–100%	75%–89%
Rb1 mutation	0	55%
KRAS mutation	0	49%
p53 mutation	0	78%
Loss of DAXX/ATRX expression	40%–60%	0
Possible coexisting neoplastic component	NET G1-G2	Adenocarcinoma

Abbreviations: G1, grade 1; G2, grade 2; G3, high grade; NEC, neuroendocrine carcinoma; NEN, neuroendocrine neoplasm.
[a] Based on a very low number of cases.
Data from Refs.[7–10,14,17,18,21,26,27,30,31,33]

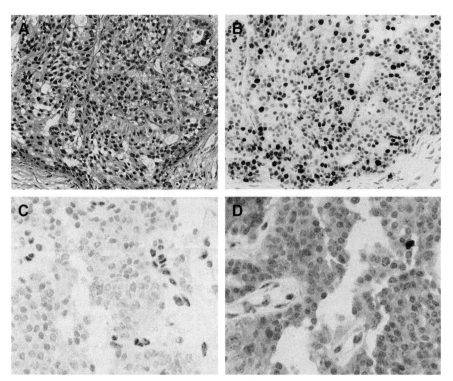

Fig. 2. High-grade neuroendocrine tumor of the pancreas. (*A*) Organoid growth pattern of a NET (stain: hematoxylin and eosin; original magnification ×40). (*B*) A 40% Ki-67 labeling index (original magnification ×40). (*C*) Loss of nuclear ATRX expression (note positively staining nonneoplastic cells) (original magnification ×40). (*D*) Retention of nuclear DAXX expression (original magnification ×40).

Molecular data show a clear genomic separation of NET and NEC: NET G3 carry driver mutations of NET (*MENIN, DAXX, ATRX*). Immunohistochemical tools can be used to get a hint on the genetic status of NEN using antibodies against DAXX, ATRX, p53, and Rb1 (see **Fig. 3, Table 3**). Mutations in *TP53* and Rb1 seem to be good markers of poor differentiation and can help to differentiate NEC from NET G3.[7,17,26] In a study of 70 patients, pancreatic NET G3 showed no abnormal Rb1 or *KRAS* alterations, whereas in pancreatic NEC 55% had Rb1 loss and 49% *KRAS* mutations.[17] In another study, abnormal p53 and Rb1 staining was found in 29 of 37 and 22 of 37 of cases with poorly differentiated GEP NEC, whereas all NET G3 showed normal expression.[26] In different organs, the mutational signature in NEC seems to be similar to their adenocarcinoma of same primary tumor location, rather than having a common neuroendocrine signature.[27–30] NEC frequently carry mutations of adenocarcinomas such as *KRAS* and *BRAF* in addition to either p53 or Rb1 mutations.[8,27,30,31] Even if therapy of GEP NEC is widely defined by analogy to lung NEC, the mutational frequencies differ: GEP NEC seems to have a lower rate of *TP53* and alteration Rb1 than small cell lung cancer and other genes were more frequently altered.[32] One-half of small cell pancreatic NEC have a *KRAS* mutation, in contrast with small cell lung cancer, where *KRAS* mutations are rarely found.[17,33] Small cell lung cancer has further a 90% Rb1 loss compared with 60% in pancreatic small cell NEC. At this time, the clinical

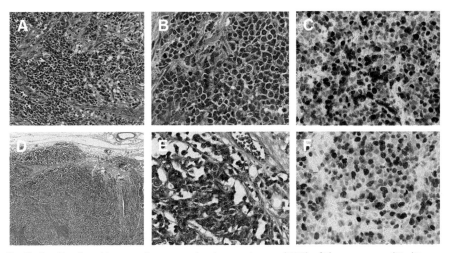

Fig. 3. Small cell and large cell neuroendocrine carcinoma (NEC) of the pancreas. (*Top*) Large cell NEC. (*A*) Solid growth (stain: hematoxylin and eosin; original magnification ×2). (*B*) Large nuclei, only small nucleoli, more abundant cytoplasm (stain: hematoxylin and eosin; original magnification ×20). (*C*) p53 overexpression (original magnification ×40). (*F*) Ki-67 of 40% in large cell NEC (original magnification ×40). (*Bottom left*) Small cell NEC. (*D*) Note geographic necrosis, very crowded nuclei (stain: hematoxylin and eosin; original magnification ×2). (*E*): Small nuclei, very fine chromatin, nuclear molding (stain: hematoxylin and eosin; original magnification ×2).

relevance of a distinction between small cell and large cell GEP NEC is uncertain. No difference was seen in Rb1 or *KRAS* mutations concerning small cell versus large cell pancreatic NEC.[17] Decreased Rb1 expression was found in 56% of colorectal NEC and high expression of p16 and BCL-2 was also seen.[29] Recently, expression of the programmed death-ligand 1 in NET tissue was significantly associated with NEN G3 (differentiation not specified), especially when the Ki-67 was greater than 60%.[34,35]

Imaging

A relevant question is whether imaging can help in separating NET G3 from NEC. Concerning computed tomography (CT) scans, pancreatic NET G3 compared with pancreatic NEC, cases tended to have a significantly maintained vascularity on contrast-enhanced CT.[17] However, only 33% of NET G3 had hypervascularity on a CT scan compared with 5% in NEC. PET with 18F-fluorodexyglucose is known to be positive in most GEP NEC: in a recent study, 110 of 119 cases were positive.[14] However, also most NET G3 also seem to have a positive PET 18F-fluorodexyglucose; in 1 study, 9 of 12 NET G3 cases (75%) were positive compared with 56 of 64 GEP NEC cases (88%).[10] GEP NET G3 usually have a high uptake on somatostatin receptor imaging (SRI), although NEC may also show an uptake as recently shown in 15 of 37 cases (37%).[14] Using immunohistochemistry, somatostatin receptor 2A expression was not limited to NET G3, as 16% of NEC had such expression.[26] Two studies have directly compered SRI in GEP NET G3 and NEC. SRI was positive in 21 of 24 (88%) and 13 of 15 (87%) cases with NET G3 compared with 23 of 58 (40%) and 6 of 12 (50%) NEC cases.[10,18] Summing up, the presence of high vascularization density or high uptake at SRI may suggest NET G3 rather than NEC, reinforcing slide revision or new biopsy specimen in difficult cases.

Diagnostic Conclusions and a Proposal for New Category of High-Grade Neuroendocrine Neoplasms

For daily routine pathology workup, the morphologic separation of NET G3 and NEC may not be obvious in many cases (see **Table 3**). Ancillary immunohistochemical or genomic methods are able to classify many neoplasms, but more research is highly needed in this area. An important step will be a consensus on the minimal data needed to classify NET G3, and a reclassification will be needed for many cases after such an international standardization of diagnostic pathologic criteria. Progress in the better understanding of this category of neoplasm pass through better characterization of this group in pathologic reports as well as new categorization. Regarding MiNEN, it is important that the proportion of neuroendocrine and nonneuroendocrine components be specified in reports, whatever the proportion, as well as their nature both in the primary tumor and metastatic tissue. Although the Ki-67 index at present is not part of the categorization of NEC, some studies suggest that it may be of prognostic relevance. Based on these results, the absolute count of Ki-67 should also be specified in pathologic reports on NEC. Recent studies suggest that molecular characterization reveals organ-specific signatures that may affect response to cisplatin-based chemotherapy. If the pathology report is uncertain on differentiation, the neoplasm should be classified as an uncertain NEN G3, which should be considered a new category in which well-differentiated or poorly differentiated morphology remains undetermined. We suggest that the NEN G3 categorization in addition to MiNEN should consist of the following categories: NET G3, NEC G3, and uncertain NEN G3. Collecting further data in these categories should lead to better understand the behavior of each group as well as the added value of additional diagnostic tools in each subgroup.

TREATING HIGH-GRADE GASTROENTEROPANCREATIC NEUROENDOCRINE NEOPLASMS

The GEP NEN G3 group is a quite heterogeneous patient group concerning prognosis and treatment benefit, depending on factors such as tumor stage, primary site, differentiation, proliferation rate, and molecular data. Predictive factors for treatment benefit on patients with GEP NEC and especially NET G3 are scarce, and few prospective studies are available. Much more research is, therefore, needed to aid clinicians selecting the best therapy for the individual patient. Until further data are present, treatment of NEN G3 has to be based on several factors as differentiation, tumor stage, primary tumor location, Ki-67, and clinical course (**Fig. 4**).

Treatment of Gastroenteropancreatic Neuroendocrine Carcinomas

Treatment of GEP NEC was initially extrapolated from small cell lung cancer data; however, recent results show several differences clinically and for tumor biology regarding GEP NEC.[3,8,12,32] Therapy for GEP NEC should, therefore, be based on studies including only GEP primaries, and not on studies including small cell lung cancer or other extrapulmonary primary sites. Small cell carcinoma was the first category described in both the lungs and GEP tract, and for this reason most of the published treatment data have been focused on GEP small cell carcinoma and fewer data exist on large cell NEC.

Localized disease

Long-term relapse-free survival is possible among patients with NEC with localized disease and seems to depend on the primary site location or stage.[12,36] Treatment

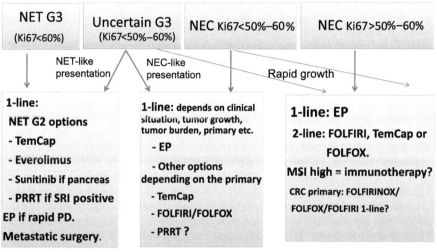

Fig. 4. Suggested treatment algorithm for advanced high-grade neuroendocrine neoplasms (G3) neuroendocrine neoplasms. CRC, colorectal cancer; EP, platinum/etoposide; MSI, microsatellite instability; NEC, neuroendocrine carcinoma; NET, neuroendocrine tumor; PD, progressive disease; PRRT, peptide receptor radionucleotide therapy; SRI, somatostatin receptor imaging; Tem/Cap, temozolomide/capecitabine.

recommendations for patients with apparently localized disease are not based on prospective data, and supporting evidence from heterogeneous retrospective studies is limited. There is consensus that surgery alone is rarely curative and that patients with limited disease should probably receive multimodality-based therapy. Surgery as part of the treatment may be curative in patients even with regional lymph node disease.[16,37–42] The 5-year survival for localized disease depends on primary site; for colorectal, stomach, and pancreas primaries, the 5-year survival is 46% to 55%, compared with 25% to 33% for anal and esophageal primaries.[12] The 5-year survival for regional disease was 22% to 30% for colorectal, stomach, and pancreas primaries compared with 9% to 15% for anal and esophageal primaries.[12] Surgery as part of the treatment could, therefore, be considered for all localized and regional patients with GEP NEC, especially when complete resection is feasible in a timely manner in fit patients. Otherwise, combined chemoradiation could be considered as an alternative. An exception to surgery seems to be an esophageal primary. Several small series confirm poor results after surgical treatment of esophageal NEC, especially for stage III disease where chemoradiation seems better.[43,44] In 1 retrospective study on esophageal NEC, patients with N1 disease had a median survival of 45 months after chemoradiation versus only 12 months with surgery and chemotherapy.[43]

The aggressive behavior of GEP NEC warrants consideration of adjuvant therapy after radical resection. Most recurrences are distant; local recurrence alone is rare.[11] Therefore, postoperative adjuvant chemotherapy seems to be more reasonable than local postoperative radiation therapy alone, assuming an R0 resection has been performed. Although there are no studies examining postoperative chemotherapy, adjuvant chemotherapy with 4 to 6 cycles of cisplatin/carboplatin and etoposide is generally recommended in most guidelines.[45–47] A neoadjuvant chemotherapy approach before surgery may also be considered early to eradicate possible metastatic microscopic disease, especially when complete resection is uncertain and or its delay more than 3 to 4 weeks; however, data are lacking.

Metastatic disease

GEP NEC are usually highly aggressive with a propensity for early metastases.[3,10,14,20] In the Surveillance, Epidemiology, and End Results database, 61% of GEP NEC were diagnosed with distant disease, compared with 27% regional and 12% with local disease.[12,14] Metastatic GEP NEC is an aggressive disease where rapid referral is necessary to consider rapid initiation of systemic treatment before the performance status deteriorates to the extent that the patient is no longer fit enough to receive chemotherapy. After a diagnosis of advanced disease, median survival is only 1 month without chemotherapy compared with 11 to 14 months with palliative chemotherapy, suggesting that the benefit from palliative chemotherapy is probably substantial.[10,11,13,14] Many patients are responsive to systemic chemotherapy, but virtually all patients progress and eventually die of their disease. Poor performance status, high tumor burden, liver metastases, a high proliferation rate, and elevated lactate dehydrogenase are usually baseline negative prognostic factors for survival in patients with metastatic disease.[4,11,13,14,48] Metastatic surgery for GEP NEC is not recommended, although published data on surgery for metastatic disease are scarce.[45,49–51] A recent retrospective study indicates that very selected patients with NEC with a few metastases at presentation or prolonged response to chemotherapy may benefit from metastatic liver surgery.[52] At present, G3 MiNEN are treated similarly to NEC, because studies are lacking to compare outcome and the natural history of the disease seems to be determined by the NEC component.[25]

Based on retrospective data, most guidelines recommend the use of platinum-based chemotherapy combined with etoposide as a first-line palliative treatment.[45,47,53] Recent large retrospective studies show quite similar results on first-line treatment with cisplatin/carboplatin and etoposide. They show a response rate of 30% to 50%, a median progression-free survival of 4 to 6 months and a median overall survival of 11 to 16 months.[10,11,13,14] In all studies as many as one-third of patients have immediate disease progression at first evaluation, indicating no benefit at all of platinum-based therapy. In the Nordic study, no differences in outcomes were seen comparing patients treated with cisplatin-based versus carboplatin-based treatment,[11] which has led to more frequent use of carboplatin owing to its better tolerability for the patients. In the Nordic study, cases with a Ki-67 of less than 55% had a significantly longer survival; however, no data separation between NEC and NET G3 has yet been published. Several studies have shown that a Ki-67 proliferation rate in the lower range (<60%) may predict less benefit from platin-based chemotherapy, although further validation is necessary to clarify the role of morphologic differentiation, large cell versus small cell subtype, and molecular markers.[11,54–56] In 258 patients with poorly differentiated GEP NEC, the response rate and survival were numerically better for irinotecan/etoposide compared with cisplatin/etoposide, but the treatment regimen was not an independent predictive factor for survival.[13] In 2 studies on poorly differentiated pancreatic NEC, the response rate to platinum-based 1-line treatment was 37% to 51% and overall survival 8.5 to 10 months, and Rb1 loss seemed to predict response to platinum-based chemotherapy.[17,18]

After first-line treatment, no further standard therapy has been established for GEP NEC. Patients that progress more than 3 months after discontinuation of platinum-based treatment may still be platinum sensitive.[11] Several small retrospective studies suggest that patients with GEP NEC can benefit from further lines of chemotherapy after failure of platinum/etoposide treatment. Temozolomide-based chemotherapy in 24 patients resulted in a 33% response rate and a progression-free survival of 6 months with most benefit seem for patients with a Ki-67 of less than 60%; however, differentiation was not specified in this study.[55] Monotherapy with temozolomide seems to have no benefit in NEC.[54] Irinotecan- and oxaliplatin-based chemotherapy may benefit as second-line treatments with response rates of 16% to 31% and progression-free survival of 2.3 to 6.2 months.[56,57] A recent retrospective study with FOLFIRI or FOLFOX after first-line treatment resulted in a very short median progression-free survival (<3 months) and overall survival (<6 months).[14] The benefit of peptide receptor radionuclide therapy (PRRT) in patients with NEC with a high uptake on SRI is unknown. A recent retrospective study reported data on 29 patients with GEP NEN G3 treated with PRRT where the majority had failed prior chemotherapy.[58] The primary tumor was located in the pancreas in 17 of the 28 cases and 22 cases had a Ki-67 of less than 55%. A partial response 3 months after PRRT was seen in 8 of 23 patients, progression-free survival was 9 months, and overall survival was 21 months. The median progression-free survival and overall survival for patients with Ki-67 of 55% or less was 12 and 41 months, compared with 4 and 7 months if the Ki-67 was greater than 55%. As for surgery, this option may be kept in mind for a very selected subgroup of patients with a less aggressive natural history.

Treatment of High-Grade Gastroenteropancreatic Neuroendocrine Tumors

Because the NET G3 subgroup has been recently defined, there are few data on how to treat NET G3; however, several studies are ongoing.

Localized disease
Specific data on surgery in NET G3 are lacking. In 1 study on pancreatic NEN G3, survival was much better for NET G3, but the study did not separate survival according to both stage and morphology.[16] It has been suggested that NET G3 patients should receive the same approach to surgery of the primary and metastatic disease as patients with NET G2.[15,16] A new and unanswered question is whether NET G3 patients should receive adjuvant chemotherapy or should be treated as patients with NET G2 without any adjuvant therapy, as recommended in a recent review.[15]

Metastatic disease
Again, most chemotherapy studies are a mixture of NET G3 and patients with NEC and specific data on the NET G3 subgroup are few and based on a very small number of patients. The optimal first-line palliative treatment for patients with metastatic NET G3 is, therefore, unclear.[15] Several recent retrospective studies suggest relatively low response rates to platinum/etoposide regimens in patients with a NET G3.[9,10,17] Among 12 NET G3 cases, the response rate to platinum-based chemotherapy was 17%, 50% had immediate disease progression, and progression-free survival was 2.4 months.[10] In another study, 10 patients with pancreatic NET G3 given platinum-based chemotherapy had a response rate of 10%, and 40% had immediate progession.[18] In the same study, 12 patients received second-line alkylating agents (temozolomide, etc); the response rate was 50% and 25% had immediate disease progression, but no progression-free survival data were given. Among 16 patients with pancreatic NET G3 given chemotherapy (8 given platinum first-line), the response rate was 0% without progression-free survival data given.[17] It has been suggested that patients with NET G3 may benefit from medical

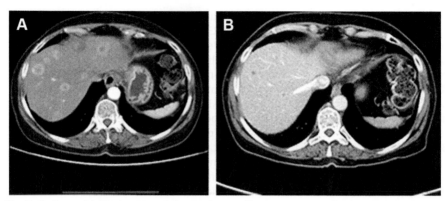

Fig. 5. Patient with liver metastasis from a large cell gastric neuroendocrine carcinoma Ki-67 41% (*A*). Near complete response after 2 months of treatment with temozolomide/capecitabine (*B*).

treatments used in NET G2, and temozolomide/capecitabine is frequently used, but data from larger prospective studies are lacking[10] (**Fig. 5**). Everolimus was given to 15 patients with pancreatic NET G3 with a Ki-67 of 55% or less (median, 30%), mainly after first-line treatment.[59] A median progression-free survival of 6 months and overall survival 28 months was found after everolimus initiation and 40% had disease stabilization for at least 12 months. PRRT is regularly used for G1-G2 NET with a high uptake on SRI and a recent small retrospective study on PRRT treatment in GEP NEN G3 patients showed promising results.[58] Most of these patients in this study had a Ki-67 of less than 55% and a primary tumor in the pancreas, so many of these cases might have been NET G3. An Australian-led multicenter randomized phase II study is under development to examine the benefit of PRRT in patients with GEP NET G3 or NEC with a Ki-67 of 55% or less. To summarize, the current literature suggests that, owing to an unfavorable risk over benefit ratio, platin-based chemotherapy is not recommended in this subgroup of patients (see **Fig. 4**). A NETG2 like strategy seems to be more appropriate, taking into account an expected more aggressive behavior of NET G3 patients.

SUMMARY

The treatment of GEP NEG G3 is challenging and difficult owing to the lack of high-quality large data. An international consensus on morphologic/molecular classification and a systematic expert pathologic review will be critical to avoid misinterpretation of new study results and to better understand the place of new therapeutic options within the new subgroups of NEN G3. Generation of large studies with clinical and molecular data is necessary to better define tumor classification and prognosis, and to aid in the individualization of therapy for future patients. Until further data are present, the treatment of NEN G3 has to be based on several factors as differentiation, tumor stage, primary tumor location, Ki-67, and clinical course.

REFERENCES

1. Bosman FT, Carneiro F, Hruban RH, et al. WHO classification of tumours of the digestive system. 4th edition. Lyon (France): IARC Press; 2010.
2. Klöppel G, Couvelard A, Hruban RH, et al. Neoplasms of the neuroendocrine pancreas. 4th edition. Lyon (France): IARC Press; 2017.

3. Sorbye H, Strosberg J, Baudin E, et al. Gastroenteropancreatic high-grade neuroendocrine carcinoma. Cancer 2014;120(18):2814–23.

4. Milione M, Maisonneuve P, Spada F, et al. The clinicopathologic heterogeneity of grade 3 gastroenteropancreatic neuroendocrine neoplasms: morphological differentiation and proliferation identify different prognostic categories. Neuroendocrinology 2017;104(1):85–93.

5. Fazio N, Milione M. Heterogeneity of grade 3 gastroenteropancreatic neuroendocrine carcinomas: new insights and treatment implications. Cancer Treat Rev 2016;50:61–7.

6. La Rosa S, Marando A, Furlan D, et al. Colorectal poorly differentiated neuroendocrine carcinomas and mixed adenoneuroendocrine carcinomas: insights into the diagnostic immunophenotype, assessment of methylation profile, and search for prognostic markers. Am J Surg Pathol 2012;36(4):601–11.

7. Tang LH, Basturk O, Sue JJ, et al. A practical approach to the classification of WHO Grade 3 (G3) well-differentiated neuroendocrine tumor (WD-NET) and poorly differentiated neuroendocrine carcinoma (PD-NEC) of the pancreas. Am J Surg Pathol 2016;40(9):1192–202.

8. Girardi DM, Silva ACB, Rêgo JFM, et al. Unraveling molecular pathways of poorly differentiated neuroendocrine carcinomas of the gastroenteropancreatic system: a systematic review. Cancer Treat Rev 2017;56(Supplement C):28–35.

9. Velayoudom-Cephise FL, Duvillard P, Foucan L, et al. Are G3 ENETS neuroendocrine neoplasms heterogeneous? Endocr Relat Cancer 2013;20(5):649–57.

10. Heetfeld M, Chougnet CN, Olsen IH, et al. Characteristics and treatment of patients with G3 gastroenteropancreatic neuroendocrine neoplasms. Endocr Relat Cancer 2015;22(4):657–64.

11. Sorbye H, Welin S, Langer SW, et al. Predictive and prognostic factors for treatment and survival in 305 patients with advanced gastrointestinal neuroendocrine carcinoma (WHO G3): the NORDIC NEC study. Ann Oncol 2013;24(1):152–60.

12. Dasari A, Mehta K, Byers LA, et al. Comparative study of lung and extrapulmonary poorly differentiated neuroendocrine carcinomas: a SEER database analysis of 162,983 cases. Cancer 2017. https://doi.org/10.1002/cncr.31124.

13. Yamaguchi T, Machida N, Morizane C, et al. Multicenter retrospective analysis of systemic chemotherapy for advanced neuroendocrine carcinoma of the digestive system. Cancer Sci 2014;105(9):1176–81.

14. Walter T, Tougeron D, Baudin E, et al. Poorly differentiated gastro-entero-pancreatic neuroendocrine carcinomas: are they really heterogeneous? Insights from the FFCD-GTE national cohort. Eur J Cancer 2017;79:158–65.

15. Coriat R, Walter T, Terris B, et al. Gastroenteropancreatic well-differentiated grade 3 neuroendocrine tumors: review and position statement. Oncologist 2016; 21(10):1191–9.

16. Crippa S, Partelli S, Bassi C, et al. Long-term outcomes and prognostic factors in neuroendocrine carcinomas of the pancreas: morphology matters. Surgery 2016; 159(3):862–71.

17. Hijioka S, Hosoda W, Matsuo K, et al. Rb Loss and KRAS mutation are predictors of the response to platinum-based chemotherapy in pancreatic neuroendocrine neoplasm with grade 3: a Japanese multicenter pancreatic NEN-G3 study. Clin Cancer Res 2017;23(16):4625–32.

18. Raj N, Valentino E, Capanu M, et al. Treatment response and outcomes of grade 3 pancreatic neuroendocrine neoplasms based on morphology: well differentiated versus poorly differentiated. Pancreas 2017;46(3):296–301.

19. Basturk O, Tang L, Hruban RH, et al. Poorly differentiated neuroendocrine carcinomas of the pancreas: a clinicopathologic analysis of 44 cases. Am J Surg Pathol 2014;38(4):437–47.

20. Korse CM, Taal BG, van Velthuysen ML, et al. Incidence and survival of neuroendocrine tumours in the Netherlands according to histological grade: experience of two decades of cancer registry. Eur J Cancer 2013;49(8): 1975–83.

21. Basturk O, Yang Z, Tang LH, et al. The high-grade (WHO G3) pancreatic neuroendocrine tumor category is morphologically and biologically heterogenous and includes both well differentiated and poorly differentiated neoplasms. Am J Surg Pathol 2015;39(5):683–90.

22. Tang LH, Untch BR, Reidy DL, et al. Well-differentiated neuroendocrine tumors with a morphologically apparent high-grade component: a pathway distinct from poorly differentiated neuroendocrine carcinomas. Clin Cancer Res 2016; 22(4):1011–7.

23. Perren A, Couvelard A, Scoazec JY, et al. ENETS consensus guidelines for the standards of care in neuroendocrine tumors: pathology: diagnosis and prognostic stratification. Neuroendocrinology 2017;105(3):196–200.

24. La Rosa S, Sessa F, Uccella S. Mixed neuroendocrine-nonneuroendocrine neoplasms (MiNENs): unifying the concept of a heterogeneous group of neoplasms. Endocr Pathol 2016;27(4):284–311.

25. de Mestier L, Cros J, Neuzillet C, et al. Digestive system mixed neuroendocrine-non-neuroendocrine neoplasms. Neuroendocrinology 2017;105(4):412–25.

26. Konukiewitz B, Schlitter AM, Jesinghaus M, et al. Somatostatin receptor expression related to TP53 and RB1 alterations in pancreatic and extrapancreatic neuroendocrine neoplasms with a Ki67-index above 20%. Mod Pathol 2017;30(4): 587–98.

27. Furlan D, Sahnane N, Mazzoni M, et al. Diagnostic utility of MS-MLPA in DNA methylation profiling of adenocarcinomas and neuroendocrine carcinomas of the colon-rectum. Virchows Arch 2013;462(1):47–56.

28. Woischke C, Schaaf CW, Yang HM, et al. In-depth mutational analyses of colorectal neuroendocrine carcinomas with adenoma or adenocarcinoma components. Mod Pathol 2017;30(1):95–103.

29. Takizawa N, Ohishi Y, Hirahashi M, et al. Molecular characteristics of colorectal neuroendocrine carcinoma; similarities with adenocarcinoma rather than neuroendocrine tumor. Hum Pathol 2015;46(12):1890–900.

30. Karkouche R, Bachet JB, Sandrini J, et al. Colorectal neuroendocrine carcinomas and adenocarcinomas share oncogenic pathways. A clinico-pathologic study of 12 cases. Eur J Gastroenterol Hepatol 2012;24(12):1430–7.

31. Sahnane N, Furlan D, Monti M, et al. Microsatellite unstable gastrointestinal neuroendocrine carcinomas: a new clinicopathologic entity. Endocr Relat Cancer 2015;22(1):35–45.

32. Bergsland EK, Roy R, Stephens P, et al. Genomic profiling to distinguish poorly differentiated neuroendocrine carcinomas: a new clinicopathologic entity. ASCO Annual Meeting 2016. J Clin Oncol 2016;34(Suppl). Abstract 4020.

33. George J, Lim JS, Jang SJ, et al. Comprehensive genomic profiles of small cell lung cancer. Nature 2015;524(7563):47–53.

34. Cavalcanti E, Armentano R, Valentini AM, et al. Role of PD-L1 expression as a biomarker for GEP neuroendocrine neoplasm grading. Cell Death Dis 2017; 8(8):e3004.

35. Kim ST, Lee SJ, Park SH, et al. Genomic profiling of metastatic gastroentero-pancreatic neuroendocrine tumor (GEP-NET) patients in the personalized-medicine era. J Cancer 2016;7(9):1044–8.
36. Fitzgerald TL, Mosquera C, Lea CS, et al. Primary site predicts grade for gastro-enteropancreatic neuroendocrine tumors. Am Surg 2017;83(7):799–803.
37. Haugvik SP, Janson ET, Osterlund P, et al. surgical treatment as a principle for patients with high-grade pancreatic neuroendocrine carcinoma: a Nordic multi-center comparative study. Ann Surg Oncol 2016;23(5):1721–8.
38. Shafqat H, Ali S, Salhab M, et al. Survival of patients with neuroendocrine carci-noma of the colon and rectum: a population-based analysis. Dis Colon Rectum 2015;58(3):294–303.
39. Mosquera C, Koutlas NJ, Fitzgerald TL. Localized high-grade gastroenteropancre-atic neuroendocrine tumors: defining prognostic and therapeutic factors for a dis-ease of increasing clinical significance. Eur J Surg Oncol 2016;42(10):1471–7.
40. Shen C, Chen H, Chen H, et al. Surgical treatment and prognosis of gastric neuroendocrine neoplasms: a single-center experience. BMC Gastroenterol 2016;16:111.
41. Ishida M, Sekine S, Fukagawa T, et al. Neuroendocrine carcinoma of the stom-ach: morphologic and immunohistochemical characteristics and prognosis. Am J Surg Pathol 2013;37(7):949–59.
42. Xie JW, Sun YQ, Feng CY, et al. Evaluation of clinicopathological factors related to the prognosis of gastric neuroendocrine carcinoma. Eur J Surg Oncol 2016; 42(10):1464–70.
43. Meng MB, Zaorsky NG, Jiang C, et al. Radiotherapy and chemotherapy are asso-ciated with improved outcomes over surgery and chemotherapy in the manage-ment of limited-stage small cell esophageal carcinoma. Radiother Oncol 2013; 106(3):317–22.
44. Deng HY, Ni PZ, Wang YC, et al. Neuroendocrine carcinoma of the esophagus: clinical characteristics and prognostic evaluation of 49 cases with surgical resec-tion. J Thorac Dis 2016;8(6):1250–6.
45. Strosberg JR, Coppola D, Klimstra DS, et al. The NANETS consensus guidelines for the diagnosis and management of poorly differentiated (high-grade) extrapul-monary neuroendocrine carcinomas. Pancreas 2010;39(6):799–800.
46. Garcia-Carbonero R, Sorbye H, Baudin E, et al. ENETS consensus guidelines for high-grade gastroenteropancreatic neuroendocrine tumors and neuroendocrine carcinomas. Neuroendocrinology 2016;103(2):186–94.
47. Janson ET, Sorbye H, Welin S, et al. Nordic guidelines 2014 for diagnosis and treatment of gastroenteropancreatic neuroendocrine neoplasms. Acta Oncol 2014;53(10):1284–97.
48. Lamarca A, Walter T, Pavel M, et al. Design and validation of the GI-NEC score to prognosticate overall survival in patients with high-grade gastrointestinal neuro-endocrine carcinomas. J Natl Cancer Inst 2017;109(5).
49. Oberg K, Knigge U, Kwekkeboom D, et al. Neuroendocrine gastro-entero-pancreatic tumors: ESMO clinical practice guidelines for diagnosis, treatment and follow-up. Ann Oncol 2012;23(Suppl 7):vii124–30.
50. Pavel M, O'Toole D, Costa F, et al. ENETS consensus guidelines update for the management of distant metastatic disease of intestinal, pancreatic, bronchial neuroendocrine neoplasms (NEN) and NEN of unknown primary site. Neuroendo-crinology 2016;103(2):172–85.
51. Frilling A, Modlin IM, Kidd M, et al. Recommendations for management of pa-tients with neuroendocrine liver metastases. Lancet Oncol 2014;15(1):e8–21.

52. Galleberg RB, Knigge U, Tiensuu Janson E, et al. Results after surgical treatment of liver metastases in patients with high-grade gastroenteropancreatic neuroendocrine carcinomas. Eur J Surg Oncol 2017;43(9):1682–9.
53. Garcia-Carbonero R, Rinke A, Valle JW, et al. ENETS consensus guidelines for the standards of care in neuroendocrine neoplasms. Systemic therapy 2: chemotherapy. Neuroendocrinology 2017;105(3):281–94.
54. Olsen IH, Knigge U, Federspiel B, et al. Topotecan monotherapy in heavily pretreated patients with progressive advanced stage neuroendocrine carcinomas. J Cancer 2014;5(8):628–32.
55. Welin S, Sorbye H, Sebjornsen S, et al. Clinical effect of temozolomide-based chemotherapy in poorly differentiated endocrine carcinoma after progression on first-line chemotherapy. Cancer 2011;117(20):4617–22.
56. Hadoux J, Malka D, Planchard D, et al. Post-first-line FOLFOX chemotherapy for grade 3 neuroendocrine carcinoma. Endocr Relat Cancer 2015;22(3):289–98.
57. Hentic O, Hammel P, Couvelard A, et al. FOLFIRI regimen: an effective second-line chemotherapy after failure of etoposide-platinum combination in patients with neuroendocrine carcinomas grade 3. Endocr Relat Cancer 2012;19(6):751–7.
58. Thang SP, Lung MS, Kong G, et al. Peptide receptor radionuclide therapy (PRRT) in European Neuroendocrine Tumour Society (ENETS) grade 3 (G3) neuroendocrine neoplasia (NEN) - a single-institution retrospective analysis. Eur J Nucl Med Mol Imaging 2018;45(2):262–77.
59. Panzuto F, Rinzivillo M, Spada F, et al. Everolimus in pancreatic neuroendocrine carcinomas G3. Pancreas 2017;46(3):302–5.

Lung and Thymic Carcinoids

Christine L. Hann, MD, PhD*, Patrick M. Forde, MB BCh

KEYWORDS

- Carcinoid • Lung carcinoid • Lung neuroendocrine • Thymic neuroendocrine
- Thymic carcinoid

KEY POINTS

- Lung carcinoid tumors are indolent cancers with a good prognosis; after appropriate staging, tumors localized to the lung are treated with surgical resection. The role of adjuvant therapy after surgical resection has not been clearly defined.
- Definitive radiation or chemoradiation may be considered for patients with unresectable atypical carcinoid, although evidence to support this approach is limited.
- Somatostatin analogue therapy should be considered for patients with advanced thoracic carcinoids that expresses somatostatin receptors.
- Everolimus is the only approved systemic therapy for patients with advanced pulmonary carcinoid.
- Chemotherapy agents, including temozolomide with or without capecitabine, may be options for patients whose tumors progress despite these approaches. Lutetium-177–dotatate has demonstrated efficacy in gastrointestinal neuroendocrine tumors and, where available, may be considered for patients with advanced somatostatin receptor–positive lung carcinoid.

The goal of early stage disease management is definitive surgical resection. Definitive radiation or chemoradiation may be considered for locally advanced pulmonary carcinoids or thymic neuroendocrine tumors, although evidence to support this approach is limited.

Systemic therapy for advanced or metastatic pulmonary carcinoids generally follows a similar paradigm to low-grade carcinoid tumors of the gastrointestinal (GI) tract. Somatostatin analogue therapy is an option for receptor-positive tumors. Similarly, peptide receptor radionuclide therapy (PRRT) with lutetium-177 (^{177}Lu)–octreotide may be considered. Everolimus has been approved for treatment of patients with

Disclosures: C.L. Hann: consulting/advisory role: AbbVie, BMS, Genentech; research funding (to institution): GSK, Merrimack, AbbVie, BMS. P.M. Forde: consulting/advisory role: BMS, AstraZeneca, Novartis, Merck, Abbvie; research funding (to institution): BMS, AstraZeneca, Novartis, Kyowa.
Upper Aerodigestive Cancer Program, Department of Oncology, Sidney Kimmel Comprehensive Cancer Center, Johns Hopkins University School of Medicine, Baltimore, MD 21231, USA
* Corresponding author. Viragh Building, Room 8123, 201 N. Broadway, Baltimore, MD 21287.
E-mail address: chann1@jhmi.edu

advanced pulmonary carcinoid, and systemic chemotherapy has shown responses in small series.

LUNG CARCINOIDS
Introduction

Neuroendocrine tumors (NETs) account for approximately 20% of all cancers arising in the lung and include a spectrum of pathologies from well-differentiated tumors (typical and atypical carcinoids) to poorly differentiated carcinomas (small cell lung cancer [SCLC] and large cell neuroendocrine carcinoma [LCNEC]). The classification of NETs is based on microscopic, macroscopic, and immunohistochemical staining. Despite similarities in morphologic and biochemical characteristics, the behavior and natural history of carcinoid tumors are dramatically different from that of SCLC and LCNEC. This review focuses on the low-grade NETs of the lung and thymus, also known as carcinoid tumors.

Incidence and Epidemiology

The lung is the second most common site of carcinoid tumors, accounting for 25% of overall cases. Pulmonary carcinoids, however, are considered rare lung neoplasms, estimated at 1% to 2% of all primary lung cancers.[1] Typical carcinoids are more common than atypical carcinoids (85% vs 15% cases) and have a lower likelihood of metastatic spread or relapse after surgery; therefore, they carry an overall better prognosis.[2–4] The average age of diagnosis for lung carcinoids is 60 years; patients with typical carcinoids usually present a decade earlier than those with atypical carcinoids.[5–7] Pulmonary carcinoids occur more commonly in women than in men and are not clearly attributed to tobacco exposure.[2,5,8] Pulmonary carcinoids can rarely occur in association with multiple endocrine neoplasia type 1 (MEN-1) syndrome.

Presentation

Most carcinoid tumors arise from the proximal airways, and presenting symptoms may be due to local obstruction (cough, dyspnea, atelectasis); hemoptysis presents in 10% to 20%.[2,9] NETs can produce a variety of biologically active peptides and hormones, some of which lead to clinically relevant syndromes. The carcinoid syndrome, due to the production of serotonin and bioactive amines, is less common in patients with lung carcinoids (<10% of cases) than in patients with midgut (small bowel, appendix, and ascending colon) NETs.[10] A detailed discussion and recommendations on the management of the carcinoid syndrome is covered in Paul Benjamin Loughrey and colleagues' article, "New Treatments for the Carcinoid Syndrome," in this issue. Lung NETs are the most common cause of ectopic adrenocorticotropic hormone (ACTH) production; thus, Cushing syndrome may be a presenting symptom of this disease, though the overall incidence in lung carcinoids is rare (1%–2% of cases).[11] Lung carcinoids are also the most common site of extrapituitary secretion of growth hormone–releasing hormone; thus, patients with lung NETs may rarely present with acromegaly.[12]

Diagnosis and Staging

Core biopsies are preferred for histopathologic diagnosis, as a definitive diagnosis may be difficult to ascertain in cytology samples, particularly in differentiating typical versus atypical carcinoid tumors. Pulmonary carcinoids are categorized as typical or atypical corresponding to well differentiated, low grade (G1) and well differentiated, intermediate grade (G2), respectively. Histologically, typical carcinoids have less than 2 mitoses per square millimeter and lack necrosis, whereas atypical carcinoids have 2 to

10 mitoses per square millimeter and may have focal necrosis.[13] Once a diagnosis of carcinoid has been confirmed, additional radiologic and serologic examinations may be helpful. The Ki-67 is usually less than 5% in typical carcinoid tumors and ranges from 5% to 20% in atypical carcinoids.[14] Diffuse idiopathic pulmonary neuroendocrine cell hyperplasia (DIPNECH), a very rare quasi-neoplastic condition affecting lung neuroendocrine cells, is defined as lung involvement by multiple carcinoid tumorlets and widespread proliferation of neuroendocrine cells within the airways.[15]

Radiographic Imaging

Approximately 5% to 20% of typical carcinoid tumors are associated with local-regional lymphadenopathy, which may be due to a local inflammatory reaction rather than tumor involvement. The positive predictive value of computed tomography (CT) in assessing hilar and mediastinal metastases from lung carcinoid tumors is reportedly low (20%–45%).[16,17] By immunohistochemistry, 60% to 80% of pulmonary carcinoids express somatostatin receptors; thus, somatostatin receptor-based imaging may be useful in staging this disease. Indium-111 (^{111}In)-DTPA-D-Phe-1-octreotide (used in *Octreoscans*) or gallium-68 (^{68}Ga)-dotatate–based PET imaging are helpful in assessing the disease extent of NETs and may assist in decisions on therapeutic management. Recent data support that ^{68}Ga-dotatate PET has higher sensitivity than does ^{111}In pentetreotide imaging.[18] In addition, PET/CT-based imaging allows for better spatial resolution of areas of tracer avidity. Atypical carcinoids are usually positive on fluorodeoxyglucose (FDG)-PET imaging, whereas typical carcinoids are usually not; therefore, FDG-PET may be most useful in staging patients with somatostatin-receptor negative atypical carcinoid tumors. Brain metastases occur relatively frequently in atypical pulmonary carcinoid tumors, and contrast-enhanced MRI brain imaging should be used for such patients who have neurologic symptoms or present with widely metastatic disease.

Staging and Prognosis

Pulmonary carcinoid tumors are staged according to the TNM classification by the American Joint Committee on Cancer used for other bronchogenic lung cancers. In general, the prognosis for pulmonary carcinoid is excellent compared with other primary lung cancers. A review of pulmonary carcinoid cases submitted to the National Cancer Institute's Surveillance, Epidemiology, and End Results registry and the International Association for the Study of Lung Cancer's database reported a 5-year overall survival (OS) for patients with stage I to IV lung carcinoids of 93% (stage I), 74% to 85% (stage II), 67% to 75% (stage III), and 57% (stage IV).[19]

Survival is significantly better for patients with typical carcinoids, with 5- and 10-year survival rates of 87% and 87%, respectively. Patients with atypical carcinoids have 5- and 10-year survival rates of 56% and 35%, respectively.[20] Overall, predictors of survival include stage, tumor size, mitotic rates, and age.[5,8,21] A nomogram using age, sex, tumor location, stage, Eastern Cooperative Oncology Group Performance Status, and prior malignancy to predict the 5-year survival after resection of typical carcinoid of the lung has been proposed and subsequently validated by an independent cohort.[22,23] Also noted was that patients with multiple nodules had a favorable prognosis, and it is possible that these individuals have a more indolent disorder of neuroendocrine cell proliferation or DIPNECH.[19]

Genetics

Recent genomic analyses of pulmonary carcinoids have revealed that mutations in chromatin remodeling genes are common. Further, mutations of *TP53* and *RB1*, two tumor suppressor genes commonly altered in SCLC, are rare in pulmonary carcinoids. A large-scale genomic study of lung carcinoids, including copy number analysis (CNA; n = 54), genome/exome sequencing (n = 44), and transcriptome sequencing (n = 69), reported an overall low mutation burden (0.4 mutations per megabase). Mutations in chromatin-remodeling genes were frequently observed, whereas TP53 and RB1 mutations were rare, suggesting that pulmonary carcinoids arise through mechanisms distinctly different than SCLC.[24] Whole-exome sequencing and high-coverage targeted sequencing of 148 lung NETs, including 88 carcinoids, and 60 high-grade NETs similarly reported mutations in chromatin-remodeling genes in 45% and mutations in TP53, RB1, and ATM in approximately 10% of the carcinoid tumors. Other rare alterations included mutations in the phosphoinositide 3 kinase/AKT/mammalian target of rapamycin (mTOR) pathway (2.3%). MEN-1 alterations were almost exclusively seen in the carcinoid tumors, and CNA prevalence was significantly lower in carcinoids than in the high-grade NE tumors.[25] Given the consistent finding of mutations in chromatin-remodeling genes, epigenetic approaches to the treatment of carcinoid tumors may be a path forward in seeking new therapies in this cancer.

MANAGEMENT BY STAGE
Stages I, II, and III Resectable

Surgery is the primary treatment modality and the only curative option for patients with pulmonary carcinoids. Because carcinoids often present in central airways, pneumonectomy or bilobectomy can be required; but most patients undergo lobectomy.[1,8] For patients with favorable prognostic features, such as typical histology and absence of lymph node involvement, more limited resection has been proposed. Patients with atypical carcinoids should be resected using the same principles guiding surgery for non-SCLC, including complete mediastinal lymph node dissection.[9,26–28]

Adjuvant chemotherapy after surgical resection for patients with typical carcinoids with or without regional lymph node metastases (stages I, II, and III) is not recommended, as the risk of recurrence is low and the impact of adjuvant chemotherapy is unknown.[28] In a series of 291 resected typical carcinoids, only 3% of patients developed recurrence.[6,29] Similarly, following surgical resection, patients with stage I and II atypical carcinoid should be followed expectantly.

As systemic recurrence occurs more frequently in patients with atypical carcinoids with mediastinal lymph node involvement (stage III), adjuvant platinum plus etoposide with or without radiation has been recommended; but it is unknown whether this is beneficial.[28] The use of adjuvant radiation therapy for nodal disease is also of undefined utility, but it has also been recommended for locally advanced atypical carcinoids.[28]

Unresectable Disease

Patients with peripheral pulmonary carcinoids who are not surgical candidates can be considered for stereotactic external beam radiotherapy. In patients with unresectable typical carcinoids, the use of radiotherapy or concurrent chemoradiotherapy is a category 3 recommendation, as chemoradiotherapy is likely to be more effective in tumors with atypical histology or a higher mitotic rate. It has not been established whether chemoradiotherapy is superior to definitive radiotherapy alone. Patients with unresectable atypical carcinoids should be offered chemoradiotherapy, though the response rates are lower than in patients with limited-stage SCLC.[30,31]

Stage IV Disease

The risk of distant metastases is significantly higher for atypical carcinoid compared with typical carcinoids (21% vs 3%); the most common site of dissemination is the liver.[2] For asymptomatic advanced pulmonary carcinoid patients with low tumor burden, close surveillance with routine imaging and clinical assessment is a reasonable option. Systemic therapy can be initiated at the time of symptomatic progression. For patients with liver-dominant metastatic disease, liver-directed treatment following a GI NET paradigm are often used for pulmonary carcinoids. Options include resection of isolated metastases, transarterial chemo-embolization, or radiofrequency ablation; liver-directed therapy is discussed in detail in Andrea Frilling and Ashley Kieran Clift's article, "Surgical Approaches to the Management of Neuroendocrine Liver Metastases," in this issue.

Data regarding the efficacy of systemic therapy in pulmonary carcinoid are generally lacking. Most recommended therapies for pulmonary carcinoids are derived from clinical trials that predominantly enrolled patients with GI NETs. Currently there is only one therapy approved by the Food and Drug Administration (FDA) for pulmonary carcinoid, the mTOR inhibitor, everolimus, based on the result of the RADIANT-4 trial, which showed improvements in progression-free survival (PFS).[32] No therapies have been shown to consistently induce regression. Various chemotherapeutic agents have been used, including temozolomide with or without capecitabine, doxorubicin, 5-fluorouracil, dacarbazine, cisplatin, carboplatin, etoposide, streptozocin, and interferon-alpha.[33,34]

Somatostatin Receptor–Targeted Therapies

Retrospective reviews including small numbers of patients with pulmonary carcinoids have reported on the use of somatostatin analogues with improvement in symptoms of carcinoid syndrome as well as prolonged disease control and survival despite very low objective response rates.[35–37] These results are similar to the experience with octreotide in GI carcinoids.[38] The PROMID study demonstrated that long-acting–release (LAR) octreotide acetate (Somatostatin LAR) significantly prolonged time to tumor progression compared with placebo in patients with well-differentiated midgut NETs (14.3 vs 6.0 months).[39] A randomized double-blind phase 3 study of lanreotide autogel versus placebo in patients with advanced, well-differentiated pulmonary NETs is ongoing (SPINET study, NCT02683941). The estimated enrollment in this study will be 216 patients, and the primary end point is PFS.

Peptide Receptor Radionuclide Therapy

Another option for patients with somatostatin receptor positive tumors is PRRT with radiolabeled somatostatin analogues. Since the early 1990s, several small studies have shown promising results with PPRT using ^{111}In-DTPA-octreotide, yttrium-90 (^{90}Y)-DOTATOC and ^{177}Lu-dotatate. radiolabeled somatostatin primarily in gastroenteropancreatic (GEP) NETs.[40–43] The largest study of PRRT in lung carcinoids was a retrospective analysis of 114 patients treated with ^{90}Y-DOTATOC, ^{177}Lu-dotatate, or both. This study reported an OS and median PFS of 59 months and 28 months, respectively. Patients treated with ^{177}Lu-dotatate had the highest 5-year OS of 61.4%, whereas those treated with the combination of ^{90}Y-DOTATOC and ^{177}Lu-dotatate had increased hematologic toxicity.[44]

The largest experience (more than 1200 patients) with ^{177}Lu-dotatate reported an overall response rate (ORR) of 39%, stable disease (SD) in 43%, with PFS and OS of 29 months and 63 months, respectively.[45] This study included 23 patients with lung NETs who had an ORR of 30% and PFS of 20 months. A phase II study of 34 consecutive patients with pulmonary carcinoid treated with ^{177}Lu-dotatate reported a disease control rate of 80%, a response rate of 33%, and a median PFS (mPFS) of 15.7 months.[46] A randomized phase 3 trial of ^{177}Lu-dotatate in midgut NETs (the NETTER-1 study) has recently been reported. This study randomized 229 patients with progression during first-line somatostatin analogue therapy to ^{177}Lu-dotatate plus 30 mg octreotide LAR or 60 mg octreotide LAR alone. The study met its primary end point of PFS; treatment with ^{177}Lu-dotatate was associated with a statistically significant reduction in the risk of disease progression or death versus high-dose octreotide.[47] Based on the NETTER-1 results and the results of a phase 1/2 study of ^{177}Lu-dotatate including more than 1200 patients, ^{177}Lu-dotatate has received FDA approval for the treatment of somatostatin receptor-positive GEP-NETs in adults.

Mammalian Target of Rapamycin –Directed Therapy

The mTOR pathway regulates cell growth, proliferation, and metabolism and has been implicated in the pathogenesis of NETs.[48]

A randomized placebo-controlled phase 3 study of everolimus plus octreotide LAR (RADIANT-2) included 429 patients with low-grade or intermediate-grade carcinoids, of which 44 were of pulmonary histology.[48] The mPFS was 16.4 months (95% confidence interval [CI]: 13.7–21.2 months) for the group receiving the combination compared with 11.3 months (95% CI: 8.4–14.6 months) in the octreotide LAR only group (hazard ratio [HR] 0.77, 95% CI: 0.59–1.0, $P = .026$); thus, the study met its primary end point. For the 44 patients with pulmonary carcinoids, the mPFS was 13.6 and 5.6 months in the everolimus plus octreotide LAR group versus the octreotide LAR only group, respectively.[48]

The RADIANT-4 study was a double-blinded phase 3 study that randomized 302 patients 2:1 with nonfunctional lung or GI NETs to receive everolimus or placebo.[32] The mPFS was 11.0 months in the everolimus arm and 3.9 months in the placebo arm. The HR for progression or death was 0.48 favoring everolimus. Grade 3/4 drug-related toxicities included stomatitis, infections, diarrhea, and anemia, all of which occurred in less than 10% of patients.[32]

A post hoc analysis of the pulmonary NET subgroup from RADIANT-4 reported a benefit from therapy with everolimus.[49] Of the 90 patients with pulmonary NETs enrolled on RADIANT-4, 63 received everolimus and 27 placebo. The mPFS was 9.2 with everolimus versus 3.6 months with placebo. Tumor shrinkage of 58% versus 13% was observed in the everolimus and placebo arms, respectively.[49]

Chemotherapy

Typical and atypical carcinoid are less chemosensitive than SCLC; however, for lack of alternatives, regimens used for SCLC often are considered for patients with symptomatic or rapidly progressive metastatic pulmonary carcinoid though with limited evidence to support their use.[50,51] In 2 small series that included 26 patients treated with chemotherapy (mostly etoposide and cisplatin, EP), the ORR was approximately 20%.[30,33] EP was administered to 18 patients with lung and thymus carcinoids after progression on first- or second-line therapy. Radiographic response was noted in 2 of 5 patients with atypical and in 5 of 13 with typical carcinoid. The median duration of response was 9 months.[52]

Similarly, among 17 patients with pulmonary carcinoids treated with etoposide plus platinum (cisplatin or carboplatin), 23.5% had a radiologic response (2 patients each with atypical and typical carcinoid) and a mPFS of 7 months.[37]

Temozolomide has been evaluated either alone or in combination with other agents, including capecitabine. Thirteen patients with pulmonary carcinoids (10 typical, 3 atypical) were included in a retrospective study of temozolomide monotherapy. Four of 13 patients (31%) had a partial response (PR).[53] In a larger retrospective study of 31 patients with pulmonary carcinoids, PR and SD were reported in 3 (14%) and 11 (52%) patients, respectively.[54] The combination of capecitabine plus temozolomide has been reported in multiple studies. The highest response rates (up to 70% in some series) have been reported in pancreatic NETs.[55–57] Responses have been reported in lung NETs. Of 4 patients with lung carcinoids reported in a retrospective analysis, 3 of 4 patients with pulmonary carcinoid attained a clinical benefit with at least stable disease.[58] Larger confirmatory studies are needed to evaluate the potential benefit of temozolomide-based therapies in pulmonary carcinoids.

Thymic Neuroendocrine Tumors

NETs of the thymus are much rarer than primary lung carcinoids with a reported incidence of 0.02 to 0.04 per 100,000 population per year; as a consequence, optimal management is even less well defined.[59] Although pathologic features of thymic NETs may resemble pulmonary carcinoids, the natural history of these tumors tends to be more aggressive with late presentation, frequent metastases, and occurrence as a component of MEN-1 in approximately 25% of cases.[60]

Pathologic classification of thymic NET follows the World Health Organization's 2015 pulmonary NET system as described earlier in this article.[13]

In contrast to lung NETs, recommended staging of thymic NETs should follow the Masaoka system used for thymic epithelial tumors.[61]

Thymic NETs have a 3:1 male/female sex distribution and approximately 40% to 50% secrete hormones, principally ACTH; secretion of ACTH is associated with a poorer prognosis.[59,60]

Most thymic NETs are somatostatin positive, and ^{111}In-octreotide–single-photon emission CT imaging is useful; data on ^{68}Ga-DOTATOC PET/CT are limited, but given the receptor positivity it is likely to be of use.

The treatment of thymic NETs involves definitive oncologic resection of the primary tumor and associated lymph node staging, and this offers the only potential for a long-term cure. There are currently no data to support adjuvant therapy, and recurrences are often late.

Systemic therapy for thymic NETs is generally undefined; however, it is likely that somatostatin analogue therapy and PRRT, where available, may have benefit. Systemic chemotherapy has been described in case reports, most frequently using temozolomide.

SUMMARY

In the approach to metastatic pulmonary carcinoid tumors, somatostatin analogue therapy is a reasonable first-line treatment of patients with a low tumor burden and somatostatin-receptor positive disease. For patients who progress on somatostatin analogues, treatment with ^{177}Lu-dotatate, if available, may be considered. Everolimus is currently the only FDA-approved systemic therapy for advanced pulmonary carcinoid and improves PFS. Chemotherapy should be considered for those with more rapidly progressing and symptomatic tumors or those who have progressed on less toxic treatments. Prospective randomized studies are needed for both traditional cytotoxic and molecularly targeted agents in this disease, and inclusion of both pulmonary and thymic NETs in larger clinical trials for carcinoid tumors is imperative.

REFERENCES

1. Harpole DH, Feldman JM, Buchanan S Jr, et al. Bronchial carcinoid tumors: a retrospective analysis of 126 patients. Ann Thorac Surg 1992;54(1):50–4 [discussion: 54–5].
2. Fink G, Krelbaum T, Yellin A, et al. Pulmonary carcinoid: presentation, diagnosis, and outcome in 142 cases in Israel and review of 640 cases from the literature. Chest 2001;119(6):1647–51.
3. Kulke MH, Mayer RJ. Carcinoid tumors. N Engl J Med 1999;340(11):858–68.
4. Davini F, Gonfiotti A, Comin C, et al. Typical and atypical carcinoid tumours: 20-year experience with 89 patients. J Cardiovasc Surg (Torino) 2009;50(6): 807–11.
5. Asamura H, Kameya T, Matsuno Y, et al. Neuroendocrine neoplasms of the lung: a prognostic spectrum. J Clin Oncol 2006;24(1):70–6.
6. Thomas CF Jr, Tazelaar HD, Jett JR. Typical and atypical pulmonary carcinoids: outcome in patients presenting with regional lymph node involvement. Chest 2001;119(4):1143–50.
7. Skuladottir H, Hirsch FR, Hansen HH, et al. Pulmonary neuroendocrine tumors: Incidence and prognosis of histological subtypes. A population-based study in Denmark. Lung Cancer 2002;37(2):127–35.
8. McCaughan BC, Martini N, Bains MS. Bronchial carcinoids. Review of 124 cases. J Thorac Cardiovasc Surg 1985;89(1):8–17.
9. Chughtai TS, Morin JE, Sheiner NM, et al. Bronchial carcinoid–twenty years' experience defines a selective surgical approach. Surgery 1997;122(4):801–8.
10. Halperin DM, Shen C, Dasari A, et al. Frequency of carcinoid syndrome at neuroendocrine tumour diagnosis: a population-based study. Lancet Oncol 2017; 18(4):525–34.
11. Limper AH, Carpenter PC, Scheithauer B, et al. The Cushing syndrome induced by bronchial carcinoid tumors. Ann Intern Med 1992;117(3):209–14.
12. Athanassiadi K, Exarchos D, Tsagarakis S, et al. Acromegaly caused by ectopic growth hormone-releasing hormone secretion by a carcinoid bronchial tumor: a rare entity. J Thorac Cardiovasc Surg 2004;128(4):631–2.
13. Travis W, Brambilla E, Burke AP, et al. WHO classification of tumours of the lung, pleura, thymus and heart. In: Bosman F, Jaffe ES, Lakhani SR, et al, editors. World Health Organization classification of tumours. 4th edition. Lyon (France): IARC Press; 2015. p. 73–7.
14. Pelosi G, Papotti M, Rindi G, et al. Unraveling tumor grading and genomic landscape in lung neuroendocrine tumors. Endocr Pathol 2014;25(2):151–64.
15. Rossi G, Cavazza A, Spagnolo P, et al. Diffuse idiopathic pulmonary neuroendocrine cell hyperplasia syndrome. Eur Respir J 2016;47(6):1829–41.
16. Divisi D, Crisci R. Carcinoid tumors of the lung and multimodal therapy. Thorac Cardiovasc Surg 2005;53(3):168–72.
17. Granberg D, Sundin A, Janson ET, et al. Octreoscan in patients with bronchial carcinoid tumours. Clin Endocrinol (Oxf) 2003;59(6):793–9.
18. Buchmann I, Henze M, Engelbrecht S, et al. Comparison of 68Ga-DOTATOC PET and 111In-DTPAOC (Octreoscan) SPECT in patients with neuroendocrine tumours. Eur J Nucl Med Mol Imaging 2007;34(10):1617–26.
19. Travis WD, Giroux DJ, Chansky K, et al. The IASLC lung cancer staging project: proposals for the inclusion of broncho-pulmonary carcinoid tumors in the forthcoming (seventh) edition of the TNM classification for lung cancer. J Thorac Oncol 2008;3(11):1213–23.

20. Travis WD, Rush W, Flieder DB, et al. Survival analysis of 200 pulmonary neuro-endocrine tumors with clarification of criteria for atypical carcinoid and its separation from typical carcinoid. Am J Surg Pathol 1998;22(8):934–44.
21. Pietanza CM, Krug LM, Wu AJ, et al. Small cell and other neuroendocrine tumors of the lung. In: DeVita VT, Hellman S, Rosenberg SA, editors. Cancer: principles & practice of oncology. Lippincott, Williams, and Wilkins; 2015.
22. Filosso PL, Guerrera F, Evangelista A, et al. Prognostic model of survival for typical bronchial carcinoid tumours: analysis of 1109 patients on behalf of the European Association of Thoracic Surgeons (ESTS) Neuroendocrine Tumours Working Group. Eur J Cardiothorac Surg 2015;48(3):441–7 [discussion: 447].
23. Cattoni M, Vallières E, Brown LM, et al. External validation of a prognostic model of survival for resected typical bronchial carcinoids. Ann Thorac Surg 2017; 104(4):1215–20.
24. Fernandez-Cuesta L, Peifer M, Lu X, et al. Frequent mutations in chromatin-remodelling genes in pulmonary carcinoids. Nat Commun 2014;5:3518.
25. Simbolo M, Mafficini A, Sikora KO, et al. Lung neuroendocrine tumours: deep sequencing of the four World Health Organization histotypes reveals chromatin-remodelling genes as major players and a prognostic role for TERT, RB1, MEN1 and KMT2D. J Pathol 2017;241(4):488–500.
26. Yendamuri S, Gold D, Jayaprakash V, et al. Is sublobar resection sufficient for carcinoid tumors? Ann Thorac Surg 2011;92(5):1774–8 [discussion: 1778–9].
27. Marty-Ane CH, Costes V, Pujol JL, et al. Carcinoid tumors of the lung: do atypical features require aggressive management? Ann Thorac Surg 1995;59(1):78–83.
28. (NCCN), N.C.C.N. NCCN clinical practice guidelines in oncology: neuroendo-crine tumors version 3.2017. 2017. Available at: https://www.nccn.org/.
29. Lou F, Sarkaria I, Pietanza C, et al. Recurrence of pulmonary carcinoid tumors after resection: implications for postoperative surveillance. Ann Thorac Surg 2013; 96(4):1156–62.
30. Wirth LJ, Carter MR, Jänne PA, et al. Outcome of patients with pulmonary carci-noid tumors receiving chemotherapy or chemoradiotherapy. Lung Cancer 2004; 44(2):213–20.
31. Mackley HB, Videtic GM. Primary carcinoid tumors of the lung: a role for radio-therapy. Oncology (Williston Park) 2006;20(12):1537–43 [discussion: 1544–5, 1549].
32. Yao JC, Fazio N, Singh S, et al. Everolimus for the treatment of advanced, non-functional neuroendocrine tumours of the lung or gastrointestinal tract (RADIANT-4): a randomised, placebo-controlled, phase 3 study. Lancet 2016; 387(10022):968–77.
33. Granberg D, Eriksson B, Wilander E, et al. Experience in treatment of metastatic pulmonary carcinoid tumors. Ann Oncol 2001;12(10):1383–91.
34. Moertel CG, Hanley JA. Combination chemotherapy trials in metastatic carcinoid tumor and the malignant carcinoid syndrome. Cancer Clin Trials 1979;2(4):327–34.
35. Filosso PL, Ruffini E, Oliaro A, et al. Long-term survival of atypical bronchial car-cinoids with liver metastases, treated with octreotide. Eur J Cardiothorac Surg 2002;21(5):913–7.
36. Srirajaskanthan R, Toumpanakis C, Karpathakis A, et al. Surgical management and palliative treatment in bronchial neuroendocrine tumours: a clinical study of 45 patients. Lung Cancer 2009;65(1):68–73.
37. Forde PM, Hooker CM, Boikos SA, et al. Systemic therapy, clinical outcomes, and overall survival in locally advanced or metastatic pulmonary carcinoid: a brief report. J Thorac Oncol 2014;9(3):414–8.

38. Modlin IM, Kidd M, Latich I, et al. Current status of gastrointestinal carcinoids. Gastroenterology 2005;128(6):1717–51.
39. Rinke A, Müller HH, Schade-Brittinger C, et al. Placebo-controlled, double-blind, prospective, randomized study on the effect of octreotide LAR in the control of tumor growth in patients with metastatic neuroendocrine midgut tumors: a report from the PROMID Study Group. J Clin Oncol 2009;27(28):4656–63.
40. Krenning EP, de Jong M, Kooij PP, et al. Radiolabelled somatostatin analogue(s) for peptide receptor scintigraphy and radionuclide therapy. Ann Oncol 1999; 10(Suppl 2):S23–9.
41. Valkema R, Pauwels S, Kvols LK, et al. Survival and response after peptide receptor radionuclide therapy with [90Y-DOTA0,Tyr3]octreotide in patients with advanced gastroenteropancreatic neuroendocrine tumors. Semin Nucl Med 2006;36(2):147–56.
42. van der Zwan WA, Bodei L, Mueller-Brand J, et al. GEPNETs update: radionuclide therapy in neuroendocrine tumors. Eur J Endocrinol 2015;172(1):R1–8.
43. Gridelli C, Rossi A, Airoma G, et al. Treatment of pulmonary neuroendocrine tumours: state of the art and future developments. Cancer Treat Rev 2013;39(5):466–72.
44. Mariniello A, Bodei L, Tinelli C, et al. Long-term results of PRRT in advanced bronchopulmonary carcinoid. Eur J Nucl Med Mol Imaging 2016;43(3):441–52.
45. Brabander T, van der Zwan WA, Teunissen JJM, et al. Long-term efficacy, survival, and safety of [(177)Lu-DOTA(0),Tyr(3)] octreotate in patients with gastroenteropancreatic and bronchial neuroendocrine tumors. Clin Cancer Res 2017; 23(16):4617–24.
46. Ianniello A, Sansovini M, Severi S, et al. Peptide receptor radionuclide therapy with (177)Lu-DOTATATE in advanced bronchial carcinoids: prognostic role of thyroid transcription factor 1 and (18)F-FDG PET. Eur J Nucl Med Mol Imaging 2016; 43(6):1040–6.
47. Strosberg J, El-Haddad G, Wolin E, et al. Phase 3 trial of (177)Lu-dotatate for midgut neuroendocrine tumors. N Engl J Med 2017;376(2):125–35.
48. Pavel ME, Hainsworth JD, Baudin E, et al. Everolimus plus octreotide long-acting repeatable for the treatment of advanced neuroendocrine tumours associated with carcinoid syndrome (RADIANT-2): a randomised, placebo-controlled, phase 3 study. Lancet 2011;378(9808):2005–12.
49. Fazio N, Buzzoni R, Delle Fave G, et al. Everolimus in advanced, progressive, well-differentiated, non-functional neuroendocrine tumors: RADIANT-4 lung subgroup analysis. Cancer Sci 2018;109(1):174–81.
50. (NCCN), N.C.C.N. NCCN clinical practice guidelines in oncology. Small Cell Lung Cancer Version 1. 2018. 2017. Available at: https://www.nccn.org/.
51. Detterbeck FC. Management of carcinoid tumors. Ann Thorac Surg 2010;89(3): 998–1005.
52. Fjallskog ML, Granberg DP, Welin SL, et al. Treatment with cisplatin and etoposide in patients with neuroendocrine tumors. Cancer 2001;92(5):1101–7.
53. Ekeblad S, Sundin A, Janson ET, et al. Temozolomide as monotherapy is effective in treatment of advanced malignant neuroendocrine tumors. Clin Cancer Res 2007;13(10):2986–91.
54. Saranga-Perry V, Morse B, Centeno B, et al. Treatment of metastatic neuroendocrine tumors of the thymus with capecitabine and temozolomide: a case series. Neuroendocrinology 2013;97(4):318–21.
55. Kotteas EA, Syrigos KN, Saif MW. Profile of capecitabine/temozolomide combination in the treatment of well-differentiated neuroendocrine tumors. Onco Targets Ther 2016;9:699–704.

56. Strosberg JR, Fine RL, Choi J, et al. First-line chemotherapy with capecitabine and temozolomide in patients with metastatic pancreatic endocrine carcinomas. Cancer 2011;117(2):268–75.

57. Saif MW, Kaley K, Brennan M, et al. A retrospective study of capecitabine/temozolomide (CAPTEM) regimen in the treatment of metastatic pancreatic neuroendocrine tumors (pNETs) after failing previous therapy. JOP 2013;14(5):498–501.

58. Fine RL, Gulati AP, Krantz BA, et al. Capecitabine and temozolomide (CAPTEM) for metastatic, well-differentiated neuroendocrine cancers: the pancreas center at Columbia University experience. Cancer Chemother Pharmacol 2013;71(3): 663–70.

59. Gaur P, Leary C, Yao JC. Thymic neuroendocrine tumors: a SEER database analysis of 160 patients. Ann Surg 2010;251:1117–21.

60. Jia R, Sulentic P, Xu JM, et al. Thymic neuroendocrine neoplasms: biological behaviour and therapy. Neuroendocrinology 2017;105(2):105–14.

61. Masaoka A, Monden Y, Nakahara K, et al. Follow-up study of thymomas with special reference to their clinical stages. Cancer 1981;48:2485–92.

The Genesis of the Neuroendocrine Tumors Concept: From Oberndorfer to 2018

Kjell Öberg, MD, PhD

KEYWORDS

- NET • Biomarker • Imaging • Somatostatin analogues • Chemotherapy • PRRT
- Targeted agents

KEY POINTS

- Immunohistochemistry with specific antibodies for recognizing the neuroendocrine phenotype was introduced in the 1970s and 80s (chromogranin A, synaptophysin).
- The World Health Organization classification system established in 2000 was upgraded in 2004; 2010; and, finally, in 2017.
- Ki-67 was instituted as a reliable proliferation marker for neuroendocrine tumors (NETs) during the last decades.
- Plasma chromogranin A was confirmed as a general tumor marker over the past decades.
- Somatostatin analogues were developed in the early 1980s and have remained as the main therapy for treatment of hormone-related syndromes in NETs.

INTRODUCTION

The concept of neuroendocrine tumors (NETs) started to develop in the early 1900s with a description of carcinoid tumors by Oberndorfer[1] in 1907; followed by specific cytotoxic agents (streptozotocin); and, finally, the identification of somatostatin as a central regulator in neuroendocrine cell physiology but also an inhibitor of clinical symptoms related to NETs. The diagnosis of a NET was further confirmed by the World Health Organization (WHO) classification systems, which were introduced in 2000, and refined in 2010 and 2017. Histopathology now included immunohistochemistry with specific antibodies and chromogranin A was established as a general marker for NETs, both in cytochemistry and in circulation, working as a biomarker. The imaging was further refined during the 1980s and 1990s with the introduction of molecular imaging, first with somatostatin receptor (SSTR) scintigraphy and later with PET using

Disclosure Statement: No disclosure.
Department of Endocrine Oncology, Uppsala University Hospital, Entrance 40:5, SE-75185, Uppsala, Sweden
E-mail address: kjell.oberg@medsci.uu.se

Endocrinol Metab Clin N Am 47 (2018) 711–731
https://doi.org/10.1016/j.ecl.2018.05.003
0889-8529/18/© 2018 Elsevier Inc. All rights reserved.

endo.theclinics.com

gallium (Ga) labeled radiochemicals. Somatostatin analogues were introduced in the early 1980s for treatment of patients with clinical symptoms related to NETs, such as carcinoid syndrome, and are still the leading agents for controlling clinical symptoms from NETs related to hormone production. New therapies were developed during the last 2 decades, including peptide receptor radiotherapy (PRRT) and targeted agents, and were evaluated in prospective randomized controlled trials. The combination of progress in diagnoses and treatment of NETs established the current concept of NETs. The increasing interest in these tumors, which were previously suggested to be rare, is shown in their increased incidence and prevalence. Friedrich Feyter[2] introduced the concept of the diffuse endocrine cell system, recognizing the regulatory system of internal control of various body functions. Between 1960 and 1970, the true NET-concept was established with the development of radioimmunoassays for peptides and hormones, and imaging with computerized tomography (CT) was introduced in clinics.

THE EARLY DAYS AND ATTEMPTS TO UNDERSTAND THE REGULATION OF ORGAN AND BODY FUNCTIONS

Based on research in the 1860s and 1870s, Ivan Pavlov[3–5] (1849–1936) introduced the concept of nervism in 1883. His work on dogs supported his theory that the nervous system plays a dominant role in the regulation of all body functions. As late as 1935, when endocrine cells were already detected and discussed, he wrote that the more developed the nervous system becomes in an animal, the more centralized it is, and the more its highest division acts as a director and distributor of all functions of the organism. Although revolutionary, Pavlov's[3–5] work was incomplete in his failure to recognize the effect of the endocrine system in the regulation of organs. William Bayliss (1860–1924) and Ernest Starling[6] (1866–1927), challenged the concept of nervism. In a series of experiments conducted on the small intestines of animals, they demonstrated that agents in the blood could be responsible for pancreatic secretion. Based on this observation by Bayliss and Starling[6] (1902), the concept of hormones and secretin stimulated an extensive research to find the cells responsible for releasing these chemical messengers. In 1867, Paul Langerhans (1847–1888), a German pathologist and physiologist, discovered a previously unrecognized clusters of pancreatic cells embedded within sheets of acinar cells.[7] Although Langerhans recognized these as novel structures, he did not identify their endocrine function. Édouard Laguesse (1861–1927), a French pathologist, studied these pancreatic cell clusters, postulated that they produce an internal secretion, and coined the term, islets of Langerhans. In 1922, 30 years later, Frederick Banting (1891–1941) and Charles Best[8] (1899–1978) discovered the secretion of the hormone called insulin from these islets.[9] Enterochromaffin (EC) cells in the gastric mucosa of rabbits and dogs were first described in 1870 by Rudolf Peter Heidenhain[10] (1834–1897). He noted that the cells contained acidophilic granules and, 2 years later, he identified small granular yellow staining cells on the surface of gastric glands that are now understood to be histamine-secreting EC-like (ECL) cells. In 1891, Adolphe Nikolas[11] (1861–1939) reported the wide distribution of EC cells throughout the gastrointestinal (GI) tract. In 1897, Nikolai Kulchitsky[12] (1856–1925) noted similar cells with granules with acidophilic properties in the crypts of Lieberkühn and intestinal mucosa of cats and dogs. He noticed that the cells had something to do with digestion. In 1906, Ciaccio[13] identified the same cell type in the GI tract of humans and coined the term EC cells. In 1914, André Gosset (1872–1944) and Pierre Masson[14] (1880–1959) described argentaffin silver staining of the cells and tumors developing from these cell systems, and outlined the existence of a diffuse endocrine system. In 1938, Friedrich Feyter[2] (1895–1973), described the helle Zellen (clear cells) of the pancreas and GI tract, and proposed the concept of a diffuse neuroendocrine cell system with the integration of the gut within a neural and endocrine frame work. The concept facilitated the development of neuroendocrinology, integrating 2 previously separate distinct philosophies of neural and hormonal regulation. A paradigm shift of organ function and regulation based on a diffuse neuroendocrine regulatory system was suggested. Feyter[2] also proposed an integrated effect to a system at the cellular level (paracrine, neurocrine, and endocrine regulation) and provided the basis for the investigation and advances of much of the twentieth century gut and neuroendocrine physiology and biology.

Building on the theory of the diffuse neuroendocrine cell system by Feyter,[2] A.G.E. Pearse[15] (1915–2003) developed the amine precursor uptake and decarboxylation (APUD) concept, linking together endocrine cells with common cytochemical characteristics. The APUD concept suggested that all neuroendocrine cells are APUD cells. Pearse[15] postulated that they derive from the neural crest. However, the neural crest origin of the diffuse neuroendocrine system proved to be wrong and has been replaced by the concept of the endodermal origin of the neuroendocrine cells of the GI tract.[16]

OBERNDORFER AND THE CARCINOID DISEASE

At the same time as the gastroenteropancreatic (GEP) neuroendocrine cell system was described, a German pathologist reported a series of unusual tumors. Siegfried Oberndorfer (1876–1944) recognized the difference between cancerous tumors of the ileocolonic junction (carcinomas) and a group of more benign-behaving lesions of the ileum (carcinoids). Oberndorfer first presented his observation on carcinoid tumors at the German Pathologic Society Convention in Dresden, Germany, 1907. In December of the same year, he published a similar article titled "*Carcinoid Tumors of the Small Intestine*" in the *Frankfurt Journal of Pathology*.[1] This article was the first to describe and characterize the tumor that previously had been referred to as a carcinoma; it was based on 6 similar cases with multiple pea-sized tumors. Oberndorfer used the term karzinoide (carcinoma-like) because at that time he considered these lesions as benign and not malignant tumors. In 1928, he revised this observation in a review indicating that these small intestinal tumors could be malignant and metastasize.[17] However, Oberndorfer was not the first to describe these small intestinal tumors. Before his observation, Theodor Langhans[18] (1839–1915) in Germany (1867), Otto Lubarsch[19] (1860–1933) in Germany (1888), and William B Ransom[20] (1860–1909) in England (1890) had all commented on similar lesions in the small intestine. Ransom[20] described a 50-year-old woman who presented with 2 egg-sized lumps in the lower part of the abdomen with severe diarrhea. The diarrhea persisted for 2 years, during which time she presented with a large abdominal mass and cachexia. Particularly interesting was the observation of severe attacks of flushing after eating, which might be the first reported presentation of the carcinoid syndrome.[20] The death autopsy revealed several small nodules in the ileum. That the EC cell is the cell of origin for carcinoid tumors was strongly argued by Friedrich Feyter[2] in 1938. EC cells were chemically active and Alden B. Dawson[21] (1948) developed a technique (silver nitrate) for staining of EC and ECL cells. The same year, serotonin was isolated and described by Rapport and colleagues.[22] In 1953, Lembeck[23] biochemically confirmed the presence of serotonin in an ileal carcinoid tumor, confirming the assumption that human EC cells contain this bioactive amine. In 1952, Biörck and colleagues[24] established the relationship of carcinoid heart disease to carcinoid tumors and the secretion of serotonin. In 1954, B. Pernow and J. Waldenström[25] added that paroxysmal flushing was part of the syndrome. I.A. Oates and colleagues[26] demonstrated the release of kallikrein from some carcinoid tumors. In 1986, Norheim and colleagues[27] published the concept that tachykinins in carcinoid tumors were possibly involved in the carcinoid flush. In 1956, B.J. Haverback and A. Sjoerdsma[28] reported on the presence of the serotonin metabolite 5-hydroxyindoleacetic acid in the urine.

THE NEUROENDOCRINE CELL CONCEPT AND NEUROENDOCRINE TUMORS

The second NET to be described after recognition of the carcinoid tumor was an insulin-producing tumor, described in 1927 by Wilder and colleagues,[29] who presented a case with hypoglycemia and a pancreatic tumor. The hepatic metastases were shown to express insulin. In 1935, 157 cases of hyperinsulinism and islet cell tumors were reported by Whipple,[30] who presented the well-known Whipple triad, symptoms of hypoglycemia with low plasma glucose, and symptoms relieved after glucose infusion. In 1955, Robert Zollinger and Edvin Ellison[31] described 2 cases with intractable abdominal pain, diarrhea, jejunal ulceration, and gastric hypersecretion that failed multiple surgical procedures. The syndrome, recognized as the triad of primary peptic ulceration in an unusual location, gastric hypersecretion, and the presence of a nonspecific islet cell tumor of the pancreas, was named the Zollinger-Ellison syndrome in 1956.[32] In 1967, J.R.P. Gregory and colleagues[33] identified a substance in the pancreatic tumor in patients with the Zollinger-Ellison syndrome that might be responsible for the gastric ulcerations. After injection of extracts from a Zollinger-Ellison-associated pancreatic tumor in 2 fasting dogs, they observed prolonged acid secretory response resembling the response induced by gastrin, which was isolated and identified as a major acid-producing hormone by S. Komarov[34] in 1942. In 1968, McGuigan and Trudeau[35] developed a radioimmunoassay technique to measure serum gastrin levels that confirmed gastrin to be the hormone responsible for the clinical syndrome. In 1958, Verner and Morrison[36] described in 2 patients a syndrome that included diarrhea, hypokalemia, hypochlorhydria, and metabolic acidosis. The syndrome was also called watery diarrhea, hypokalemia, achlorhydria and vipoma syndrome, and the responsible hormone was found to be vasoactive intestinal polypeptide (VIP).

The glucagonoma syndrome was first reported by Becker[37] in a patient with skin rash associated with pancreatic tumor in 1942. In 1966, McGavran and colleagues[38] reported the first case of a patient with the glucagonoma syndrome who had elevated plasma immunoreactive glucagon levels, diabetes mellitus, skin rash, and a pancreatic NET. In 1974, Mallinson and colleagues[39] reported the association of the skin rash with hyperglucagonemia, diabetes mellitus, unexplained weight loss, and thromboembolism.

A somatostatinoma was first described in 1977; since then approximately 6 cases per year have been reported. They are the fifth most common NETs in the pancreas but they are more commonly located in the duodenum. The clinical symptoms are sometimes diffuse but might include diabetes and gall bladder stones.[40,41]

INHERITED FORMS OF NEUROENDOCRINE TUMORS

Although most NETs are sporadic, multiple inherited syndromes associated with NETs exist, including multiple endocrine neoplasia (MEN) types 1 and 2, von Hippel-Lindau (VHL) disease, neurofibromatosis 1 (NF1), and tuberous sclerosis. In 1903, J. Erdheim[42] was the first to describe a patient with tumors in 2 different endocrine organs (pituitary and parathyroid tumors). In 1953, L. Underdahl and colleagues[43] published 8 cases featuring tumors in the pituitary, parathyroids, and pancreatic islets. In 1954, Paul Wermer[44] was the first to report that the cases reported by Underdahl and colleagues[43] must be genetic disorders with autosomal dominant inheritance (MEN1) or Wermer syndrome. It was not until 1988 that the research group of Larsson and colleagues[45] (including the current author) localized the gene to chromosome 11q13. Finally, in 1997, the group at the National Institutes of Health isolated the gene, a tumor suppressor.[46] In 1959, J.H. Sipple[47] reported on an association between carcinoma of the thyroid and pheochromocytoma. In 1987, the causative gene was mapped to chromosome 10, the receptor tyrosinekinase gene protooncogene.[48,49] In 1904, Eugen von Hippel[50] first described retinal angiomas. In 1927, David Vilhelm Lindau[51] described hemangiomas of the central nervous system. VHL disease includes hemangioblastomas, clear cell renal carcinoma, pancreatic NETs, pheochromocytomas, and endolymphatic sac tumors of the middle ears. The VHL gene is a tumor suppressor gene located on chromosome 3p 25–26.

In 1882, Friedrich Daniel von Recklinghausen[52] first described NF1, which is characterized by neurofibromas, pheochromocytomas, and periampullary somatostatinomas. The NF1 gene is located on chromosome 17q11.2. Tuberous sclerosis complex (TSC) is a multisystem autosomal dominant disease described by D.M. Bourneville[53] (1880) that includes pancreatic NET. TSC is caused by mutations in 2 genes TSC1 (chr 9q39) and TSC2 (chromosome 16p13.3). The mutations result in an upregulation of the phosphoinositide 3-kinase–serine kinase–mammalian target of rapamycin (mTOR) pathway.

THE NEW ERA OF DIAGNOSTICS AND TREATMENT OF NEUROENDOCRINE TUMORS (1960–2018)
Progress in Diagnostics

Before 1970, NETs were considered an extremely rare condition and generated very little interest in the surgical, oncological, or endocrinological community. The recognition that the GI tract contained plenty of endocrine cells, producing more than 50 peptides and amines, started a rally in gut physiology, as well as NETs. The development of specific antibodies to secreted peptides from the endocrine cells of the GI tract has been fundamental for the development of the field. Key persons in the development of specific antibodies to GI peptides were Professor Victor Mutt and K. Tatemoto[54] at the Karolinska institute in Sweden. By boiling tons of pig intestines, they could extract small amounts of a large number of different peptides (VIP, gastric inhibitory peptide, gastrin-releasing peptide, cholecystokinin, gastrin, peptide YY, pancreastatin, neuropeptide Y, neuropeptide K) (**Fig. 1**), which were distributed to various research centers globally, where they developed specific antibodies. These specific antibodies were not only a prerequisite for the development of specific radioimmunoassays and enzyme-linked immunosorbent assays (ELISAs) for measurement of different peptides and hormones in the plasma but also for immunohistochemistry for the pathologist to clarify the content of different peptides and hormones in NETs. In 1960, the development of radioimmunoassays by Rosalyn Yalow and Solomon Berson[55] (for which they were awarded the 1977 Nobel Prize) was a very important step for diagnosing NETs. During later decades, several new peptides and amines were isolated (**Fig. 2**). These amines and peptides identified in the circulation served as biomarkers for the detection and follow-up of NETs during treatment. In the early 1970 to 1980s, much work by researchers was devoted to the detailed profiling of cells with endocrine properties disposed in different organs. These efforts resulted in the definition of at least 14 cell types in the GI tract. The identification of novel hormones and peptides were

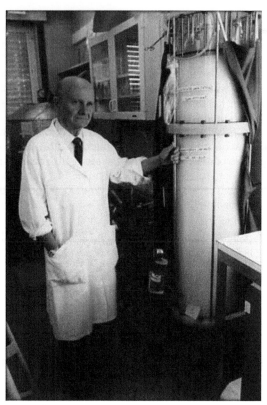

Fig. 1. Professor Viktor Mutt of Karolinska Institute, who has been instrumental in the isolation of gut peptides or hormones.

based on immunohistochemical techniques on tissue samples or at the ultrastructural level by the use of a transmission electron microscope for looking at size and the forms of secretory granules. Important contributions to these studies were made by Steven Bloom and colleagues[56] at the Hamersmith Hospital, London, and Rolf Hakanson and colleagues[57] at Lunds University, Sweden. Similar techniques were applied to tumor specimens, which made it possible to define subtypes of NETs in different organs, showing that these tumors present a family of malignant diseases with different localization, clinical presentation, and biological behavior.[58–60] In the beginning of the 1980s, silver impregnation techniques were still in use because they were cheap and effective[61] but were later replaced by specific antibodies and immunocytochemistry. Chromogranin A and synaptophysin were identified and became reliable and effective markers of neuroendocrine differentiation.[62–64] Chromogranin A is localized in large dense core granules in neuroendocrine cells, whereas synaptophysin is located in small synaptic vesicles.

In the 1980s, there was a specific classification of neoplasms of the diffuse endocrine system of the gut, including the carcinoid.[65] Classification was separated from a similar classification for the pancreatic tumors. These 2 classification systems were combined and formed the basis for the WHO classification system in 2000.[66] The major novelty of this concept was that the tumors were different at different anatomic sites, depending on the tumor cell type. The tumors were defined as

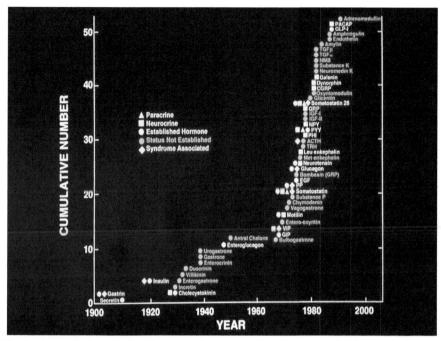

Fig. 2. The explosion of identified peptides in the gut and pancreas thanks to specific antibodies and radioimmunoassay's.

well-differentiated endocrine tumors or endocrine carcinomas, the most malignant being the poorly differentiated endocrine carcinomas. This classification system was later refined in the 2010 WHO classification system,[67] which introduced a grading system: grade (G)1, G2, and G3, based on proliferation capacity of the tumor cells according to the Ki-67 index and mitotic count.[68] Ki-67, or MIB-1, is an antibody that recognizes tumor cells in proliferation.[69,70] This antibody was first introduced in 1992 by Chaudhry and colleagues[71] (including the current author) in Uppsala in a small series of subjects with various types of NETs. After its discovery, it took almost 10 years to be widely accepted as a proliferation marker for NETs. Worldwide, it was introduced into clinical use by the European Neuroendocrine Society (ENETS).[72] Later, it was picked up by the WHO for the 2010 classification.[67] Currently, staining for Ki-67 in tumor specimens is required at all centers and continues to form the basis for the 2017 WHO classification system[73] (**Fig. 3**). Furthermore, a specific staging system has been developed using the classic tumor-node-metastases (TNM) scheme.[72] Important key points currently in the diagnosis of NETs are the WHO classification system and the TNM staging, which form the basis for decision of treatment. The WHO 2017 classification is similar to the 2010 classification system but has now introduced a new group of tumors. NET-G3 with a proliferation greater than 20% (Ki-67) is not as malignant as the NEC-G3 with higher proliferation, usually greater than 50%. This new classification with a new group of tumors will refine the future treatment of patients with NETs.[73] To further refine the diagnoses and management of patients with NETs, the application of high-throughput molecular techniques for molecular profiling will be an important adjunct in selecting the right treatment for the patient. A better understanding of the molecular events leading to neuroendocrine cancer development is still needed, specifically those driving invasion and metastases.[74–76]

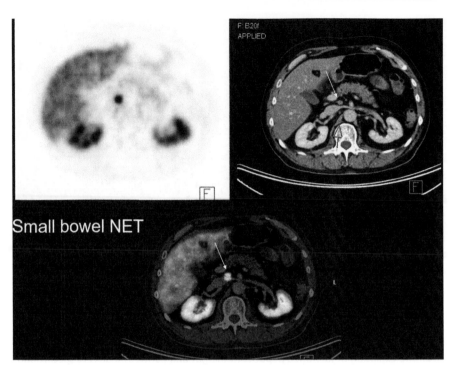

Fig. 3. Ga-68-DOTATOC-PET imaging of patients with small intestinal NETs (NETs). Localization of the primary tumor.

In parallel with the improvement in histopathology and immunohistochemistry, many specific radioimmunoassays for the measurement of the different peptide hormones and amines in the circulation were developed. Many patients with NETs, particularly in the pancreas but even at other locations, required analysis of all the different well-known hormones and peptides found in normal cells in these organs. It can be very expensive, and the radioimmunoassays and ELISAs are not specific because the tumors have the capacity to modify the secreted peptides and hormones at the genetic level, and the product circulating is not recognized by the current radioimmunoassay. Some tumors can use different splice variants of the hormone; the most well-known is gastrin, which may appear in 4 to 5 different forms in the circulation.[77] The clinically available radioimmunoassays could not detect some of the variants. The search for a general marker was ongoing during the 1980s, similar to the general tumor marker in immunohistochemistry (chromogranin A). The first publication on a radioimmunoassay for chromogranin A was in 1986 by O'Connor and Deftos.[78] In 1989, Eriksson and colleagues[79] (including the current author) managed to establish the first chromogranin A assay in Europe. Rapidly, several commercial radioimmunoassays were developed for its use in patients with NETs. This protein became the most important general tumor marker over the years. Recently, pitfalls have been discussed with regard to the nonspecificity of chromogranin A assays; nevertheless, it is the work horse of the management and follow-up of patients with NETs. Other general biomarkers include pancreatic polypeptide, neuron-specific enolase, and beta-human chorionic gonadotropin subunits.[80] Currently, chromogranin A and NSE are the most applied general biomarkers for NETs. NSE has a special role in patients with more malignant tumors and, particularly, lung NETs. Recently, measurements of circulating DNA and tumor cell RNA cells are under development in clinical practice in patients with NETs.[81] One commercial test, the NETest, is now in clinical trials with promising results.[82] The NETest measures 56 gene transcripts by measuring RNA in the circulation. The preliminary data indicate that it might outperform current available biomarkers, such as chromogranin A and NSE.

Progress in Imaging

A new era in diagnosis and follow-up of patients with NETs started during the 1970s. When CT was developed, it was the beginning of a new radiological era. The technique was developed by Godfrey Hounsfield,[83] who received the 1979 Nobel Prize in physiology and medicine in for his invention. The CT technique has been improved over the years. Spiral (helical CT) has been the standard technique for many years and modern multidetector (MD)-CT scanners are currently available in most radiology departments. MD-CT techniques allow the use of intravenous contrast media with acquisition of several contrast-enhancement phases. CT scanning is currently the standard radiology method for diagnosis and follow-up of NETs.[84] Other techniques, such as ultrasonography of the abdomen and MRI, are also used in the diagnosis and follow-up of NET patients. MRI is building on the phenomenon of nuclear spin resonance that has been known since the 1940s. However, it was not until the 1970s that the imaging technique started to be developed. In the 1980s it was implemented into health care. The chemist Paul Lauterbur[85] and the physician Peter Mansfield[86] developed the technique for clinical use and received the 2003 Nobel Prize in physiology and medicine. For imaging of the abdomen, bone, and brain, MRI is generally better than CT and is, therefore, preferred if available. It may also be complementary to a CT investigation. The MRI technique has been improved during the last decades and the current available scanners have high field strengths, generally between 1.5 T and 3 T. Diffusion-weighted imaging (DWI) is an MRI technique that is receiving much attention in oncology. DWI offers high lesion-to-background contrast for tumor imaging, including NETs. No contrast administration is needed.[87]

Radiolabeled peptides have been used for targeting specific receptors on NETs for more than 20 years.[88] The overexpression of peptide receptors in various tumor cells opened a new chapter in molecular imaging. Somatostatin analogues labeled with different radionuclides is an example of these peptides that have been used with high efficiency in the diagnosis of NETs. The first radiolabeled somatostatin analogue approved for scintigraphy of NET was indium (In)-111, DTPA-octreotide (Octreoscan), which was introduced by Eric Krenning and colleagues[89] in 1989. Clinical results have demonstrated that this radiopharmaceutical is ideally suited for localizing primary, as well as metastatic, NETs. The next-generation somatostatin analogues, DOTATOC, DOTATATE, and DOTANOC, were developed and labeled with different radionuclides (Ga-68, yttrium [Y]-90, lutetium [Lu]-177) for imaging, as well as for therapy.[90,91] DOTATATE showed the highest affinity for the SSTR2 and became the standard.[92,93] The next developments were the third-generation somatostatin analogues, such as DOTANOC, which improved affinity for SSTR2, as well as for SSTR3 and SSTR4.[91] To further improve molecular imaging, single-photon emission CT-PET was developed during the 1980s and 1990s. There is a clear superiority of PET-imaging compared with imaging by gamma camera.[94] Therefore, currently, Ga-68–labeled DOTATATE-TOC-NOC is the standard of care for patients with NETs and is now replacing the old In-111 (Octreoscan) (see **Fig. 3**). 18F-fluorodeoxyglucose (FDG) is also an important radiopharmaceutical for imaging of NETs, particularly those of higher grade.[95] Other agents with high sensitivity and specificity for NETs are 18F-LDOPAMIN and C11-5-hydroxytryptophan.[96,97] Sometimes there are mixtures or subclones of tumor cells with different tumor biology and expression of SSTRs. Therefore, it has been increasingly common to combine FDG and Ga-68 PET-scans. Hybrid imaging is currently the standard with combined machines, both PET-CT scan and MRI, to obtain better anatomic localization.

Development and Advances in Neuroendocrine Cell Therapy

Surgery is the cornerstone in the management of patients with NETs (**Fig. 4**). In patients with localized disease, curative surgery can be performed. However, more than 50% of the patients present with metastatic disease and, therefore, most patients cannot be cured by surgery. Nevertheless, during the last decades, more extensive surgery has emerged using local resection, debulking procedures, and radiofrequency ablations. Currently, more patients undergo surgery to improve clinical symptoms and to facilitate forthcoming medical or radioactive treatment.[98] Surgery is not specifically discussed in this article.

Chemotherapy has been attempted in the treatment of patients with NETs since the early 1960s. Streptozotocin, an alkylating agent, has been used since 1968 when Murray-Lyon and colleagues[99] reported improvement in hypoglycemic symptoms and tumor load in a malignant pancreatic NET. The US Food and Drug Administration approved the use of streptozotocin for islet cell carcinoma in 1982. Other past-generation cytotoxic DNA damaging agents are 5-fluorouracil (5FU) and doxorubicin, which have been tried with rather low efficacy.[100,101] Combinations of 5FU or doxorubicin with streptozotocin have demonstrated significant efficacy in pancreatic NETs.[102,103] Temozolomide is an alkylating agent that shares its active metabolite with dacarbazine with rapid penetration through the blood–brain barrier. It was first introduced for treatment of gliomas and malignant melanoma in the early 2000s. The first patient with NET treated with temozolomide in the author's department was in 1999; the patient had recurrent brain metastases from a thymic NET after conventional radiotherapy of the brain.[104] Temozolomide has been used as a single drug but currently it is most commonly used in combination with capecitabine, with promising results in pancreatic NETs.[105–107] For patients with poorly differentiated NETs or high-grade tumors with a proliferation (Ki-67) greater than 50%, cisplatinum-carboplatin plus etoposide has been the standard of care and is still considered

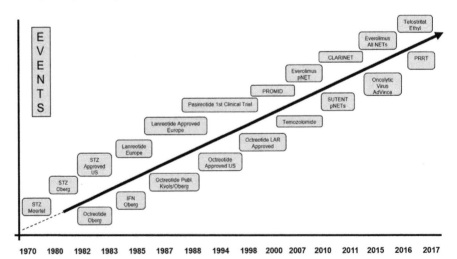

Fig. 4. Development of therapies for NETs over the last decades.

first-line treatment.[108] Temozolomide plus capecitabine has been used as second-line therapy in NEC-G3.[109]

Somatostatin and Its Analogues

Biotherapy for NETs emerged in the 1980s, and somatostatin analogues and interferons were investigated in small series of subjects with malignant carcinoid syndrome[110,111] (**Fig. 5**). Native human somatostatin is a cyclic peptide hormone that exists in 2 natural forms consisting of 14 and 28 amino-acids. It is widely distributed in multiple tissues, including the central nervous system, pancreas, and GI tract. It has been involved in regulation of secretion in pancreatic and intestinal hormones, including gastrin, glucagon, and serotonin. The physiologic action of somatostatin is mediated through 5 subtypes of SSTRs (SSTR1–SSTR5), which belong to the family of G-protein couple receptors.[112,113] In 1908, Krulich and colleagues[114] isolated a substance with an action on the release of pituitary growth hormone (GH) from rat hypothalamus and called it growth hormone-release inhibitory factor (GH-RIF). In 1969, Hellman and Lernmark[115] reported on the presence of a potent inhibitor of insulin secretion in extracts from pancreatic islets. Eventually, in 1973, GH-RIF was isolated and purified from 500,000 sheep hypothalamus by Brazeau and colleagues,[116] using a new in vitro assay. This factor was named somatostatin and, shortly after its discovery, the structure of somatostatin was solved, which allowed it to be purified and synthesized.[117] The discovery of somatostatin and its effects was rewarded with the Nobel Prize in 1977 to Roger Guillemin and Andrew Schally, the same year as Rosalyn Yalow and Solomon Berson[55] received the prize for the development of radioimmunoassays. Native somatostatin is rapidly cleared in the circulation due to enzymatic cleavage, which limits its clinical utility. In 1978, Vale and colleagues[118] reported on an octapeptide analogue that displayed the full biological activity of somatostatin.

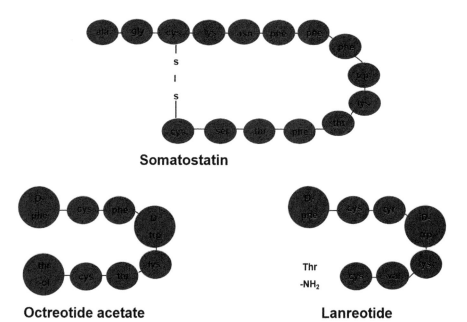

Fig. 5. Somatostatin and its analogues: clinical practice that has revolutionized the treatment of symptoms but also inhibition of tumor growth.

From 1980 to 1982, Bauer and colleagues,[119] at Sandoz, synthesized an analogue named octreotide. Shortly thereafter, other companies and research institutes became interested in somatostatin analogues and produced several other analogues, such as lanreotide and RC160, and, most recently, SOM230 (pasireotide) by Novartis. Five SSTR subtypes (SSTR1–SSTR5) have been identified by gene cloning techniques.[113] These subtypes present different binding affinity to specific somatostatin analogues, an important characteristic relevant to imaging and therapeutics. In 1987, Reubi and colleagues[120] reported on the expression of SSTR2 in NETs. In 1982, the author's group received the first analogue octreotide, which rapidly became accepted in clinical practice for treatment of severe clinical symptoms related to NETs, such as carcinoid syndrome, Verner-Morrison syndrome, and glucagonoma syndrome.[121] Since then, the synthetic analogues of somatostatin, octreotide, and lanreotide have proven to be excellent treatments to control the symptoms from NETs and are convenient to administer.[121] Over the past decades, long-acting formulations of octreotide (Octreotide LAR), as well as lanreotide (Somatuline Autogel), were developed and became standard therapies for symptomatic NETs. In recent years, strong evidence has emerged that somatostatin analogues can inhibit the growths of NETs. The tumor activity can occur via direct or indirect mechanisms. Direct mechanism involves the binding of somatostatin analogues to SSTRs on tumor cells, leading to activation of intracellular signaling transaction pathways. Indirect antiproliferative mechanisms include inhibitor of circulating growth factors, such as vascular endothelial growth factor (VEGF), and insulin-like growth factor, as well as inhibition of tumor angiogenesis through interaction with SSTRs on the endothelial cells.[122] The definitive evidence of the antiproliferative effect of somatostatin analogues emerged with the PROMID trial, the first randomized placebo-controlled study performed in small intestinal carcinoids,[123] published in 2009. Later, a randomized placebo-controlled study in nonfunctional NETs with long-acting lanreotide (Somatuline Autogel) confirmed the results in small intestinal NETs (carcinoids) and in pancreatic NETs.[124] Pasireotide is a novel somatostatin analogue that binds to 4 out of 5 SSTRs: 1, 2, 3, and 5. This analogue has been evaluated in patients with carcinoid tumors that were resistant to standard doses of octreotide, and showed improvement of flushing and diarrhea. However, in a randomized trial these data could not be confirmed and this somatostatin analogue is currently on hold for this indication.[125]

Interferon alpha was first introduced for treatment of small intestinal NETs in 1983 by the author's group.[126] Single-arm studies have supported objective tumor responses in up to 10% of the subjects, biochemical responses in about 50% of the subjects, and stabilization of the disease.[127] Interferons activate the STAT complexes, including the JAK-STAT signaling pathway, leading to signaling cascades involving the tumor cell and the host immune system. It stimulates dendritic cell proliferation or differentiation, and demonstrates inhibition of angiogenesis and exerts a direct antiproliferative effect on tumor growth through induction of cell cycle arrest.[128] Combinations of interferon alpha plus somatostatin analogues were reported in the 1990s, demonstrating additional antitumor activity but, more importantly, a reduction of interferon's side effects.[129,130] Interferon is currently usually used as a second-line treatment after somatostatin analogues for treatment of patients with G1 tumors with proliferation (Ki-67 <5%).

Peptide Receptor Radiotherapy

Based on the frequent expression of SSTR2 in GEP NETs, especially in well-differentiated NETs, and the demonstration of the ability to image this expression using radiolabeled peptide, it was a logical extension to consider treatment. Over the past 2 decades, several different radiolabeled somatostatin analogues have been used. The first treatment was published in 1994 by the Rotterdam group using In-111-DTPA-octreotide at high doses.[131] Y-90 and Lu-177 DOTA-octreotide, as well as DOTATOC-TATE, have been evaluated in multiple phase II clinical trials over the last decades.[132–135] Currently, PRRT with somatostatin analogues is an established treatment based on a new randomized controlled trial (NETTER-1) with lutetium-DOTATATE versus high-dose octreotide (Octreotide LAR) for patients with small intestinal NETs in whom PRRT demonstrated significant superiority.[136] In 2017, lutetium-DOTATATE became registered as Lutathera for treatment in Europe and it will become registered globally in 2018 for treatment of malignant metastatic GEP NETs.

Targeted Therapies

A better understanding of the mechanisms driving secretion and tumor growths in NETs has led to the development of several so-called targeted antitumor agents. The mTOR pathway has a central role in controlling functions and integrating multiple signaling pathways in response to growth factors, including cell growth, proliferation, and angiogenesis.[137,138] Inhibiting the mTOR pathway may reduce cell growth and proliferation, and reduce the metastatic potential of tumor cells. Angiogenesis is a very important regulation of tumor growth in NETs mediated via tyrosine kinase receptors, such as VEGF receptor-alpha, platelet-derived growth factor, KIT, and RET. VEGF-driven angiogenesis may play an important role in NET developed and tumor progression.[139] In NET, mTOR inhibitors and angiogenesis inhibitors have been extensively studied. The clinical value of temsirolimus and everolimus, inhibitors of the mTOR pathway, have been evaluated in different subsets of NETs. The first trial performed in pancreatic NETs (RADIANT-1) reported a significant antitumor effect,[140] which was later explored in the subsets of NETs, small intestinal NETs, and lung-NETs. In these trials, everolimus was combined with the somatostatin analogue octreotide (RADIANT-2 and RADIANT-3).[141,142] The RADIANT-4 study confirmed the antitumor efficacy of everolimus in patients with lung and small intestinal NETs.[143] Thereafter, in 2016, everolimus became registered worldwide for treatment of all types of NETs. Tyrosine kinase receptor inhibitors have been applied for treatment of pancreatic NET. Sunitinib, an oral multitargeted tyrosine kinase inhibitor, was evaluated in a phase III study showing significant antitumor efficacy compared with placebo.[144] Bevacizumab, an antibody against VEGF has been evaluated in combination with somatostatin analogues, systemic chemotherapy everolimus, and other drugs, and has demonstrated promising results.[145]

Telotristat ethyl is a newly registered agent for controlling diarrhea in patients with the carcinoid syndrome not controlled by somatostatin analogues. The agent blocks the enzyme tryptophan hydroxylase, which convert tryptophan to serotonin.[146]

Currently, several antitumor therapies in NETs exist based on several randomized controlled trials and, particularly in pancreatic NETs, there are several treatment options, such as chemotherapy, somatostatin analogues, targeted agents, and PRRT. For small intestinal NETs, the number of established therapies is smaller with somatostatin analogues, interferon, and PRRT. Currently, trials are ongoing to look at immunotherapy for patients with NETs, including oncolytic viruses, as well as PD1-antibodies, but no data are currently available .

REFERENCES

1. Oberndorfer S. Karzenoide tumoren des dünndarms. Frankf Z Pathol 1907;1: 426–32.

2. Feyter F. Ueber diffuse endokrine epithealiale organe. Zentralbl Innere Med 1938;545:31–41.
3. Pavlov I. Die innervation des pankreas. Germany: Klin Wochenzeitung; 1888. p. 667–75.
4. Pavlov I. Lectures on the work of digestive glands. London: Charles Griffin and Company; 1910.
5. Pavlov I. Poln Sobr Trudov 1940;1:410.
6. Bayliss WM, Starling EH. The mechanism of pancreatic secretion. J Physiol 1902;28:325–53.
7. Moorison H. Contributions to the microscopic anatomy of the pancreas. Baltimore: John Hopkins Press; 1869.
8. Banting FG, Best CH. The internal secretion of the pancreas. J Lab Clin Med 1922;251–66.
9. Sakura A. Paul Langerhans (1847-1888): a centenary tribute. J R Soc Med 1988; 81:414–5.
10. Heidenhain RP. Untersuchungen uber den Bau der Labdrusen. Arch Mikr Anat 1870;6:368.
11. Nikolas A. Recherches sur l'epithelium de l-intestin grele. Intern Monatssch Anat Physiol 1891;1.
12. Kulchitsky N. Zur Frage uber den Bau des Darmkanals. Arch Mikr Anat 1897;49: 7–35.
13. Ciaccio M. Sur une nouvelle espece cellulaire dans les glandes de Lieberkuhn. C R Seances Soc Biol Fil 1906;60:76–7.
14. Gosset A, Masson P. Tumeurs endocrines de l'appendice. Presse Med 1914;25: 237–9.
15. Pearse AG. 5-hydroxytroptophan uptake by dog thyroid "C"cells and its possible significance in polypeptide hormone production. Nature 1966;211:598–600.
16. Andrew A, Kramer B, Rawdon BB. The origin of gut and pancreatic neuroendocrine (APUD) cells–the last word? J Pathol 1998;186:117–8.
17. Oberndorfer S. Karzinoide handuch der speziellen. handbuch der speziellen pathologischen anatomie und histologie. Berlin: Springer; 1928. p. 814–47.
18. Langhans T. Uber einen Drusenpolyp im ileum. Virchows Arch Patohol Anat Physiol Klin Med 1867;38:550–60.
19. Lubarsch O. Uber dem primaren Krebs des ileum nebst bemerkukngen uber das gleichzeitige Vorkommen van krebs und tuberculose. Virchows Arch 1888;111:280–317.
20. Ransom W. A case of primary carcinoma of the ileum. Lancet 1890;2:1020–3.
21. Dawson A. Argentophile and argentaffin cells in gastric mucosa of rat. Anat Rec 1948;100(3):319–29.
22. Rapport M, Green A, Page I. Partial purification of the vasoconstrictor in beef serum. J Biol Chem 1948;174:735–41.
23. Lembeck F. 5-Hydroxytryptamine in carcinoid tumor. Nature 1953;172:910–1.
24. Biörck G, Axen O, Thorson A. Unusual cyanosis in a boy with congenital pulmonary stenosis and tricuspid insufficiency: fatal outcome after angiocardiography. Am Heart J 1952;44(1):143–8.
25. Pernow B, Waldenström J. Paroxysmal flushing and other symptoms caused by 5-hydroxytryptamine and histamine in patients with malignant tumours. Lancet 1954;267:951.
26. Oates JA, Melmon K, Sjoerdsma A, et al. Release of a kinin peptide in the carcinoid syndrome. Lancet 1964;1:514–7.

27. Norheim I, Theodorsson-Norheim E, Brodin E, et al. Tachykinins in carcinoid tumors: their use as a tumor marker and possible role in the carcinoid flush. J Clin Endocrinol Metab 1986;63:605–12.
28. Haverback BJ, Sjoerdsma A, Terry LL. Urinary excretion of the serotonin metabolite, 5-hydroxyindoleacetic acid, in various clinical conditions. N Engl J Med 1956;255:270–7.
29. Wilder RM, Allan FN, Power WH, et al. Carcinoma of the islands of the pancreas: Hyperinsulinism and hypoglycemia. JAMA 1927;89:348–55.
30. Whipple AO. Adenomas of the islet cells with hyperinsulinism. Ann Surg 1935; 101:1299.
31. Zollinger RM, Ellison EH. Primary peptic ulcerations of the jejunum associated with islet cell tumors of the pancreas. Ann Surg 1955;142:709–23 [discussion: 24–8].
32. Eiseman B, Maynard RM. A noninsulin producing islet cell adenoma associated with progressive peptic ulceration (the Zollinger-Ellison syndrome). Gastroenterology 1956;31(3).296–304.
33. Gregory RA, Grossman MI, Tracy HJ, et al. Nature of the gastric secretagogue in Zollinger-Ellison tumours. Lancet 1967;2:543–4.
34. Komarov S. Methods of isolation of a specific gastric secretagogue from the pyloric mucous membrane and its chemical properties. Rev Can Biol 1942;1: 191–207.
35. McGuigan JE, Trudeau WL. Immunochemical measurement of elevated levels of gastrin in the serum of patients with pancreatic tumors of the Zollinger-Ellison variety. N Engl J Med 1968;278:1308–13.
36. Verner JV, Morrison AB. Islet cell tumor and a syndrome of refractory watery diarrhea and hypokalemia. Am J Med 1958;25:374–80.
37. Becker ER. The Iowa Academy of Science. Science 1942;95:651–2.
38. McGavran MH, Unger RH, Recant L, et al. A glucagon-secreting alpha-cell carcinoma of the pancreas. N Engl J Med 1966;274:1408–13.
39. Mallinson CN, Cox B, Bloom SR. Proceedings: Plasma levels of amino acids and glucagon in patients with pancreatic glucagonomas. Gut 1974;15(4):340.
40. Ganda OP, Weir GC, Soeldner JS, et al. "Somatostatinoma": a somatostatin-containing tumor of the endocrine pancreas. N Engl J Med 1977;296:963–7.
41. Williamson J, Thorn C, Spalding D, et al. Pancreatic and peripancreatic somatostatinomas. Ann R Coll Surg Engl 2011;93:356–60.
42. Erdheim J. Zur normalen und pathologischen Histologie der Glandula thyreoidea, parathyroidea und Hypophysis. Beit Z Path Anat Z Allg Path 1903;158–236.
43. Underdahl LO, Woolner LB, Black BM. Multiple endocrine adenomas; report of 8 cases in which the parathyroids, pituitary and pancreatic islets were involved. J Clin Endocrinol Metab 1953;13:20–47.
44. Wermer P. Genetic aspects of adenomatosis of endocrine glands. Am J Med 1954;16:363–71.
45. Larsson C, Skogseid B, Oberg K, et al. Multiple endocrine neoplasia type 1 gene maps to chromosome 11 and is lost in insulinoma. Nature 1988;332:85–7.
46. Chandrasekharappa SC, Guru SC, Manickam P, et al. Positional cloning of the gene for multiple endocrine neoplasia-type 1. Science 1997;276:404–7.
47. Sipple J. The association of pheochromocytoma with carcinoma of the thyroid gland. Am J Med 1961;31:163–6.
48. Simpson NE, Kidd KK, Goodfellow PJ, et al. Assignment of multiple endocrine neoplasia type 2A to chromosome 10 by linkage. Nature 1987;328:528–30.

49. Mulligan LM, Kwok JB, Healey CS, et al. Germ-line mutations of the RET proto-oncogene in multiple endocrine neoplasia type 2A. Nature 1993;363:458–60.
50. von Hippel E. Über eine sehr seltene Erkrankung der Netzhaut. Albrecht Von Graefes Arch Ophthalmol 1904;59:83–106.
51. Lindau A. Zur frage der angiomatosis retinae und ihrer hirncomplikation. Acta Ophthal 1927;193–226.
52. von Recklinghausen F. Über die multiplen, fibrome der Haut und ihre beziehung zu den multiplen neuromen. Berlin: Festschrift für Rudolf Virchow; 1882.
53. Bourneville D. Contribution à l'étude del'idiotie; observation III: sclérose tubéreuse des circonvolutions cérébrales: idiotie et èpilepsie hémiplégique. Arch Neurol 1880;1:81–91.
54. Tatemoto K, Mutt V. Chemical determination of polypeptide hormones. Proc Natl Acad Sci U S A 1978;75:4115–9.
55. Yalow RS, Berson SA. Immunoassay of endogenous plasma insulin in man. J Clin Invest 1960;39:1157–75.
56. Bloom SR, Bryant MG, Polak JM. Proceedings: distribution of gut hormones. Gut 1975;16:821.
57. Hakanson R, Alumets J, Sundler F. Classification of peptide-hormone-producing cells. Lancet 1978;1:997.
58. Solcia E, Capella C, Buffa R, et al. Endocrine cells of the gastrointestinal tract and related tumors. Pathobiol Annu 1979;9:163–204.
59. Solcia E, Rindi G, Capella C. Histochemistry in pathology. In: Felipe MI, Lake BD, editors. New York: Churchill-Livingstone; 1990. p. 397–409.
60. Rindi G, Villanacci V, Ubiali A. Biological and molecular aspects of gastroenteropancreatic neuroendocrine tumors. Digestion 2000;62:19–26.
61. Grimelius L. A silver nitrate stain for alpha-2 cells in human pancreatic islets. Acta Soc Med Ups 1968;73:243–70.
62. Lloyd RV, Wilson BS. Specific endocrine tissue marker defined by a monoclonal antibody. Science 1983;222:628–30.
63. Lloyd RV, Mervak T, Schmidt K, et al. Immunohistochemical detection of chromogranin and neuron-specific enolase in pancreatic endocrine neoplasms. Am J Surg Pathol 1984;8:607–14.
64. Wiedenmann B, Huttner WB. Synaptophysin and chromogranins/secretogranins–widespread constituents of distinct types of neuroendocrine vesicles and new tools in tumor diagnosis. Virchows Arch B Cell Pathol Incl Mol Pathol 1989;58:95–121.
65. Williams E, Siebenmann R, Sobin L, editors. Types hystologiques des tumeurs endocriniennes. Geneve (Switzerland): Organisation mondiale de la santé; 1980.
66. Solcia E, Kloppel G, Sobin L. Histological typing of endocrine tumours. In: Verlag S, editor. World Health Organization histological classification of tumours. 2nd edition. New York: Springer; 2000. p. 38–74.
67. Bosman FT, Carneiro F. WHO classification of tumours, pathology and genetics of tumours of the digestive system. Lyon (France): IARC Press; 2010.
68. Rindi G, Arnold R, Capella C. Nomenclature and classification of digestive neuroendocrine tumours. In: Bosman F, Carneiro F, editors. Word Health Organization classification of tumours, pathology and genetics of tumours of teh digestive system. Lyon (France): IARC Press; 2010.
69. Dhall D, Mertens R, Bresee C, et al. Ki-67 proliferative index predicts progression-free survival of patients with well-differentiated ileal neuroendocrine tumors. Hum Pathol 2012;43:489–95.

70. Gerdes J, Schwab U, Lemke H, et al. Production of a mouse monoclonal antibody reactive with a human nuclear antigen associated with cell proliferation. Int J Cancer 1983;31:13–20.

71. Chaudhry A, Oberg K, Wilander E. A study of biological behavior based on the expression of a proliferating antigen in neuroendocrine tumors of the digestive system. Tumour Biol 1992;13:27–35.

72. Rindi G, Kloppel G, Alhman H, et al. TNM staging of foregut (neuro)endocrine tumors: a consensus proposal including a grading system. Virchows Arch 2006;449:395–401.

73. Lloyd R, Osamura R, Klöppel G, et al. 4th edition. WHO classification of tumours of endocrine organs, vol. 10. Lyon (France): International Agency for Research on Cancer; 2017. p. 210–39.

74. Jiao Y, Shi C, Edil BH, et al. DAXX/ATRX, MEN1, and mTOR pathway genes are frequently altered in pancreatic neuroendocrine tumors. Science 2011;331: 1199–203.

75. Banck MS, Kanwar R, Kulkarni AA, et al. The genomic landscape of small intestine neuroendocrine tumors. J Clin Invest 2013;123:2502–8.

76. Mafficini A, Scarpa A. Genomic landscape of pancreatic neuroendocrine tumours: the international cancer genome consortium. J Endocrinol 2018; 236(3):R161–7.

77. Rehfeld JF. Gastrins in serum. A review of gastrin radioimmunoanalysis and the discovery of gastrin heterogeneity in serum. Scand J Gastroenterol 1973; 8:577–83.

78. O'Connor DT, Deftos LJ. Secretion of chromogranin A by peptide-producing endocrine neoplasms. N Engl J Med 1986;314:1145–51.

79. Eriksson B, Arnberg H, Oberg K, et al. Chromogranins–new sensitive markers for neuroendocrine tumors. Acta Oncol 1989;28:325–9.

80. Oberg K. Circulating biomarkers in gastroenteropancreatic neuroendocrine tumours. Endocr Relat Cancer 2011;18(Suppl 1):S17–25.

81. Oberg K, Modlin IM, De Herder W, et al. Consensus on biomarkers for neuroendocrine tumour disease. Lancet Oncol 2015;16:e435–46.

82. Modlin IM, Drozdov I, Bodei L, et al. Blood transcript analysis and metastatic recurrent small bowel carcinoid management. BMC Cancer 2014;14:564.

83. Hounsfield GN. Computerized transverse axial scanning (tomography). 1. Description of system. Br J Radiol 1973;46:1016–22.

84. Sundin A, Arnold R, Baudin E, et al. ENETS consensus guidelines for the standards of care in neuroendocrine tumors: radiological, nuclear medicine and hybrid imaging. Neuroendocrinology 2017;105(3):212–44.

85. Lauterbur PC. NMR imaging in biomedicine. Cell Biophys 1986;9:211–4.

86. Mansfield P. NMR imaging in biomedicine: supplement 2 advances in magnetic resonance. Elsevier; 1982.

87. Mayerhoefer ME, Ba-Ssalamah A, Weber M, et al. Gadoxetate-enhanced versus diffusion-weighted MRI for fused Ga-68-DOTANOC PET/MRI in patients with neuroendocrine tumours of the upper abdomen. Eur Radiol 2013;23:1978–85.

88. Reubi JC. Regulatory peptide receptors as molecular targets for cancer diagnosis and therapy. Q J Nucl Med 1997;41:63–70.

89. Krenning EP, Kwekkeboom DJ, Bakker WH, et al. Somatostatin receptor scintigraphy with [111In-DTPA-D-Phe1]- and [123I-Tyr3]-octreotide: the Rotterdam experience with more than 1000 patients. Eur J Nucl Med 1993; 20:716–31.

90. Maecke HR, Hofmann M, Haberkorn U. (68)Ga-labeled peptides in tumor imaging. J Nucl Med 2005;46(Suppl 1):172S–8S.

91. Krausz Y, Freedman N, Rubinstein R, et al. Ga-DOTA-NOC PET/CT imaging of neuroendocrine tumors: comparison with (1)(1)(1)In-DTPA-octreotide (Octreo-Scan(R)). Mol Imaging Biol 2011;13:583–93.

92. Velikyan I, Sundin A, Sorensen J, et al. Quantitative and qualitative intrapatient comparison of 68Ga-DOTATOC and 68Ga-DOTATATE: net uptake rate for accurate quantification. J Nucl Med 2014;55:204–10.

93. Yang J, Kan Y, Ge BH, et al. Diagnostic role of Gallium-68 DOTATOC and Gallium-68 DOTATATE PET in patients with neuroendocrine tumors: a meta-analysis. Acta Radiol 2014;55:389–98.

94. Gabriel M, Decristoforo C, Kendler D, et al. 68Ga-DOTA-Tyr3-octreotide PET in neuroendocrine tumors: comparison with somatostatin receptor scintigraphy and CT. J Nucl Med 2007;48:508–18.

95. Binderup T, Knigge U, Loft A, et al. 18F-fluorodeoxyglucose positron emission tomography predicts survival of patients with neuroendocrine tumors. Clin Cancer Res 2010;16:978–85.

96. Koopmans KP, de Vries EG, Kema IP, et al. Staging of carcinoid tumours with 18F-DOPA PET: a prospective, diagnostic accuracy study. Lancet Oncol 2006;7:728–34.

97. Orlefors H, Sundin A, Garske U, et al. Whole-body (11)C-5-hydroxytryptophan positron emission tomography as a universal imaging technique for neuroendocrine tumors: comparison with somatostatin receptor scintigraphy and computed tomography. J Clin Endocrinol Metab 2005;90:3392–400.

98. Partelli S, Bartsch DK, Capdevila J, et al. ENETS consensus guidelines for standard of care in neuroendocrine tumours: surgery for small intestinal and pancreatic neuroendocrine tumours. Neuroendocrinology 2017;105(3):255–65.

99. Murray-Lyon IM, Eddleston AL, Williams R, et al. Treatment of multiple-hormone-producing malignant islet-cell tumour with streptozotocin. Lancet 1968;2:895–8.

100. Moertel CG, Lavin PT, Hahn RG. Phase II trial of doxorubicin therapy for advanced islet cell carcinoma. Cancer Treat Rep 1982;66:1567–9.

101. Eriksson B, Oberg K. An update of the medical treatment of malignant endocrine pancreatic tumors. Acta Oncol 1993;32:203–8.

102. Moertel CG, Lefkopoulo M, Lipsitz S, et al. Streptozocin-doxorubicin, streptozocin-fluorouracil or chlorozotocin in the treatment of advanced islet-cell carcinoma. N Engl J Med 1992;326:519–23.

103. Kouvaraki MA, Ajani JA, Hoff P, et al. Fluorouracil, doxorubicin, and streptozocin in the treatment of patients with locally advanced and metastatic pancreatic endocrine carcinomas. J Clin Oncol 2004;22:4762–71.

104. Ekeblad S, Sundin A, Janson ET, et al. Temozolomide as monotherapy is effective in treatment of advanced malignant neuroendocrine tumors. Clin Cancer Res 2007;13:2986–91.

105. Strosberg JR, Fine RL, Choi J, et al. First-line chemotherapy with capecitabine and temozolomide in patients with metastatic pancreatic endocrine carcinomas. Cancer 2011;117:268–75.

106. Saif MW, Kaley K, Brennan M, et al. A retrospective study of capecitabine/temozolomide (CAPTEM) regimen in the treatment of metastatic pancreatic neuroendocrine tumors (pNETs) after failing previous therapy. JOP 2013;14:498–501.

107. Fine RL, Gulati AP, Krantz BA, et al. Capecitabine and temozolomide (CAPTEM) for metastatic, well-differentiated neuroendocrine cancers: the Pancreas Center

at Columbia University experience. Cancer Chemother Pharmacol 2013;71: 663–70.

108. Go RS, Adjei AA. Review of the comparative pharmacology and clinical activity of cisplatin and carboplatin. J Clin Oncol 1999;17:409–22.

109. Welin S, Sorbye H, Sebjornsen S, et al. Clinical effect of temozolomide-based chemotherapy in poorly differentiated endocrine carcinoma after progression on first-line chemotherapy. Cancer 2011;117:4617–22.

110. Kvols LK, Moertel CG, O'Connell MJ, et al. Treatment of the malignant carcinoid syndrome. Evaluation of a long-acting somatostatin analogue. N Engl J Med 1986;315:663–6.

111. Öberg K, Norheim I, Lundqvist G, et al. Treatment of the carcinoid syndrome with SMS 201-995, a somatostatin analogue. Scand J Gastroenterol 1986;21: 191–2.

112. Reichlin S. Somatostatin. N Engl J Med 1983;309:1495–501.

113. Maurer R, Reubi JC. Somatostatin receptors. JAMA 1985;253:2741.

114. Krulich I, Dhariwal AP, McCann SM. Stimulatory and Inhibitory effects of purified hypothalamic extracts on growth hormone release from rat pituitary in vitro. Endocrinology 1968;83:783–90.

115. Hellman B, Lernmark A. Evidence for an inhibitor of insulin release in the pancreatic islets. Diabetologia 1969;5:22–4.

116. Brazeau P, Vale W, Burgus R, et al. Hypothalamic polypeptide that inhibits the secretion of immunoreactive pituitary growth hormone. Science 1973; 179:77–9.

117. Burgus R, Ling N, Butcher M, et al. Primary structure of somatostatin, a hypothalamic peptide that inhibits the secretion of pituitary growth hormone. Proc Natl Acad Sci U S A 1973;70:684–8.

118. Vale W, Grant G, Rivier J, et al. Synthetic polypeptide antagonists of the hypothalamic luteinizing hormone releasing factor. Science 1972;176:933–4.

119. Bauer W, Briner U, Doepfner W, et al. SMS 201-995: a very potent and selective octapeptide analogue of somatostatin with prolonged action. Life Sci 1982;31: 1133–40.

120. Reubi JC, Maurer R, von Werder K, et al. Somatostatin receptors in human endocrine tumors. Cancer Res 1987;47:551–8.

121. Oberg K, Kvols L, Caplin M, et al. Consensus report on the use of somatostatin analogs for the management of neuroendocrine tumors of the gastroenteropancreatic system. Ann Oncol 2004;15:966–73.

122. Grozinsky-Glasberg S, Shimon I, Korbonits M, et al. Somatostatin analogues in the control of neuroendocrine tumours: efficacy and mechanisms. Endocr Relat Cancer 2008;15:701–20.

123. Rinke A, Muller HH, Schade-Brittinger C, et al. Placebo-controlled, double-blind, prospective, randomized study on the effect of octreotide LAR in the control of tumor growth in patients with metastatic neuroendocrine midgut tumors: a report from the PROMID Study Group. J Clin Oncol 2009;27:4656–63.

124. Caplin ME, Pavel M, Cwikla JB, et al. Lanreotide in metastatic enteropancreatic neuroendocrine tumors. N Engl J Med 2014;371:224–33.

125. Kvols LK, Oberg KE, O'Dorisio TM, et al. Pasireotide (SOM230) shows efficacy and tolerability in the treatment of patients with advanced neuroendocrine tumors refractory or resistant to octreotide LAR: results from a phase II study. Endocr Relat Cancer 2012;19:657–66.

126. Oberg K, Funa K, Alm G. Effects of leukocyte interferon on clinical symptoms and hormone levels in patients with mid-gut carcinoid tumors and carcinoid syndrome. N Engl J Med 1983;309:129–33.

127. Oberg K. Interferon in the management of neuroendocrine GEP-tumors: a review. Digestion 2000;62(Suppl 1):92–7.

128. Pestka S, Langer JA, Zoon KC, et al. Interferons and their actions. Annu Rev Biochem 1987;56:727–77.

129. Faiss S, Pape UF, Bohmig M, et al. Prospective, randomized, multicenter trial on the antiproliferative effect of lanreotide, interferon alfa, and their combination for therapy of metastatic neuroendocrine gastroenteropancreatic tumors–the International Lanreotide and Interferon Alfa Study Group. J Clin Oncol 2003;21: 2689–96.

130. Arnold R, Rinke A, Klose KJ, et al. Octreotide versus octreotide plus interferon-alpha in endocrine gastroenteropancreatic tumors: a randomized trial. Clin Gastroenterol Hepatol 2005;3:761–71.

131. Krenning EP, Kooij PP, Bakker WH, et al. Radiotherapy with a radiolabeled somatostatin analogue, [111In-DTPA-D-Phe1]-octreotide. A case history. Ann N Y Acad Sci 1994;733:496–506.

132. Waldherr C, Pless M, Maecke HR, et al. The clinical value of [90Y-DOTA]-D-Phe1-Tyr3-octreotide (90Y-DOTATOC) in the treatment of neuroendocrine tumours: a clinical phase II study. Ann Oncol 2001;12:941–5.

133. Imhof A, Brunner P, Marincek N, et al. Response, survival, and long-term toxicity after therapy with the radiolabeled somatostatin analogue [90Y-DOTA]-TOC in metastasized neuroendocrine cancers. J Clin Oncol 2011;29:2416–23.

134. Kwekkeboom DJ, de Herder WW, Kam BL, et al. Treatment with the radiolabeled somatostatin analog [177 Lu-DOTA 0,Tyr3]octreotate: toxicity, efficacy, and survival. J Clin Oncol 2008;26:2124–30.

135. Baum RP, Kluge AW, Kulkarni H, et al. [(177)Lu-DOTA](0)-D-Phe(1)-Tyr(3)-Octreotide ((177)Lu-DOTATOC) for peptide receptor radiotherapy in patients with advanced neuroendocrine tumours: a phase-II study. Theranostics 2016;6: 501–10.

136. Strosberg J, El-Haddad G, Wolin E, et al. Phase 3 Trial of 177Lu-Dotatate for midgut neuroendocrine tumors. N Engl J Med 2017;376:125–35.

137. Shaw RJ, Cantley LC. Ras, PI(3)K and mTOR signalling controls tumour cell growth. Nature 2006;441:424–30.

138. Shida T, Kishimoto T, Furuya M, et al. Expression of an activated mammalian target of rapamycin (mTOR) in gastroenteropancreatic neuroendocrine tumors. Cancer Chemother Pharmacol 2010;65:889–93.

139. Scoazec JY. Angiogenesis in neuroendocrine tumors: therapeutic applications. Neuroendocrinology 2013;97:45–56.

140. Yao JC, Phan AT, Chang DZ, et al. Efficacy of RAD001 (everolimus) and octreotide LAR in advanced low- to intermediate-grade neuroendocrine tumors: results of a phase II study. J Clin Oncol 2008;26:4311–8.

141. Pavel ME, Hainsworth JD, Baudin E, et al. Everolimus plus octreotide long-acting repeatable for the treatment of advanced neuroendocrine tumours associated with carcinoid syndrome (RADIANT-2): a randomised, placebo-controlled, phase 3 study. Lancet 2011;378:2005–12.

142. Yao JC, Shah MH, Ito T, et al. RAD001 in advanced neuroendocrine tumors, third trial (RADIANT-3) study group: everolimus for advanced pancreatic neuroendocrine tumors. N Engl J Med 2011;364:514–23.

143. Yao JC, Fazio N, Singh S, et al. Everolimus for the treatment of advanced, non-functional neuroendocrine tumours of the lung or gastrointestinal tract (RADIANT-4): a randomised, placebo-controlled, phase 3 study. Lancet 2016; 387:968–77.
144. Raymond E, Dahan L, Raoul JL, et al. Sunitinib malate for the treatment of pancreatic neuroendocrine tumors. N Engl J Med 2011;364:501–13.
145. Abdel-Rahman O, Fouad M. Bevacizumab-based combination therapy for advanced gastroenteropancreatic neuroendocrine neoplasms (GEP-NENs): a systematic review of the literature. J Cancer Res Clin Oncol 2015;141: 295–305.
146. Kulke MH, Horsch D, Caplin ME, et al. Telotristat Ethyl, a tryptophan hydroxylase inhibitor for the treatment of carcinoid syndrome. J Clin Oncol 2017;35: 14–23.

Moving?

Make sure your subscription moves with you!

To notify us of your new address, find your **Clinics Account Number** (located on your mailing label above your name), and contact customer service at:

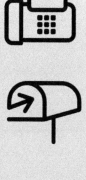

Email: journalscustomerservice-usa@elsevier.com

800-654-2452 (subscribers in the U.S. & Canada)
314-447-8871 (subscribers outside of the U.S. & Canada)

Fax number: 314-447-8029

Elsevier Health Sciences Division
Subscription Customer Service
3251 Riverport Lane
Maryland Heights, MO 63043

*To ensure uninterrupted delivery of your subscription, please notify us at least 4 weeks in advance of move.

Printed and bound by CPI Group (UK) Ltd, Croydon, CR0 4YY

08/05/2025

01864729-0001